Readers tell us that *Choose to Lose* really works . . .

"It is amazing that it can be so easy — after I've struggled so long."

Lisa M. Russell, Waxahachie. Texas

"With *Choose to Lose* I'm not hungry and I don't feel deprived — two *major* reasons for abandoning other diet and weight maintenance programs I've joined over the years. I can't say enough positive things about *Choose to Lose* and I can't find any negatives. Thank you for contributing to the betterment of the second half of my life!"

Esther Leadley, Pavilion, New York

"As an avid follower of *Eater's Choice* and a new follower of *Choose to Lose*, I must compliment the authors on their interesting and simple writing style. Their ideas and belief in those ideas are well corresponded and very contagious. I would like to thank them for helping me to turn my cholesterol count around as well as helping me to lose weight. Also, the recipes are truly delicious."

Harold Topper, Stamford, Connecticut

"I never dreamed something would come along like your plan to make weight loss easy, even enjoyable. I'm spreading the word to all my friends to go out and buy *Choose to Lose*. Any other book I'd lend them, but I wouldn't part with my copy."

R. Comparetto, Chicago, Illinois

"I've got a long way to go but I'm enjoying the trip."

Pam Ingersoll, Mason City, Iowa

"In addition to my weight loss of 45 pounds, my cholesterol level also dropped significantly, and is now below 200 for the first time. We have tried virtually all the programs in existence, and *Choose to Lose* is the only one that really works for us. Thanks again for improving our health and showing us that we can continue to enjoy a wide range of foods without worry."

Bill Rogers, Reston, Virginia

"Finally I found a book that I read and that actually made sense. [*Choose to Lose*] was such an inspiration to me, I was motivated to lose weight and to exercise. From January 25 to Jul·· ˙ ˙ lost 69 pounds and went from a size 24 to ˙ ˙ ˙ ˙ ˙ ˙ ˙ ˙ ˙ ˙ˑ ore in those six and a half months than I have my entire life put together. People see me and ask, 'What did you do to yourself? Starve yourself?' I say, 'No, I finally found the right way to lose weight without suffering.' Thanks for writing something that . . . truly has changed my way of life!!"

Marcia M. Meshak, Marshfield, Wisconsin

"I am so glad that I have found your book! It's absolutely *GREAT*! I had always been a very thin person with a high metabolism, but when I got married and became a homemaker the pounds seemed to come from nowhere. Along with that, my self-esteem plummeted and I began a search for a diet where I could: 1) prepare my own foods and not purchase expensive Weight Watchers or Jenny Craig (frozen) foods; 2) eat what I wanted to; and 3) *understand* exactly what it would take to lose weight in a safe manner. Your book fits my needs. . . . I have lost 18 pounds thanks to you."

Lillian Stevens, San Jose, California

"I just wanted to let you know how very much I enjoy the *Choose to Lose* lifestyle! As one of the thinner patients at a health spa in my native England last month, I was constantly asked what my 'secret' is. I was happy to retort 'NO FAT!' and would launch into a glowing report about *Choose to Lose* and its benefits."

Trish Maskell, Cos Cob, Connecticut

"Thank you so much for the information you made available to me through your *Eater's Choice* and *Choose to Lose* books. I am 5'10" with a small frame. I began the 'way of life' diet on March 17, 1991, weighing 181 pounds. As of today (September 12, 1991) I weigh 133 pounds. I have never felt better."

Kimberly Patterson, Lawton, Oklahoma

"My physician was correct in recommending your books to me. I trusted him to have my health foremost in . . . his mind and he has never let me down. I understand better now why he has placed his trust in your books."

Mary Riggs, APO, New York

"I want you to know that not a day goes by that I don't give thanks for having found your book."

Judith Leff, Syosset, New York

"I find your book very well written, easily understood, and extremely informative. Not only do I recommend it to my patients, I also find it an excellent gift for family and friends."

Michael E. Rubin, M.D., Des Plaines, Illinois

"Thank you. This book has really encouraged me. I have struggled with food all of my life. I feel free of the bondage. I know how to make the correct choices."

Fleta Gamble, Lindsay, California

"I've been using *Choose to Lose* as a referral for our patients to control the fat in their diet. We have been very pleased with our patients' success."

Sara H. Murphy, M.D., Indianapolis, Indiana

"This lengthy story is just to tell you how *great* we think your books are, how interesting to read and understand and how yummy the recipes are. . . . I feel like I want to convert everyone I encounter that has weight or cholesterol problems, and feel I just have to share the knowledge obtained in your books."

Nancy Paulk, Oklahoma City, Oklahoma

"A friend recently recommended *Choose to Lose* to me. I am absolutely delighted with it. I feel there is hope! I don't feel deprived! Ingredients are usually ones I have on hand. Most of the recipes are able to be made quickly which fits into my busy schedule."

Barbara Karpinski, Rockville, Maryland

Choose to Lose

Also by Dr. Ron Goor and Nancy Goor

Eater's Choice: A Food Lover's
Guide to Lower Cholesterol

Choose to Lose

A Food Lover's Guide to Permanent Weight Loss

Dr. Ron Goor and Nancy Goor

Revised Edition

HOUGHTON MIFFLIN COMPANY
Boston   New York

For information about permission to reproduce
selections from this book, write to Permissions,
Houghton Mifflin Company, 215 Park Avenue South,
New York, New York 10003.

Library of Congress Cataloging-in-Publication Data
Goor, Ron
    The choose to lose diet : a food lover's guide to
permanent weight loss / Ron Goor and Nancy Goor
        p.   cm.
    Includes bibliographical references.
    ISBN 0-395-49336-6
    ISBN 0-395-70814-1 (pbk.)
    1. Low-fat diet.   2. Food — Fat content —
Tables.   I. Goor, Nancy.   III. Title.
RM237.7.G66   1990   89-24467
613.2'5 — dc20   CIP

Printed in the United States of America

AGM   10 9 8 7 6 5

Book design by Joyce C. Weston

Recipes from *Eater's Choice* copyright © 1987, 1989,
1992, 1995, by Ronald S. Goor and Nancy Goor.
Reprinted by permission of Houghton Mifflin
Company.

Before beginning this or any diet, you should consult your physician to be sure it is safe for you.

In loving memory of Charles Goor

Acknowledgments

Ron and Nancy Goor wish to thank the many people who have contributed to the development of this book: Robert R. Betting, Dr. J. P. Flatt, Alex Goor, Dan Goor, Jeanette Goor, Anita Hamel, Genevieve Kazdin, Suzanne Lieblich, Roland Lippoldt. Helen Miller, Martin Miller, Ted Mummery, Isabelle Schoenfeld, Kendra Stemple Todd, Dawn Weddle, R.D., and all the Choose to Lose Leaders.

Contents

Food Tables

A Note on the Second Edition

WE would like to thank all of you Choosers to Lose who have written or called to tell us of your successes. It is gratifying to hear that not only have you lost weight — up to 120 pounds or more — but that you are eating healthier and feeling better than ever before. We'd love to hear from more of you about how you are progressing. Send us pictures. (We were delighted to receive a photograph of Bill Rogers's CHZ 2 LUZ license plate. What a thrill to learn of *Choose to Lose* mania in Lisco, Nebraska, where almost the whole town has embraced our plan. In 18 months they collectively lost 1600 pounds or an average of 17.7 pounds for each of their 90 inhabitants.)

Not only have you lost inches and pounds, but you have reported improved health. Blood cholesterols have plummeted (some by as much as 100 points), blood pressures have gone down, blood sugars have normalized, and people report that their ankles are no longer swollen. These short-term changes predict a healthier future — reduced risks of heart disease, stroke, cancer, and diabetes.

We love hearing how *Choose to Lose* has helped you feel good about yourselves. Readers tell us they are able to take control of their diet for the first time. The resulting self-esteem has given them the confidence to take control and succeed in other areas of their life.

Readers tell us it is easy to be a success with *Choose to Lose* because *Choose to Lose* asks you only to do something natural — eat lots of delicious, nutritious food and never be hungry. As one Chooser to Lose from Bigfork, Minnesota, wrote, "Eating has become a normal life function and not an obsession."

Gone are the feelings of failure. You will soon realize it was not you who failed. Starvation diets and the American high-fat food system failed you. Armed with tools and knowledge from *Choose to Lose*, you will be equipped to make better choices, enjoy yourselves, and reach and maintain your desirable and healthy weight.

What's new about the second edition of *Choose to Lose*? With five years of experience come insight and better understanding. (We have also incorporated comments and suggestions from our Choose to Lose Leaders and readers throughout the country.) We originally thought the major impediment to following *Choose to Lose* would be an inability to cut the fat. We warned about stuffing in as many high-fat foods as your Fat Budget would allow. It turns out that this is not the big difficulty. The widespread problem is fear of eating. The mythology that you should limit the amount (portion size) of food you eat to control your weight has so taken root in the American subconscious that it is difficult to overcome. Even overweight people eat too little food. When they claim they eat no more than their thin friends, they are telling the truth in terms of quantity (but of course not in terms of fat). One Wisconsin reader aptly described herself as an obese anorexic — she ate too little food but too much fat. In this edition, we have put a greater emphasis on the importance of eating enough calories to lose weight. We have stressed the fact that the total caloric intake you use to determine your Fat Budget is a floor. **You must eat above it.** Let us assure you that not only won't you gain weight by eating lots of low-fat, high-carbohydrate, high-fiber foods, you will probably not lose weight if you don't. If that seems like a logical inconsistency to you, Chapter 1 should convince you it isn't. The experience of thousands of Choosers to Lose should also convince you.

New food labels are in the stores. In the summer of 1994 all food labels changed to conform with the new FDA and USDA labeling laws. We have updated the information on food labels to help you understand them. We discuss the pluses — that almost all foods have a legible, standardized nutrition label; that the label includes fat calories, grams of saturated fat, and dietary fiber; and that serving sizes are now more standardized, which makes comparisons between similar products easier. We also clarify the minuses — the confusing Daily Value and % Daily Value.

We have included a new chapter to help you with your overweight children. As children spend more and more time sitting in front of the television and video game monitor and consuming more and more high-fat junk, obesity in children is becoming a common problem. This chapter gives you tips on how to change your child's food environment to facilitate his fat loss. *Choose to Lose* is perfect for teens and some mature preteens because it makes their fat loss their problem. It isn't Mother's problem, Father's problem, Grandma's problem, Uncle Harry's problem. It is theirs. They have their own Fat Budget and they keep track of their own food intake. One particularly gratifying story came from Colorado, where an overweight ten-year-old boy took *Choose to Lose* to heart. (He carried the book around wherever he went.) The chunky kid who was always picked last when teams were chosen became the slim, "most improved athlete" in less than a year.

Good news on the recipe front. We have reduced the fat content of many of the recipes in the book and we have added a few new recipes, such as *Cheesecake!* and *Ted Mummery's Turkey Barbecue* (Ron's favorite lunch). Also, those of you who cook (and we hope more and more of you will) should know that *Eater's Choice* has 290 low-fat recipes (from which 72 of the 74 in *Choose to Lose* were selected) and that we have just reduced the fat in most of those recipes. If you have an old copy of *Eater's Choice,* you may want to check out the new one.

We have also updated and expanded the Food Tables in *Choose to Lose,* which will help you choose foods to stay within your budget. We have added more fast foods, updated the commercial frozen foods, and added some restaurant foods.

All in all, *Choose to Lose* is the same book, but even better! We hope it brings a lot of joy and good health into your life.

Introduction

Choose to Lose is an outgrowth of our book *Eater's Choice: A Food Lover's Guide to Lower Cholesterol.* Soon after *Eater's Choice* was published we began receiving letters from ecstatic readers. Not only were they lowering their cholesterol, they were losing weight — typically 10 to 15 pounds and some up to 40 or more pounds. This was not the intention of the cholesterol-lowering plan, but it was a side effect that was appreciated as much (or more!).

Readers tell us that they find the *Eater's Choice* method simple, direct, and flexible. It gives them the tools and knowledge to take control of their diet for the first time. And it is positive. All foods are allowed. No exchanges, no two-week meal plans to follow for the rest of your life. *You* determine which foods you eat.

Choose to Lose uses essentially the same approach that was successfully utilized in *Eater's Choice.* But while *Eater's Choice* limits only saturated fat intake, *Choose to Lose* limits *total* fat consumption. Saturated fat is the chief culprit in the diet that raises blood cholesterol, but all three types of fat — saturated, monounsaturated, and polyunsaturated — in the foods you eat make you gain weight. In recent years scientific research has shown that dietary fat, not carbohydrates or total calories, is the primary cause of weight gain. Furthermore, the researchers note that weight loss can be achieved simply by limiting fat intake. That is why *Choose to Lose* uses a Fat Budget and the total fat content of foods to help you make food choices that satisfy your palate and help you to lose weight.

Like *Eater's Choice, Choose to Lose* helps you adopt a new eating lifestyle. After all, permanent weight loss, like permanent cholesterol lowering, requires a new lifelong eating pattern, not just a two-week crash diet. Whatever changes are made to lower cholesterol and weight must be continued. The diet plan must therefore be palatable and practical.

Not only is *Choose to Lose* easy to follow, it is also enjoyable. Most people eat a limited number of foods and are probably bored with their diet. This new low-fat way of eating will broaden your culinary horizons and add spice and variety to your life. You will explore new foods and new food preparations. To discover a world of new taste treats, try the 74 mouth-watering recipes in *Choose to Lose* — as well as 216 more in *Eater's Choice* — recipes for real foods, such as *Tortilla Soup, Cajun Chicken, Broiled Ginger Fish, Cinnamon Sweet Cakes, Honey Whole-Wheat Bread, Calzone, Divine Buttermilk Pound Cake,* and *Deep-Dish Pear Pie,* to mention just a few favorites.

Any change in eating patterns takes commitment and motivation. *Choose to Lose* provides you with the tools and knowledge to make food choices to keep you lean for a lifetime. You will find you are eating more food and enjoying it more. And most important, you will also lose weight.

Good luck and good health.

1. Fat's the One

"With *Choose to Lose*, eating has become a normal life function and not an obsession."

Joey Jacobson, Bigfork, Minnesota

TAKE A LOOK in the mirror — a good look. Is the person staring out at you a little pudgier than you would like? Has the muscle turned to flab? Are the seams and buttons on the verge of splitting and popping? Don't turn away in disappointment. Give yourself a smile. Already you are making a big change in *you*. You are starting *Choose to Lose*. Soon you will see a trim version of what you see now. The trim version will be beaming. No suffering will have made the pounds melt away. Only good, abundant food, including your all-time favorites. *Choose to Lose* is not a miracle diet. In fact, it's not even a diet. It's a new way of eating that is easy, healthy, and delicious. And it works.

The key to *Choose to Lose* is FAT.

FAT MAKES FAT

The word is FAT. FAT is what you don't want to be and FAT is what you ate to become FAT. So, the way to become NOT FAT is to reduce fat in your diet. Don't focus on total calories . . . or sugar . . . or starch. Focus on FAT.

Until recently, most diet formulators based their weight loss methods on reducing *total calories*. Sugar and starch were always forbidden. These approaches pinpointed the wrong culprit. The reason that foods containing sugar make you gain weight is not because they contain sugar. It is because they contain *fat* and sugar. It is the fat in the cheesecake, not the sugar, that puts dimples in your knees. It is the fat in the

1

sour cream, not the starch in the potato, that rounds your belly. It is your fat tooth, not your sweet tooth, that gets you into trouble.

CARBOHYDRATES: WEIGHT LOSS FOOD

Carbohydrates are the good guys. They increase your energy without increasing your girth. You can eat them with gusto* and, as you will see, you *must* eat lots of carbohydrates to keep up your metabolism to burn fat. *Choose to Lose* encourages you to eat fruit and complex carbohydrates — vegetables and whole grains and even some simple sugars. *Choose to Lose* focuses on reducing the nutrient that is making you fat — FAT.

You may find this recommendation hard to accept. After all, you have probably been trying to cut *total calories* and limit carbohydrates for years. Please. Don't accept this advice on faith. Read the following section, which explains simply how the fats and carbohydrates you eat affect your weight. The science behind *Choose to Lose* is fascinating, illuminating — and motivating!

FOOD — MORE THAN JUST PLEASURE

This is a book about fat, food, and you. Ice cream sundaes, chicken soup, T-bone steaks, potato chips — for most people food offers more than gustatory satisfaction. Food may represent love (you want to please those you love; therefore you feed them); status (with your raise you can afford to eat filet mignon and caviar); comfort (you feel lonely or frustrated so you console yourself with a bowl of ice cream); nostalgia (the aroma of hot dogs conjures up visions of baseball games and family picnics); or something just plain wonderful to eat. Food fulfills a different need in each person, but for everyone, no matter how thin, fat, young, old, rich, poor — food is energy.

---

*A note to diabetics: *Choose to Lose* is a healthy diet for diabetics to follow because a low-fat, high-fiber diet will help to reduce your risk of heart disease and may help to control your blood sugar. However, *Choose to Lose* does not limit sugar or carbohydrates. You must consult with your physician for guidelines on sugar and carbohydrate consumption suited to your individual needs.

ENERGY EXPENDITURE

BMR

Your body needs a certain amount of energy to function. The amount of energy you use when you are completely at rest is called your basal metabolic rate, BMR. This is the energy needed to power your heart, lungs, brain, kidneys, and other organs and keep them in good repair, and for children, the energy to grow.

Physical Activity

You also need energy for physical activity — walking, running, moving. This is an expandable amount depending on how active you are.

So, the total amount of energy you expend is equal to the sum of your BMR and your physical activity.

ENERGY INTAKE

Food — Source of Energy

Where does your body get this energy? Energy is stored in fats, proteins, and carbohydrates in the foods you eat. More calories are stored in fat than in carbohydrates or proteins. One gram of fat has 9 calories (some scientists say 11!). One gram of carbohydrate or protein has 4 calories. Fat is so densely caloric that when you eat a little, you've eaten a lot of calories. For example, when you eat 1½ ounces of fat-laden potato chips you are consuming the same number of calories as when you eat 12 ounces of potatoes (two medium-large potatoes).

To release energy stored in fats, carbohydrates, and protein they must be burned. Picture a stack of logs blazing in a fireplace. The burning of nutrients and the burning of wood in a fireplace are similar chemical processes. In both cases the chemicals are combined with oxygen (burned or oxidized) and the energy stored in them is released. In the case of wood, the energy is released all in one step as heat. In the body, the oxidation goes on at a lower temperature (98.6°F) in small steps controlled by enzymes. In this way, most of the energy stored in the food is captured for growth, maintenance, repair, and physical activity, and less is wasted as heat.

What Is a Calorie?

Energy is stored in fats, proteins, and carbohydrates in units called calories. Total calories are the sum of the fat calories, protein calories, and carbohydrate calories you eat.

$$
\begin{array}{r}
\text{Fat calories} \\
\text{Carbohydrate calories} \\
+ \ \text{Protein calories} \\
\hline
\text{Total calories}
\end{array}
$$

All Calories Are Not Equal

You may have thought that everything you ate ended up as those rolls of fat rippling down your belly. You may even have been avoiding carbohydrates in the belief that they are fattening. But you were misguided.

In the past it was believed that calories from all foods contributed equally to weight gain. Recent scientific evidence has shown that fats, carbohydrates, and proteins are metabolized (burned and stored) differently. Fat calories are fattening while carbohydrate and protein calories (consumed in reasonable amounts) are not. In fact, eating nutrient-rich carbohydrates can help you lose weight. To understand why, read on.

CARBOHYDRATES

The body has a limited capacity to store carbohydrates (about 800–1000 calories or approximately one day's intake). Consequently, when you eat a meal, the carbohydrates are either burned immediately (for quick energy) or temporarily stored and then burned within a few hours to make room for the next day's intake. A small amount of carbohydrate always remains stored as glycogen* in muscle and liver as a source of quick energy.

How does this need to dispose of carbohydrates affect your weight?

---

*Carbohydrate is stored in the body as glycogen, long chains of the simple sugar glucose.

Under normal circumstances, *the carbohydrate you eat is never stored as fat* — that soft padding that currently covers too much of your frame.

Thermogenesis

To prevent overloading the body's limited storage capacity for carbohydrates, any carbohydrate consumed in excess of your immediate energy needs (BMR + physical activity) is burned and the energy is converted to heat. **It is not stored as fat.** This process of producing heat from burning carbohydrate is called the thermogenic effect of food. When you feel warm during or after a meal you're feeling the thermogenic effect.

Won't I Gain Weight If I Overeat Carbohydrates?

It is almost impossible to overeat carbohydrates because the body has developed mechanisms to prevent it.

1. Within normal limits the body burns off almost all the carbohydrate you eat. Only if you were to eat more than 2200 calories of pure carbohydrate over your normal daily total caloric intake for 5 to 6 days in a row might the excess carbohydrates possibly turn to fat. This is called glycogen loading and is difficult to do if the sources of carbohydrates you are eating are mainly fruit, vegetables, and whole-grains.
2. As an additional safeguard against overloading the body with too much carbohydrate, eating carbohydrates triggers a feeling of satiety. You feel full so you stop eating, thus limiting the amount of carbohydrates you consume.
3. If you overeat carbohydrates one day, you tend to undereat them the next so that your average intake remains constant.
4. In addition, carbohydrates* provide so much bulk, it is difficult to overeat them. Imagine eating 990 calories of air-popped popcorn: 33 cups! You would never want to chew again. Compare this with a Dairy Queen large chocolate shake, which also has 990 calories.

---

*That is, fiber-rich carbohydrates, such as fruit, vegetables, and whole-grains.

Four Reasons Why *Choose to Lose* Encourages You to Eat Carbohydrates

1. To maximize your metabolic rate;
2. To ensure an adequate intake of vitamins, minerals, and fiber* for long-term good health;
3. To keep you full, satisfied, and content;
4. To increase your energy and stamina.

FAT: WHY *CHOOSE TO LOSE* FOCUSES ON IT

In contrast to carbohydrates, the fats that you eat are not burned right away but are immediately and completely stored in the adipose tissue, where they promptly become the soft, squishy blubber that pads your body. Imagine a cheeseburger being slapped onto your hips and you've got the picture. The adipose tissue contains enormous stores of fat. A normal lean person stores about 140,000 calories, but there is no upper limit. Thus a person who weighs 300 pounds may be storing 200 pounds of fat.

Eating fat neither causes the body to burn it quickly — or burn it at all, for that matter — nor does it trigger satiety. You can eat and eat fat without feeling full and, since all the fat is stored, overeating fat makes you fatter and fatter. When you overeat fat one day, your body has no mechanisms for limiting your fat consumption the next. You feel just as hungry for fat as you did the day before. So you can overeat fat one day and the next and the next. And given the high-fat food system in the U.S., that is exactly what Americans do.

The Secret to Weight Loss: Raiding the Fat Stores

Now you know why the carbohydrates you eat don't become fat on your body and the fats you eat do. But what can you do about the fat that already rounds your edges? How can you make your body mobilize the fat out of the fat stores so you can lose weight?

Each day fat from the foods you eat is added to the fat stores. Some is removed to furnish energy not supplied by the carbohydrate and protein you eat. Your weight is determined by how much fat you add to the fat depots versus how much you remove.

---

*See page 94 for a discussion of fiber.

If you eat just the amount of fat needed to furnish the energy not supplied by the carbohydrate and protein, your weight will remain the same. If you eat more fat than is needed, the excess will go into the fat stores and you will gain weight. If you eat less fat than is required to satisfy your energy needs, then the body will have to make up the deficit by burning additional fat. And where does this fat come from? The fat is removed from the fat stores and **you lose weight.**

It all makes sense. You became fat because you ate *more* fat than you burned. To lose weight, you have to eat *less* fat than you burn so that your body will use up the excess fat luxuriating in your adipose tissues to help supply your energy needs.

THREE STRATEGIES TO SHRINK THE FAT STORES

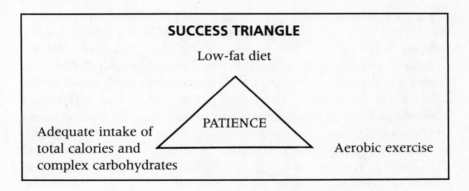

SUCCESS TRIANGLE

Low-fat diet

PATIENCE

Adequate intake of
total calories and
complex carbohydrates

Aerobic exercise

Strategy #1: Low-fat Diet — Put Less Fat into the Fat Stores

Obviously the less fat you add to the fat stores, the less you will need to take out later. The way to do this is to eat a low-fat diet. *Choose to Lose* provides a powerful tool, the Fat Budget, and an effective method (see Chapter 2) to help you follow a low-fat diet.

Maximizing Fat Loss. Eating less fat is essential for weight loss, but you can't stop there. To shrink the fat stores faster, you must not only add less to them, you need to remove fat that is already there. The next two strategies are aimed at removing stored fat. Strategy #2 you are not going to believe.

Strategy #2: Adequate Intake of Total Calories and Complex Carbohydrates — You Have to Eat to Lose Weight

Can you imagine a weight loss program insisting that you eat an abundance of food to lose weight? It's not a dream — only a dream diet! You need to eat enough calories to keep your BMR chugging along at a maximum rate so you will burn fat at a maximum rate and thus help reduce your fat stores. Of course, you must eat a lot of the right foods. This does not mean a bowl of fat-laden peanuts or a box of fat-free cookies. It does mean replacing much of the fat in your diet with nutritious low-fat food — fruits, vegetables, whole-grains, nonfat dairy, poultry, fish, shellfish. Don't fear that those potatoes and bread and carrots and tangerines and nonfat yogurt will end up as double chins. Remember, the body is great at burning up carbohydrates but quite inefficient at storing them.

Eating Too Little Can Be Hazardous to Your Diet. Have we convinced you? After years of following low-calorie diets, you probably have a mindset against eating. You may still think that a nifty way to force your body to burn fat from its fat stores is to reduce your total energy intake drastically. How about an 800-calorie-a-day crash diet for three weeks to turn you into a string bean? The problem is that not only are 800-calorie-a-day diets dangerous and sometimes even fatal, deficient in vital nutrients, and impossible to follow for more than a few weeks, but starvation diets depress your basal metabolic rate. If you eat fewer than 1500 total calories a day, you will find that your weight loss will *slow down.* Your body doesn't know that you are starving just to lose weight. It reacts to the intake of too few calories by burning food more

---

Important Message!!!

Although you just read that you can eat as many total calories as you want as long as you limit fat, we know in your heart of hearts you don't *really* believe it. You will limit your fat, but you will still be afraid to eat a lot of food — even low-fat, nutritious food. DON'T BE AFRAID! Limiting total calories has not been successful for you in the past, at least not in the long term. You can't lose anything (but weight!) by trying a different approach. So TRY IT! (But be sure the foods you eat in abundance are nutritious, low-fat foods, not fiber-free, sugar-filled, nutritionally empty calories.)

slowly, by lowering the BMR to conserve stored energy. That's a great help if food is really scarce, but if you are trying to lose weight, burning stored energy (fat) more slowly means losing weight more slowly. Conclusion: Starving makes you a loser, eating makes you a winner. Repeat to yourself 1000 times each day, "I must eat to lose weight. I must eat to lose weight . . ."

Strategy #3: Aerobic Exercise — Build Muscle to Burn Fat

This third strategy to maximize fat removal may not be your favorite. But it is absolutely essential and you may learn to enjoy, even love, it. The third strategy is daily aerobic exercise. Plain, old-fashioned walking is just fine. You don't have to strain and sweat to make it work. **The main value of aerobic exercise is to build and preserve muscle. Muscle burns fat.** The more muscle you have, the more fat-burning capacity you have. Muscle is metabolically active (burns energy at a high rate) and the more you have of it, the higher your BMR and the faster you burn everything, including fat. Not only will aerobic exercise help you lose weight, it will help you keep it off. That doesn't mean you have to exercise until you look like Arnold Schwarzenegger. Thirty minutes of walking each day is fine. It doesn't even have to be fast, just nonstop. See Chapter 11 for more information on exercise.

Preserving Muscle: Another Good Reason to Exercise. You think of your muscles as being permanent, but they aren't. When you don't use your muscle, it breaks down and the protein is burned. (Have you ever had your leg in a cast for 5 or 6 weeks? When the cast comes off, the muscle is withered and wasted from disuse. Much of the protein has been burned for energy. But as soon as you start walking again, the muscle begins rebuilding and within a short time your leg looks normal.) When you use your muscles, some of the protein you eat is used to build them up again.

When you are in energy deficit, that is, when you are using more energy than you are taking in, you must make up for the deficit by using energy stored in the body. The two major sources of stored energy are fat in the adipose tissues and protein in the muscle. Wouldn't it be great if the body automatically burned fat from the fat stores? No such luck. Unfortunately, fat is the stored energy of last resort. The body prefers to burn protein from the muscle — if you are *not* exercising. YOU DO NOT WANT YOUR BODY TO BURN PROTEIN INSTEAD OF FAT. **To protect your muscle from being broken down and** burned for energy, and to force your body to burn stored fat instead, you must exercise aerobically* (not in intensive bursts and spurts but steadily and continuously).

Yo-Yoing: Starvation Diets Make You Fatter

Almost all diets are a combination of starvation and no exercise. Now that you know about the importance of exercise, you'll understand why this duo can be so destructive to your weight loss goals.

People who go on low-calorie diets rarely exercise. They believe the ads that show a beautiful, slender young woman sipping a diet shake as she languishes on the beach. If this were reality, the next picture would show her hungry, bored, and fatigued, leaving her chaise lounge to find a hamburger stand. The immediate and natural response to a week or two of deprivation is to overeat. After all, so much suffering deserves a reward. But now, because of a lowered BMR and less muscle mass, the reward sits on hips and thighs instead of being burned off. And since the dieters haven't learned new low-fat eating habits and still don't exercise, the combination of a lower BMR and their old high-fat diet results in new pounds of fat being added back at a faster rate. This is the famous yo-yo effect. With each cycle of weight loss and gain, you lose more muscle, your weight comes off more slowly and is re-gained more quickly and you end up fatter (fat being a higher percent-age of your body weight) and heavier. Starvation plus no exercise equals a system destined to fail.

Breaking the Cycle

If you are a former yo-yoer, don't be discouraged. You don't have to be trapped in the cycle. By eating a diet low in fat and high in complex carbohydrates and doing a moderate amount of exercise, you will build new muscle and get your metabolism going again.

A Related Word about Dieting and Guilt

Eating only 500–1000 calories a day is like holding your breath for 20 minutes. It's impossible. After a few minutes of not breathing you

---

*Aerobic exercise is exercise which is steady, repetitive, uses large muscle masses, and requires a steady supply of oxygen. Example: walking.

gasp for breath. You don't feel guilty. Why should you? But if you quit your diet after a few weeks of starving, you think you have failed — you are bad. Don't blame yourself. Blame the diet. What you need is an eating plan that works, and *Choose to Lose* is it. With *Choose to Lose* you will not starve. Rather you will eat more than you ever ate before. You will be full and satisfied. You will learn to make choices that will make and keep you lean. You will be in control. And you will be able to follow *Choose to Lose* forever.

Throw Away Your Scale!

The only weight loss that is meaningful and permanent and has long-term health benefits is loss of fat. If you reduce your intake of fat, eat lots of total calories, and exercise aerobically every day to build and preserve your muscle, you will lose fat. Don't weigh yourself every half hour. In fact, THROW AWAY YOUR SCALE. Give it to an enemy. *Choose to Lose* is not about weight loss. It is about fat loss. (Rest assured, if you lose fat, you will lose weight.)

The scale does not distinguish among water loss,* muscle loss, and fat loss. A more accurate and positive way to measure your progress is to take note of the way you fit into your clothes. Fitting into a smaller pair of pants or dress indicates that you are losing fat and building lean muscle mass, which is just as important as losing pounds. In fact, it is more important because the greater your muscle mass, the greater your metabolic capacity to burn fat and the more weight you will lose in the future. Changes in size are more likely to occur if you exercise aerobically every day.

In the first few weeks of following *Choose to Lose*, you will be replacing the fat you are losing with the muscle you are building from exercising. This muscle has weight. Actually, muscle is heavier than fat. In the long run, added muscle will help you burn fat. In the short run, because the muscle you are building may weigh as much as the fat you are losing, you may not see the loss registered on the scale. This is another reason not to measure your progress by stepping on the scale fifteen times a day.

---

*It takes 4 grams of water to store 1 gram of carbohydrate. When you follow a low-carbohydrate diet, you reduce your carbohydrate stores and thus the weight you lose is mostly water.

Patience Is at the Center

You'll notice that the word *patience* lies at the center of the triangle on page 16. Patience is the byword of *Choose to Lose*. People lose weight at different rates. You may be one of the fortunate people whose fat melts away like butter in the summer sun. Or you may find that fat clings to you like an adoring friend. In either case, if you follow *Choose to Lose*, you will lose weight. One reader wrote to us after she had lost 45 pounds, "My goal is to lose another 50 lbs. I don't worry about losing weight any longer, because I know that living this lifestyle will put me there in the next year or so."

Telling It Like It Is

That's it. You are overweight

not because you eat too much food, but because you eat too much fat (more than you are burning) and the excess is going directly into your fat stores;

not because you eat too much carbohydrate, but because you eat too little;

not because you are not a marathon runner, but because you are not exercising regularly to protect your muscle and force your body to burn fat from the fat stores.

So, to lose weight, you must eat less fat and more carbohydrates, and also exercise aerobically, which includes walking.

CHOOSE TO LOSE WORKS AND KEEPS ON WORKING

Choose to Lose Is Livable

Choose to Lose is an eating plan for life. It is not a quick fix. Many people think of a diet as a dreadful, but short-term endeavor. They decide to lose weight. They jump on Diet Island, where they starve, are deprived, eat powders, drink liquids, or balance exchanges. Everything they do is totally unnatural. And then, when they have lost weight (or given up), they jump off the island and return to their old eating habits. They gain back all the weight they lost because they made no permanent lifestyle changes. Sound familiar?

Choose to Lose is not an island. It is not temporary (or dreadful, either) because you are full and satisfied and can follow it forever.

But if your goal is to lose 40 pounds in the next three weeks so you can fit into your bathing suit or the fancy silk dress that you haven't been able to zipper for 20 years, then you may be disappointed. Following *Choose to Lose*, you will lose that 40 pounds, but it will take longer than three weeks. And the results will last. You will learn to love a low-fat diet so you can maintain your weight loss for your lifetime, as well as improve your long-term health prospects.

Choose to Lose Gives You the Tools and Skills to Take Control

You now know the science behind *Choose to Lose*. Next you will learn the details, the specifics that will help you apply *Choose to Lose* in your life. For instance, you know that *fat* is the culprit that is making you fat, but do you know the sources of fat in your diet? You know that cheesecake and ice cream sundaes are full of fat, but how about whole milk and granola bars? Are steaks high-fat or high-protein? You want to reduce the fat in your diet but by how much? *Choose to Lose* has the answers.

Choose to Lose provides insight, so you know where fat lurks in your diet and what changes you need to make to lose weight.

Choose to Lose helps you determine a FAT BUDGET, so you know how much fat you can "afford" to eat and still reach and maintain your desirable and healthy weight.

Choose to Lose shows you how to keep track of the fat you eat, so you know that you are making enough changes to reach your goal.

Choose to Lose puts you in control.

Choose to Lose Gives You a New Outlook on Food

Choose to Lose is not restrictive. It is an eating plan you can follow for a lifetime because it is palatable, practical, and flexible. You can choose to eat anything you want as long as it fits into your Fat Budget.

You're the boss. No one can tell you what you can or cannot eat. But knowing that you can eat high-fat favorites gives you the freedom not to eat them. Do you regard every high-fat goodie as a last-chance opportunity? When you see a piece of cheesecake, do you view it as the last cheesecake on earth? You know you shouldn't eat it, but it's your last chance to eat it — so you eat it. This reasoning is not logical; it is a gut reaction. Knowing that the cheesecake has 160 fat calories and that you can fit it into your Fat Budget (albeit you will have to eat a low, low-fat diet for a few days to compensate) frees you. Maybe you'll have it another day.

You won't believe it now, but having a Fat Budget and knowing the "cost" of foods will change you. You will go to a wedding and instead of frantically eating everything in sight because you'll never have the chance again, you will say, "Yuk, that greasy chicken wing isn't worth 120 fat calories," or "Yum, that slice of Black Forest cake is worth a major (but temporary) dent in my Fat Budget." Knowing you can eat the way others do relieves the pressure to gorge yourself whenever enticing food appears.

The goal of *Choose to Lose* is for you to move from a high-fat taste to a delicious, low-fat taste. Today you may say, "Not me. I'll never lose my fat tooth," but in a short time you may be repelled by food you once thought you couldn't live without.

Tastes Change

One Chooser to Lose told us he had given up fast food altogether, but for his birthday, he decided to treat himself to a Quarter Pounder. He bought the burger, but couldn't stomach eating it. He had made the lifestyle switch. This is not unusual. Scientific studies have shown it takes about 12 weeks to change from a high-fat to a low-fat taste. It may (and probably will) happen to you.

Choose to Lose Makes a Healthier You

Overweight people have all sorts of health problems, which they might have avoided had they followed *Choose to Lose*. By eating a diet low in fat and high in carbohydrates and fiber you can reduce your risk of diabetes, heart disease, stroke, kidney disease, cancer of the breast, prostate, and colon, bone and joint disorders, female sterility, pregnancy problems, and premature death. You will also improve your regularity.

People following *Choose to Lose* have reported major reductions in blood cholesterol (some as much as 100 points), significant reductions in blood pressure, and normalization of blood sugar. Some have told us they no longer suffer from swollen ankles. These short-term changes are just the tip of the iceberg. They predict vastly improved health in the future.

Focus on Health

Studies have shown that the people who are most successful at losing weight and keeping it off are those whose prime motivation is their health rather than their appearance. They know that by reducing their intake of fat and eating nutritious foods they are reducing their risks of many chronic diseases. Weight loss will come as a side effect. Think of *Choose to Lose* first as your ticket to good health.

Choose to Lose Improves the Quality of Your Life

Changing the way you eat will give you a new lease on life. You will be introduced to a whole new variety of delicious, tasty low-fat foods. Freed from the bonds of limited calories, you will be able to enjoy a baked potato, a bowl of cereal, half a cantaloupe, whenever your heart desires. Encouraged by the many benefits of home-cooked meals, you may find you love to cook and are a talented chef.

More Energy and Stamina. Low-fat/high-carbohydrate eating will keep your glycogen stores filled up. As a result you will have more energy and more stamina. No more dragging yourself around from hour to hour after no breakfast and lunch, and a high-fat dinner. With your new infusion of energy, you may have to make a new set of friends twenty years younger who are able to keep up with the new you.

If you are obese now, you will find that such simple activities as walking are a lot easier after losing weight. No more huffing and puffing. No more embarrassment at stuffing yourself into chairs or navigating through narrow passages. What's more, you'll feel good about yourself.

Enough Talking — Let's Get Started

Read the next chapter to see how you can make *Choose to Lose* work for you.

Remember:

1. Not all calories contribute equally to weight gain or loss.
2. Carbohydrates are not fattening because
    a. you have a limited capacity to store carbohydrates, so almost all the carbohydrates you eat are burned within a few hours.
    b. the more carbohydrates you eat, the higher is your basal metabolic rate and thus the faster you burn everything, including stored fat.
    c. under normal conditions, carbohydrate is never converted to fat and thus never leads to weight gain.
3. Fat calories are fattening because
    a. all the fat you eat is immediately stored.
    b. the capacity to store fats is essentially unlimited.
    c. fat is the stored energy of last resort.

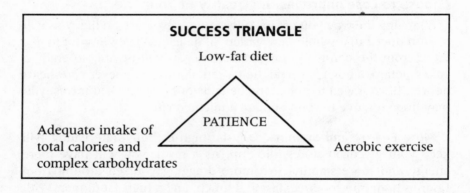

4. *Choose to Lose* is a simple, practical, and flexible plan based on three strategies for maximizing weight loss (Success Triangle):
    a. reduce your intake of fat because the less fat you add to the fat stores, the less you will have to remove.
    b. eat lots of vegetables, fruits, low-fat whole-grains, and low- and nonfat dairy to:
        (1) maximize your metabolic rate;
        (2) ensure that you consume enough vitamins, minerals, and fiber for long-term good health;
        (3) keep you full, satisfied, and content;
        (4) increase your energy and stamina.
    c. engage in regular aerobic exercise to:
        (1) build and maintain muscle;

(2) force the body to burn fat rather than protein from muscle;

(3) maximize your BMR.

5. *Choose to Lose* puts you in control and teaches you to make food choices that will keep you thin for life.

6. *Choose to Lose* is a healthy way of eating and will reduce your risks of many chronic diseases.

2. The *Choose to Lose* Plan

"Counting fat calories is much easier than counting anything else."

Jennie Pagano, Metuchen, New Jersey

"The two concepts in your books that spurred me to action were
(1) choices amongst alternatives and (2) keeping track of essentially
one thing: fat calories. They made sense, didn't markedly interfere
with my lifestyle, and allowed me to say to myself, 'I can do that.'"

Carl Iseli, Silver Spring, Maryland

THE *Choose to Lose* plan is simple. You need to know:

1. Your personal **Fat Budget** — the maximum number of fat calories
   you can eat each day and still reach and maintain your desirable
   and healthy weight. This is yours alone. It is based on the total number of calories needed to satisfy *your* basal metabolic rate (BMR) at
   your goal weight.
2. The number of **fat calories** in foods.

YOUR FAT BUDGET: THE KEY TO SUCCESS

Your Fat Budget is a powerful tool. It gives you a framework for making
choices. It is like your salary. If you went shopping and didn't know
your salary, how could you make choices? How could you decide
whether you could afford a $250 television set or a $40 pair of shoes?
The same is true of food. The reason that so many Americans are overweight is not because they all have psychological difficulties. They are
fat because they have no idea how much fat is in the food they eat and
they have no way of judging if they can afford it. Your Fat Budget puts
all foods into perspective so you can make choices. If you know that a
3-ounce bag of Fritos contains 270 fat calories and your Fat Budget is
315 for the whole day, you can decide whether you want to blow your
day's fat intake on a tiny bag of chips.

Knowing your Fat Budget and the calories of fat in different foods, **you can choose to eat any combination of foods** — even your high-fat favorites — **as long as you stay within your Fat Budget.**

DETERMINING YOUR VERY OWN FAT BUDGET

Choose to Lose is based on a Fat Budget that is tailored to you. It is based on your sex, height, frame size, and goal weight. You probably know what your goal weight is without looking at the following tables. Skip to Table 2, pages 21–22, if you know what you should weigh. Otherwise, if you want to determine your desirable weight or just want to see if the weight table agrees with your perception of perfection, consult Table 1.

Step 1: Determine Your Desirable Weight

Table 1 lists desirable weights according to sex, height, and frame size — small, medium, or large. (To determine your frame size, see the box below.) Find your height along the left-hand column of Table 1 under the heading *Women* or *Men.* Look across to the weight range listed under your frame size and choose the weight within the range that is right for you. Fill in Step 1 of the worksheet on page 27.

How to Determine Your Frame Size

Place your left thumb and middle finger around your right wrist and squeeze your fingers together. If the thumb and finger overlap, you have a small frame. If they just touch, your frame size is medium. If they do not touch, you have a large frame. This method is crude, but adequate for our purposes. (If you know you have a smaller or larger frame than this method shows, use your actual frame size and ignore the results of the wrist test.)

Step 2: Determine your ⬭Minimum⬭ Daily Total Caloric Intake

Table 2 lists minimum daily total caloric intakes for various goal weights. This is the number of calories needed to satisfy your basal metabolism at your goal weight. In other words, this is the minimum amount of calories (energy) you need each day to maintain your vital functions when you are *completely* at rest. This is a MINIMUM. We repeat. THIS IS A MINIMUM! THIS IS A FLOOR. Your body needs more

Table 1. Desirable Weights for Adults Age 25 and Over
(weight in pounds without clothing)

HEIGHT WITHOUT SHOES		FRAME		
(FEET)	(INCHES)	SMALL	MEDIUM	LARGE
Women				
4	8	92–98	96–107	104–119
4	9	94–101	98–110	106–122
4	10	96–104	101–113	109–125
4	11	99–107	104–116	112–128
5	0	102–110	107–119	115–131
5	1	105–113	110–122	118–134
5	2	108–116	113–126	121–138
5	3	111–119	116–130	125–142
5	4	114–123	120–135	129–146
5	5	118–127	124–139	133–150
5	6	122–131	128–143	137–154
5	7	126–135	132–147	141–158
5	8	130–140	136–151	145–163
5	9	134–144	140–155	149–168
5	10	138–148	144–159	153–173
5	11	142–152	148–163	157–177
6	0	146–156	152–167	161–181
Men				
5	1	112–120	118–129	126–141
5	2	115–123	121–133	129–144
5	3	118–126	124–136	132–148
5	4	121–129	127–139	135–152
5	5	124–133	130–143	138–156
5	6	128–137	134–147	142–161
5	7	132–141	138–152	147–166
5	8	136–145	142–156	151–170
5	9	140–150	146–160	155–174
5	10	144–154	150–165	159–179
5	11	148–158	154–170	164–184
6	0	152–162	158–175	168–189
6	1	156–167	162–180	173–194
6	2	160–171	167–185	178–199
6	3	164–175	172–190	183–204
6	4	168–179	177–195	188–209

Courtesy of Metropolitan Life Insurance Company, New York, N.Y., 1959
For persons between 18 and 25 years of age, subtract 1 pound for each year under 25.

Table 2. Minimum Total Caloric Intake and Fat Budget
Based on Goal Weight and Sex

GOAL WEIGHT	MINIMUM DAILY TOTAL CALORIC INTAKE*	FAT CALORIES		
		20% BUDGET	17% BUDGET	15% BUDGET
Women				
90	1053	211	179	158
95	1111	222	189	167
100	1170	234	199	176
105	1228	246	209	184
110	1287	257	219	193
115	1345	269	229	202
120	1404	281	239	211
125	1462	292	248	219
130	1521	304	258	228
135	1579	315	268	237
140	1638	328	278	246
145	1696	339	288	254
150	1755	351	298	263
155	1813	363	308	272
160	1872	374	318	281
165	1930	386	328	290
170	1989	398	338	298
175	2047	409	348	307
180	2106	421	358	316
185	2164	433	368	325
190	2223	445	378	334
195	2281	456	388	342
200	2340	468	398	351
Men				
110	1430	286	243	215
115	1495	299	254	224
120	1560	312	265	234
125	1625	325	276	244
130	1690	338	287	254
135	1755	351	298	263
140	1820	364	309	273
145	1885	377	320	283
150	1950	390	332	292
155	2015	403	343	302
160	2080	416	354	312
165	2145	429	365	322
170	2210	442	376	332
175	2275	455	387	341
180	2340	468	398	351
185	2405	481	409	361

Table 2. (continued)

GOAL WEIGHT	MINIMUM DAILY TOTAL CALORIC INTAKE	FAT CALORIES		
		20% BUDGET	17% BUDGET	15% BUDGET
Men (cont'd)				
190	2470	494	420	370
195	2535	507	431	380
200	2600	520	442	390
205	2665	533	453	400
210	2730	546	464	410
215	2795	559	475	419
220	2860	572	486	429
225	2925	585	497	439
230	2990	598	508	449
235	3055	611	519	458
240	3120	624	530	468
245	3185	637	541	478
250	3250	650	552	488

*From *The DINE System* by Dr. Darwin Dennison

than this MINIMUM total caloric intake to operate. Remember BMR + physical activity. You walk, you climb steps, some of you even run, bike, or swim. You need more calories than this minimum amount in order to power your physical activity. How many more depends on how much physical activity you do each day. For most people 400 to 600 total calories in addition to the minimum total caloric intake will be sufficient. But if you eat a few hundred total calories beyond even that amount as fiber-rich carbohydrates, don't worry. They will be burned off and not be stored as fat.

So if you are a woman who wants to weigh 140 pounds, you need to eat a *minimum* of 1638 calories a day. You should actually be eating about 2000 or 2100 total calories a day. That's right. You won't gain weight if you eat more than 2000 calories a day. In fact, if your minimum total caloric intake is 1638 and you eat less than that, you will probably not lose weight. (See Chapter 1 to understand the science.)

You may wonder why we ask you to determine total calories when *Choose to Lose* is based on limiting fat, not total calories, and we insist that you do not limit your total calories. This is why: knowing your minimum total caloric intake is important so you don't eat *too few* total calories. (See the box on page 25.)

To determine your minimum total daily caloric intake, first find your goal weight along the left-hand column of Table 2 under the heading *Women* or *Men*. Look across to the column labeled Minimum Daily Caloric Intake to find your number. Fill in Step 2 of your worksheet.

Why You Must Eat MORE than Your Minimum Total Caloric Intake

1. To ensure that you get enough energy (calories) to fuel your basal metabolic rate (the rate at which you burn calories at rest) + physical activity.
2. To keep up your basal metabolic rate. If your total caloric intake falls below the minimum amount you determined, your basal metabolic rate will decrease and you will lose fat more slowly.
3. To ensure that you consume enough vitamins, minerals, and fiber for long-term health.
4. To ensure you will not be hungry. Hunger leads to bingeing and eating foods that work against your healthy-eating/fat-loss goals.

Step 3: Determining Your Fat Budget

Choosing a Percentage. You will notice that three Fat Budgets are listed under the column Fat Calories: 20 percent, 17 percent, and 15 percent. We advise you to start your Fat Budget at 20 percent, meaning that you will eat no more than 20 percent of your minimum total calories as fat. If you are now consuming a typical American diet (about 35 to 40 percent of total calories from fat), 20 percent will represent a substantial change in your diet. Actually, because you will be eating more total calories than the minimum total on which you based your Fat Budget, the 20 percent Fat Budget is really more like 17 percent. Reducing fat intake to 17 percent of calories will easily create a new slim you.

Going Lower. If, after three or four weeks, you find that the 20 percent Fat Budget allows you more fat than you feel necessary to achieve your desirable and healthy weight, lower your Fat Budget to 17 or 15 percent. Be careful. You are going to follow *Choose to Lose* for life so you shouldn't choose a Fat Budget that is so bare-bones that you can follow it for only a few weeks. You want to choose a budget that lowers your fat intake but one that you can follow without suffering pangs of martyrdom.

Losing by Stages. On the other hand, you may feel that the 20 percent Fat Budget for your goal weight is too restrictive. For example, if you weigh 190 pounds and want to weigh 120, the 20 percent Fat Budget for 120 pounds is 281 fat calories. If a limit of 281 fat calories a day seems impossible to achieve, pick an attainable weight somewhere between 190 pounds and 120 pounds — perhaps 155 pounds. Determine a 20 percent Fat Budget for the intermediate weight (363 fat calories) and adhere to it until you weigh 155 pounds. When you attain that weight, adopt the Fat Budget for your next goal, 120 pounds. (This will be your Fat Budget for the rest of your life.) Your weight loss may be somewhat slower this way, but if you feel more comfortable working in stages, you are more likely to follow *Choose to Lose* until you reach your final goal. After all, a weight loss plan works only if it fits your individual needs and you stick with it.

Calories, Not Grams

Choose to Lose uses calories rather than grams for three reasons. First, grams are a mystery while calories are familiar. You have lived with calories all your life. You probably even know approximately how many total calories you should be eating. If you see that a chocolate bar contains 99 fat calories of fat, familiarity helps you judge how fattening it is. What does the same amount of fat in grams (11 grams) mean to you?

Second, since your Fat Budget is a percentage of your minimum daily total caloric intake it makes more sense to express your Fat Budget in the same units as your total intake — that is, calories. Calories are units of energy. Grams are units of weight.

Third, expressing fat content as grams has less impact than expressing it as calories since each gram of fat equals 9 calories. "Only 5 grams of fat per cookie," you say as you cram 5 cookies in your mouth. But would you eat them with abandon if you knew each cookie contained 45 fat calories?

To determine your Fat Budget, find your goal weight again and look across to the column labeled 20% BUDGET. Fill in Step 3 of your worksheet.

Now you have a Fat Budget. Engrave it in your mind. This number is your key to success.

Important: Your Fat Budget is a part of your daily total caloric intake, not an addition to it.

Your Fat Budget Is a Ceiling

Remember, your Fat Budget is a ceiling, *not* a goal. If, at the end of the day, you have eaten only 150 fat calories and your Fat Budget is 315, don't, we repeat DON'T, run out to Kentucky Fried Chicken and order a fried chicken wing to boost up your fat intake so it equals your Fat Budget. Rather, pat yourself on the back and smile because you will reach your fat-loss goal that much sooner.

A CASE STUDY

Meet Ellen. Ellen is trying to lose weight. Her example should clarify each step of the *Choose to Lose* system for you.

Here's how Ellen figures out her Fat Budget. (See Ellen's worksheet, page 26.) Ellen is 5 feet 5 inches tall and weighs 185 pounds. She determines by the wrist test that she has a medium frame. To find her desirable weight, she locates her height (5'5") in the left-hand column of Table 1 under the heading *Women*. Reading across to the Frame column labeled Medium, she finds that her weight range is 124–139. Ellen knows that she will look and feel great at 135 pounds.

Table 1

HEIGHT WITHOUT SHOES		DESIRABLE WEIGHTS FRAME		
(FEET)	(INCHES)	SMALL	MEDIUM	LARGE
Women				
5	4	114–123	120–135	129–146
5	**5**	118–127	**124–139**	133–150
5	6	122–131	128–143	137–154

Worksheet to Determine Your Daily Fat Budget

Name ___ELLEN_____ Date ___1/9/94_____

STEP 1:   DETERMINE YOUR GOAL WEIGHT.

      A. Sex: Male _____ Female ___X_____

      B. Height: ___5____ feet ___5____ inches

      C. Frame (wrist method):

           Small _____ Medium ___X_____ Large _____

      D. Weight Range (Table 1): __124-139_____

      E. Goal Weight: ___135_____

STEP 2:   DETERMINE YOUR MINIMUM DAILY TOTAL CALORIC INTAKE.

      Minimum daily total caloric intake (use Table 2): __1579_____

STEP 3:   DETERMINE YOUR FAT BUDGET.

      FAT BUDGET (use Table 2):

      Choose one:

      20% of _____1579_____ = ____315____
             (your minimum daily caloric intake)   (your Fat Budget)

      17% of _____ = _____
             (your minimum daily caloric intake)   (your Fat Budget)

      15% of _____ = _____
             (your minimum daily caloric intake)   (your Fat Budget)

Worksheet to Determine Your Daily Fat Budget

Name _____ Date _____

STEP 1:   DETERMINE YOUR GOAL WEIGHT.

    A. Sex: Male _____ Female ___✓___

    B. Height: ___5___ feet _10 ½_ inches

    C. Frame (wrist method):

       Small ___✓___ Medium _____ Large _____

    D. Weight Range (Table 1): _140 - 150_

    E. Goal Weight: _145_

STEP 2:   DETERMINE YOUR MINIMUM DAILY TOTAL CALORIC INTAKE.

    Minimum daily total caloric intake (use Table 2): _1696_

STEP 3:   DETERMINE YOUR FAT BUDGET.

    FAT BUDGET (use Table 2):

    Choose one:

    20% of _____ = _339_
          (your minimum daily caloric intake)   (your Fat Budget)

    17% of _____ = _2-88_
          (your minimum daily caloric intake)   (your Fat Budget)

    15% of _____ = _254_
          (your minimum daily caloric intake)   (your Fat Budget)

Next, Ellen needs to determine her minimum daily caloric intake. She locates her goal weight (135) in Table 2 under the heading *Women*. Looking across to the column labeled Minimum Daily Caloric Intake, she finds her number — 1579. Ellen remembers that this number is a floor. She must eat more than 1579 total calories if she wants to lose weight.

Ellen chooses the 20 percent Fat Budget. Looking across to the column labeled 20% Budget, Ellen finds her daily Fat Budget — 315 fat calories.

Table 2

GOAL WEIGHT	MINIMUM DAILY TOTAL CALORIC INTAKE	FAT CALORIES		
		20% BUDGET	17% BUDGET	15% BUDGET
Women				
130	1521	304	258	228
135	**1579**	**315**	268	237
140	1638	328	278	246

See page 27 to fill out your own worksheet.

What Does Your Fat Budget Mean in Terms of Food?

What does Ellen's budget of 315 fat calories mean? What about your Fat Budget? How does this number translate into food choices? Here are some foods and the fat calories they contain. As you read, keep your own Fat Budget in mind.

FOOD	FAT CALORIES
Egg (yolk)	50
Potato chips (1 cup)	75
Peanut butter (1 tablespoon)	74
Baked potato with skin	0
Wendy's potato with cheese	306
Vinaigrette dressing (2 tablespoons)	128
Swiss cheese (1 oz)	70
Broiled lamb loin chop, untrimmed	144

FOOD	FAT CALORIES
Chicken breast baked without skin	13
Chicken breast, batter-dipped and fried, with skin	166
Plain white rice (1 cup), no fat added	0
Whole milk (1 cup)	73
2% milk (1 cup)	45
Skim milk (1 cup)	4
Kit Kat candy bar	110
Stouffer's Turkey Pie	300
Swanson Kids Fun Feast Frazzlin' Fried Chicken	320
Lunchables Fun Pack (bologna)	260
Margarine (1 tablespoon)	100
Hardee's Big Country Breakfast	630

Are any of these foods familiar? Do you understand now why you haven't been mistaken for a stick recently?

USING YOUR FAT BUDGET TO MAKE CHOICES

Your Fat Budget will make you food-smart. You won't eat just because a food is there. Before you pop a handful of peanuts (about 35 nuts) into your mouth, knowing that 35 peanuts cost about 125 fat calories and your Fat Budget is 315 fat calories for the entire day, you can decide if that fleeting pleasure is worth more than one-third of your budget.

Having a Fat Budget and knowing the fat calories in foods helps you make better choices. Instead of gulping down a cup of cream of mushroom soup at 155 fat calories, you might choose to start dinner with 6 large boiled shrimp (6 fat calories) dipped in cocktail sauce (0 fat calories). You might decide that Kellogg's Nutri·Grain Wheat and Raisins Cereal at 0 fat calories is a better choice than Quaker 100% Natural Oat, Honey, & Raisins Cereal at 70 fat calories per half cup.

Although your goal is to move from a high-fat/low-complex-carbohydrate diet to a low-fat/high-complex-carbohydrate diet, you may still want to include some sinful favorites. This eating plan is for life, after all. If you really want to eat a slice of Aunt Tilly's chocolate mousse pie at a cost of 250 fat calories, you can. You will just have to balance the fat calories with low, low-fat choices for several days. With *Choose to Lose* you never have to feel guilty or deprived.

Percentage of Fat in Foods: A Misinterpretation of the Guidelines

You have probably read healthy-eating articles urging you to choose only foods with less than 30 percent of their calories coming from fat or have seen foods listed according to the percentage of fat they contain so you can choose those with low percentages. This is a misunderstanding of the health guidelines that recommend that you eat less than 30 percent* of your **total** daily caloric intake as fat and could lead to eating massive amounts of fat.

Let us explain. Percentage of fat in individual foods is irrelevant. For example, a malted milk has 1060 total calories. Of those total calories, 225 or 21 percent are fat calories. While 21 percent is a relatively low percentage of fat, how do 225 fat calories fit into your Fat Budget? Drink two malteds and you consume a whopping 450 fat calories. Yet each drink is still only 21 percent fat. If a healthy diet could include any food as long as it had less than 30 percent of its calories from fat or even less than 21 percent of its calories from fat, you could drink ten of these malteds and accumulate 4500 fat calories. On the other hand, you wouldn't be allowed to eat a food if 5 of its 10 total calories came from fat because it would be 50 percent fat. Five fat calories would hardly make a flea fat.

If you eat only foods with less than 30 percent fat, not only could you accumulate enough fat calories to obliterate your Fat Budget, but your diet would be unnecessarily restricted. You could never cook with even a teaspoon of oil because all oils are 100 percent fat. Cheese, beef, and nuts would be totally verboten because they contain more than 30 percent of their calories from fat. Your food choices would be limited as would be your healthy-eating attention span.

The percentage you used to determine your Fat Budget is the only percentage that should ever concern you (and, now that you have used it to determine your Fat Budget, you can tuck it away in the back of your brain.) The only information you need to know to choose a food is the number of fat calories it contains and how it fits into your budget.

---

*All the major health agencies recommend eating less than 30 percent of your total caloric intake as fat. We think 30 percent is too high. This percentage was chosen despite the fact that many health educators agree that 20–25 percent is a healthier range because they felt the public might balk at fat intakes this low.

You will soon find that you prefer many foods that are low in fat. Knowing the "cost" of commercial foods, you will appreciate how easily and deliciously the *Choose to Lose* and *Eater's Choice* recipes fit into your Fat Budget. For example, take a dinner of *Cauliflower Soup** (7 fat calories) to begin. Then have *Cajun Chicken* (28 fat calories) on a bed of rice (0 fat calories), steamed broccoli (0 fat calories), and a baked sweet potato (0 fat calories), and for dessert a dish of nonfat frozen yogurt (0 fat calories) covered with strawberries (0 fat calories). The total cost: 35 fat calories. Compare this to a meager dinner of Stouffer's Macaroni and Cheese at a cost of 150 fat calories.

DETERMINING THE FAT CALORIES IN FOODS

Now that you have your own Fat Budget, you are probably eager to find out how much fat you have been eating. How much does that handful of innocent sunflower seeds cost you? Is the Arby's chicken breast sandwich you had for lunch a low-fat choice? To help you learn the fat calories in foods so you can make better choices, the *Choose to Lose* Food Tables list fat calories and total calories for many foods. You will want to become familiar with these tables. Not only can you use them to look up the fat calories of foods you ate or plan to eat, you can browse through them to find low-fat alternatives for high-fat foods. Read on to find out how easy it is to use the Food Tables.

THE FOOD TABLES

The Food Tables on pages 277–437 are an invaluable source of information — and surprises. They give you insight into why you did not wear a bikini last summer. Would you have thought that 15 potato chips have 90 fat calories? Four ounces of lean flank steak has 140 fat calories? Nine little cashews have 60 fat calories? Keep your Fat Budget in mind when you browse through the tables.

Organization

The Food Tables are organized alphabetically into major food groups, such as **BEVERAGES, DAIRY PRODUCTS AND EGGS, FAST**

---

*Italicized recipes come from *Choose to Lose* or *Eater's Choice: A Food Lover's Guide to Lower Cholesterol* by Dr. Ron Goor and Nancy Goor (Houghton Mifflin, 1987, 1989, 1992, 1995).

FOODS, FATS AND OILS, etc. You will find a list of Contents on page 277 to help you locate these major food groupings. You might want to put your own identifying tabs at the beginning of each group so you can turn to them quickly.

The food categories within each major group are also organized alphabetically. For example, the first subheading under **DAIRY PRODUCTS AND EGGS** is *Butter.* The next is *Cheese.*

Within each food category, foods are listed alphabetically according to type. The first entry under *Cheese* is American, then blue, then Camembert, and so on.

Quick Find: Food Tables Index

If you have difficulty locating specific foods in the Food Tables, check the Food Tables Index (pages 438–41) following the Food Tables. In this index, foods are listed alphabetically rather than by group.

How Much Did You Actually Eat? The amount that you ate and the portion size listed in the Food Tables may differ. You must adjust the numbers of total calories and fat calories listed in the tables to the amount you actually ate. For example, if a half cup of Ben & Jerry's Vanilla Bean ice cream contains 150 calories of fat, and you ate 1 cup (or 2 times as much as the listed amount), you consumed 150 × 2 or 300 fat calories. You would also double the total calories (230 total calories × 2 = 460 total calories). On the other hand, if you ate a quarter cup of the ice cream or half a serving, you consumed 150 ÷ 2 or 75 fat calories and 230 ÷ 2 = 115 total calories.

Comparison Value. Data for many foods such as cheeses and meats are given in 1-ounce amounts to help you compare fat contents so you can make informed choices. However, keep in mind that although 1-ounce portions are listed for a food, 1 ounce may be much less than you eat and you must adjust your figures accordingly.

No One Eats a 1-Ounce Piece of Steak. For instance, at first glance, the meats (beef, veal, lamb, pork, poultry, fish) all look like low-fat foods because the fat values are given for 1-ounce portions. But, as you rarely eat 1 ounce of meat, you must multiply the calories and fat calories for a 1-ounce portion by the number of ounces you actually ate. If you ate 4 ounces of lean ground beef, you would multiply the fat content of lean ground beef — 47 fat calories — by 4 to determine the number of fat calories you actually ate: $4 \times 47 = 188$ fat calories.

Find Your Favorites in the Food Tables

If you are dying to know the cost of that pecan Danish you bought at the supermarket to sustain you while you shopped or the 8-ounce bag of cheese twists you emptied while watching your favorite football team crush their perennial rival, turn to the Food Tables and take a look. You might also want to make a list of 5 to 10 of your favorite foods. Next, using the Food Tables, determine the fat calories for the amount you usually eat. Then find low-fat alternatives by scanning through the same section of the Food Tables. For example, if you have been eating trail mix as a healthy "diet" dessert, look it up in the Food Tables under **NUTS AND SEEDS** or **SNACKS.** Is it worth 80 fat calories per quarter cup? Look on a little farther in the Snacks section and you'll find air-popped popcorn at 0 fat calories. It tastes great. Perhaps at 0 fat calories, you'll find it an attractive alternative.

Coming Next . . . Before you try to discover where fat lurks in every aspect of your own diet, read on to see what Ellen eats, what it costs her, and what insights she gains from keeping track. Don't be surprised if you get the eerie feeling you are reading about yourself.

Remember:
1. *Choose to Lose* is a simple method for losing weight that limits the amount of fat you eat while still allowing you to fit in your high-fat favorites. You need to know two things:
   a. Your personal **Fat Budget,** the maximum number of fat calories you can eat each day to reach and maintain your desirable and healthy weight. Your Fat Budget provides a framework for making food choices.
      (1) Use the step-by-step guide to *Choose to Lose* to:
         (a) determine your desirable weight (Table 1).
         (b) determine your minimum daily total caloric intake (Table 2).
         (c) determine your Fat Budget (Table 2).

    (2) Your Fat Budget is the key to success because:

        (a) You can judge the "cost" of any food so you can make wise food choices.

        (b) You can eat any combination of foods as long as they fit within your budget.

        (c) You can budget in high-fat splurges.

  b. Use the Food Tables to determine the fat calories of the foods you ate.

    (1) Adjust the calories and fat calories for the actual amount you consumed

    (2) Don't forget that meat, cheese, and some other foods are listed in 1-ounce portions.

2. The minimum daily total caloric intake (Table 2) is a floor. It is the number of calories needed to sustain your body if you are completely at rest. You will need to eat additional calories to fuel your activity. If you don't eat enough calories (and complex carbohydrates), your basal metabolic rate slows down, you burn fat more slowly, and you do not consume an adequate amount of vitamins, minerals, and fiber for good health. Therefore, **YOU MUST EAT MORE THAN THIS MINIMUM NUMBER OF TOTAL CALORIES. YOU MUST EAT TO LOSE. OF COURSE, YOU MUST EAT NUTRITIOUS, LOW-FAT FOODS TO LOSE.**

3. Self-Discovery

"I never realized how much fat I take in during one day, and now that I have been cutting back on the fat calories I have lost 12 lbs in 4 weeks and yet I'm not starving myself or depriving myself of all of those 'forbidden foods' on every other diet."

Janice Douglass, Newark, Delaware

MOST all of us think we eat *no* fat and thus are mystified that we are overweight. Ellen would also insist that she eats no more fat than her thin friends and can't understand why she is fat and they are not. Let's look at her intake for a day for the real story.

ELLEN'S FOOD RECORD: AN ILLUMINATING EXAMPLE

Ellen is going to keep track of everything she eats without making changes. Before she begins altering her diet, she wants to have a picture of how much fat she currently eats and which foods are the high-fat culprits. Ellen will write down the times of day she eats as well as the exact amount of every morsel she lets slip between her lips. She will use the Food Tables on pages 277–437 and food labels to determine the fat calories of the foods she eats.

BREAKFAST: DON'T MISS IT

Ellen is supposed to be at work by 8:30 A.M., which means getting out of the house by 7:45. Ellen hates getting up in the morning, but she hates missing breakfast even more. She allows herself time to grab a muffin and a cup of coffee in the coffee shop in her building.

She records her muffin and coffee in her food record as she sits down to eat them. For the first time, Ellen questions her choice. It is a very large muffin and tastes a lot like pound cake. Perhaps she'll skip it this morning. A little voice inside her whispers, "This food record is for you alone. You are not keeping it to impress anyone with how little you eat. You need a baseline record so you can make changes — and lose weight. *Eat the muffin!*" By being honest with herself, Ellen has already made a step toward being a thin person.

Ellen's first entry in her food record looks like this.

	Ellen's Breakfast			
TIME	FOOD	AMOUNT	TOTAL CALORIES	FAT CALORIES
8:15 A.M.	Blueberry muffin	1 large	400	**140**
	Coffee	1 cup	0	**0**
	Half-and-half	1 tbsp	20	**15**
	Accumulated Fat Calories:			**155**
	Ellen's Fat Budget:			**315**

Ellen was wise to eat breakfast. Eating three meals a day (low-fat, high-carbohydrate meals, natch) is *extremely* important for weight loss. You want to start burning calories as soon as you get up. In addition, when you skip breakfast, you are apt to satisfy your midmorning cravings with a high-fat snack. However, the blueberry muffin was a poor choice. It tastes a lot like pound cake because it is made with all the same high-fat ingredients — butter, lard, or vegetable oil, and whole milk, sometimes cream. Next time, Ellen will have to decide if the blueberry muffin is worth almost half her Fat Budget.

Ellen uses half-and-half in her coffee. At 15 fat calories for each tablespoon, the fat adds up. How about 2% milk? 1% milk? Nonfat milk? Why not drink it black?

For better breakfast choices, see Chapter 6, "Putting *Choose to Lose* to Work for You."

MIDMORNING SNACK

At about 10:30, Ellen's friend Lisa often stops by with a treat. By this time, Ellen is already famished. Lisa reaches into a small white bag and, with a flourish, pulls out a glazed doughnut and a cup of coffee. Normally, Ellen eagerly eats the doughnut, considering it her splurge for the day. But today Ellen regards the doughnut with suspicion. She *knows* it's not going to look good on her food record. "How bad is it?" she wonders as she looks it up in the **SWEETS** section of the Food Tables: 130 fat calories! She sighs deeply as she records the number.

	Ellen's Morning Snack			
TIME	FOOD	AMOUNT	TOTAL CALORIES	FAT CALORIES
10:30 A.M.	Glazed doughnut	1 large	240	**130**
	Coffee	1 cup	0	**0**
	Half-and-half	1 tbsp	20	**15**
	Total Fat Calories:			**145**
	Accumulated Fat Calories:			**300**
	Ellen's Fat Budget:			**315**

Your Mother Was Right

Many adults have established the pattern of eating no breakfast and no lunch or a very light lunch. For some, the mistaken notion is that starvation is the way to lose weight. For others, breakfast and lunch may be the casualties of life in the fast lane. In either case, it is much healthier to eat three well-balanced meals than to starve yourself all day. Stuffing into one meal all the calories and nutrients needed for functioning at peak efficiency makes for very low efficiency peaks.

The chances are that if you eat no lunch, not only will you feel like a limp rag all afternoon, you will be so hungry and tired when you get home you will lose control and binge on high-fat snacks. Eating at least three meals a day is important for weight loss, too, because your body needs the fuel to maintain your basal metabolic rate (see Chapter 1).

Treat yourself like the special person you are. Take advantage of lunch to unwind and enjoy a delicious, nutritious, low-fat meal.

Instead of the doughnut, Ellen could have eaten a carton of nonfat flavored yogurt (0 fat calories), a bagel (9 fat calories) with jelly (0 fat calories), or an orange (0 fat calories), or all three.

LUNCH: SIT DOWN, CHOOSE WELL, AND ENJOY

The Fast-Food Option

Ellen looks forward to lunch. She knows she's always "good" at lunchtime. A salad should balance out the doughnut. Ellen has second thoughts about her restaurant choice — a fast-food restaurant. Next time she will have first thoughts. But it won't be easy. Friends or co-workers often choose restaurants that offer no food options for fat-conscious diners. Peer pressure is a poor excuse. Ellen has to stand up for her rights. The companionship of people who don't respect your diet wishes is not worth a lethal gash in your Fat Budget. Ellen might even convince her friends that they can enjoy a restaurant with low-fat options.

		Ellen's Lunch		
TIME	**FOOD**	**AMOUNT**	**TOTAL CALORIES**	**FAT CALORIES**
Noon	Mixed salad			
	lettuce	2 cups	20	**0**
	tomato	½	12	**0**
	cucumber	¼	10	**0**
	carrot	¼	8	**0**
	Russian dressing	4 tbsp*	308	**280**
	Sunflower seeds	1 tbsp	50	**39**
	Biscuit	1	231	**108**
	Butter	1 pat (tsp)	36	**36**
	Diet cola	8 oz	0	**0**
		Total Fat Calories:		**463**
		Accumulated Fat Calories:		**763**
		Ellen's Fat Budget:		**315**

*Two ladles = 2 ounces = 4 tablespoons

But today Ellen feels she can handle a fast-food restaurant. Her selections from the salad bar are bound to look good on her record. Ellen tops her salad with two ladles of Russian dressing and a tablespoon of sunflower seeds. Ellen notices that the ladle handle is marked 1 oz. She takes a biscuit — "so little and dry, it must be fat-free" — and a pat of butter — "just a tiny square." She chooses a diet cola.

Ellen determines the fat calories for the tiny salad and biscuit she ate. She is dismayed. She ate 463 fat calories and is hungrier after eating than she was before she started.

Salad Bar: Diet Trap

Ellen's notion that the salad bar is a good diet choice is wishful thinking. Most of the salad bar options are made with high-fat ingredients — mayonnaise salad with a macaroni or two, oil salad with a few slices of cold cuts or green beans, sour cream salad with walnuts and apple slices. Eating at a salad bar takes much care. Ellen's choice of salad vegetables — carrots, lettuce, tomatoes, and cucumbers — was diet-wise. Salad vegetables are complex carbohydrates that are high in fiber, vitamins, and minerals and almost completely fat-free. Ellen then added her favorite "vegetable": salad dressing.

Salad Dressing. Like many people who eat salad only because it is a socially acceptable way of consuming salad dressing, Ellen poured a lot — 2 ladles or 4 tablespoons of Russian dressing (70 fat calories per tablespoon or 280 calories for 4) — on her salad. A low- or reduced-calorie dressing would have been a better choice, although creamy reduced-calorie dressings at fast-food restaurants are still high in fat calories. (At Wendy's the reduced-calorie bacon-and-tomato dressing has about 32 fat calories per tablespoon.) Using 2 tablespoons of dressing instead of 4 cuts the fat calories in half, and 1 tablespoon cuts even more. Better yet, use the fork method.

The Fork Method

To reduce the amount of salad dressing you use, have the salad dressing served on the side. Then dip your fork into the dressing and spear a biteful of salad. You will get a taste of dressing, but most of the fat will remain in the bowl, not in you.

> BEWARE: The small salad dressing ladle at the salad bar holds 2 tablespoons of salad dressing. Two dunks and you have a quarter cup of dressing.

Sunflower Seeds. Ellen sprinkled a tablespoonful of sunflower seeds over her salad. That casual gesture cost her 39 fat calories. Seeds and nuts are high-fat foods.

Biscuits

Biscuits don't *look* fattening. A biscuit made in your kitchen may have about 50 fat calories, depending on the size and how much butter or shortening you add. A fast-food biscuit ranges from 63 fat calories (Denny's) to 135 (Arby's). Add a little pat of butter (36 fat calories) and your "innocent" biscuit creates a 99-to-171-calorie dent in your Fat Budget.

Diet Drinks

Ellen chose a diet drink to save calories. This choice is a throwback to the old diet mentality. While neither regular or diet sodas have any redeeming qualities, neither contains fat and thus neither is fattening. In addition, diet drinks contain unhealthy sugar substitutes. Both are poor choices. Choose skim milk, 100 percent fruit juices, or water.

Fast-Food Restaurants: The Ultimate Poor Choice

Although fast-food restaurants may lure you because they are quick, relatively inexpensive, and everywhere, the price of convenience is more than your body can afford. Think of what all that fat will cost in terms of fat calories (and your long-term health) and stay away. Even if you come with good intentions, the temptation to splurge on a Burger King Double Beef Whopper with cheese (549 fat calories), an order of Long John Silver fish and fries (432 fat calories), an order of Taco Bell Nachos Supreme (243 fat calories), or even an order of fries (126 fat calories) at Roy Rogers is hard to resist. As you can see from Ellen's food record, even the salad bar can be a disaster. Choose a sandwich shop, a real restaurant, or bring your lunch from home. For more on eating out, see Chapter 6, "Putting *Choose to Lose* to Work for You."

AFTERNOON SNACK

Ellen's lunch has left her ravenous. The grumbles from her stomach are so loud, she can hardly pay attention to her work. She has drained her trusty Big Sipper of 48 ounces of water, but she is still hungry. Finally she succumbs and opens a package of Oodles of Noodles she has squirreled away in her desk. "At least it's pasta and good for you." She smiles as she zaps the container in the office microwave. After finishing every last noodle, Ellen checks the label: 140 fat calories! "Why didn't I check the label first?" Ellen is stumped. How could 3 ounces of noodles have so much fat? The answer: the noodles are quick-fried in partially hydrogenated cottonseed oil.

	Ellen's Afternoon Snack			
TIME	FOOD	AMOUNT	TOTAL CALORIES	FAT CALORIES
3 P.M.	Oodles of Noodles (chicken)	1 package (3 oz)	400	**140**
		Total Fat Calories:		**140**
		Accumulated Fat Calories:		**903**
		Ellen's Fat Budget:		**315**

Water Is a Poor Substitute for Food

It is easy to spot dieters. They are the people walking around their worksites holding a gigantic plastic container of water. Every diet course they have taken (and there have been many) requires that they drink at least 8 glasses of water a day. Why? The first reason: Restricted-calorie diets produce toxins. Drinking water washes out the kidneys and prevents you from getting very sick. Second reason: Restricted-calorie diets make you hungry, and water helps fill you up.

Best reasons to drink water: you are thirsty and you enjoy it. But if you are doing it to lose weight, throw away your Big Sipper and start eating real, nutritious, low-fat food. Food is a lot more filling and satisfying and will really help you lose weight.

Always read the label *before* you eat the food. Repenting afterward doesn't take the fat back. Never make assumptions. Unadulterated pasta is a great, low-fat choice, but look what happened when it was turned into Oodles of Noodles.

DINNER: TAKE TIME TO EAT HEARTY

Ellen works without break until 6 P.M. By the time she leaves work she is ready to eat her handbag. On her way home, she runs into the grocery store to pick up a frozen dinner. She grabs Weight Watchers Chicken Fettucini. She always chooses Weight Watchers or some other lean or light frozen dinner. Ellen doesn't actually like the taste of frozen dinners, but she generally cooks only on weekends if she cooks at all.

Ellen doesn't even take off her coat. She immediately goes to the kitchen and sticks her meal in the microwave. While her dinner is being zapped, she cuts a head of iceberg lettuce into fourths and sticks one on her plate. She covers it with 4 tablespoons of fat-free dressing, congratulating herself that she didn't repeat her lunchtime dressing fiasco. Ellen does not linger over dinner because there is little to linger over. As she puts her dinner dishes in the sink, she is once again struck by how quickly she is finished with dinner. Is it because she is eating almost no food? Ellen is proud of her dessert choice. She had chosen low-fat yogurt. Not just any yogurt, this yogurt has chocolate fudge crunch on top. "Mmm, this is good," she says, as she licks her lips and gathers her boxes together to read the labels. The Chicken Fettucini at 80 fat calories is not much of a weight-loss buy. The salad dressing added no fat, but she sees that her "healthy" dessert cost her 45 fat calories. Read the labels *before* you buy, Ellen, and certainly before you eat.

Ellen is like millions of working people. They labor all day, spend hours in the car getting to and from work, and when they get home, they don't feel like cooking. They feel pressured for time and want food that takes no effort to prepare and seconds to cook. This mindset has created a multibillion dollar frozen-food industry. In an ideal world, one could shove a box into a microwave oven and produce delicious, healthy meals. This is the real world. Meals in a box do not taste great and they are often shot up with fat and sodium as well as artificial colors and flavors. Whether or not they are overladen with fat, they are usually underladen with food and fiber. Read the section on frozen dinners in Chapter 4, "Where's the Fat?" and check out the fat calories of frozen dinners in the Food Tables.

If you want to lose weight or are just interested in good health and sensory pleasure, you need to cook your own food using real ingredients. Ellen is cheating herself by eating plastic food. Cooking does take time, but it doesn't have to take a lot of time. Try the recipes in *Choose to Lose* or *Eater's Choice* for scrumptious proof. See Chapter 9 for ideas on cooking low-fat.

	Ellen's Dinner			
TIME	FOOD	AMOUNT	TOTAL CALORIES	FAT CALORIES
7 P.M.	Chicken Fettucini			
	(Weight Watchers)	1 meal	280	**80**
	Iceberg lettuce	¼ head	20	**0**
	Fat-free dressing (ranch)	4 tbsp	60	**0**
	Vanilla yogurt with			
	chocolate fudge crunch	6 oz	230	**45**
		Total Fat Calories:		**125**
		Accumulated Fat Calories:		**1028**
		Ellen's Fat Budget:		**315**

Frozen Dinners: Packaged Fat

The Weight Watchers Chicken Fettucini has 80 fat calories. With very little effort, Ellen could make *Apricot Chicken Divine* (page 227), which has 23 fat calories, or *Shrimp Curry* (page 237) at 35 fat calories. Both take little time to prepare and taste superb.

The Missing Vegetable

Ellen's diet is vegetable-bare. Vegetables can be steamed in minutes, add color and texture to your meal, contain fiber, vitamins, and minerals, and taste wonderful. They fill you up, improve your bowel function, and help reduce your risk of breast and colon cancer. What's more, vegetables can be eaten with abandon because they contain little or no fat. Even if you insist on eating boxed meals, enhance them with a baked plain potato or sweet potato and a steamed vegetable or two.

All Yogurts Are Not Equal

Ellen's choice of yogurt for dessert could have been weight-wise — except she chose a yogurt with a high-fat topping. (Chocolate fudge is chocolate fudge no matter what it's topping.) She could have selected any number of delicious nonfat flavored yogurts that have 0 to 9 calories of fat in 8 ounces.

HIGH-FAT SNACKS: DIETER'S DOWNFALL

The evening stretches before Ellen. She has made no plans. She settles comfortably into her favorite chair, turns on the television, and proceeds to devour the peanuts in the bowl beside her. "Aha!" she thinks. "I'll measure the amount of peanuts in the bowl before I eat them and then I'll measure the amount left when I go to bed." Good idea, Ellen. The bowl originally held three-quarters of a cup of peanuts. Ellen finds nothing in the bowl when she goes to bed. Where could all the nuts have gone? Ellen feels a bit foolish that she has consumed almost a whole cup of peanuts. She feels sick when she reads the label on the peanut jar and determines that her mindless snack cost her 482 fat calories. She adds the item to her food record.

	Ellen's Evening Snack			
TIME	FOOD	AMOUNT	TOTAL CALORIES	FAT CALORIES
9–11 P.M.	Oil-roasted salted peanuts	¾ cup	630	**482**
		Accumulated Fat Calories:		1510
		Ellen's Fat Budget:		315

Snack foods are the downfall of weight watchers. Snacks are almost always filled with fat, and they are addictive. It is impossible to eat one peanut. One peanut leads to another and another, until finally the whole bowl of peanuts has disappeared. The snacker eats without thought. When the bottom of the bowl appears, he wonders where all the peanuts, potato chips, corn chips, cheese twists, have gone.

A tip for snackers: Put out no more than you plan to eat. Another tip: Don't put out high-fat snacks at all.

THE FINAL TALLY

Ellen ate 1028 fat calories from breakfast through dinner. By the time she finished her evening snack and went to bed she had eaten 1510 calories of fat. Is it any wonder she is fat? Remember, Ellen's Fat Budget is 315. She's 1195 fat calories over her budget. You may think that her fat calorie intake is unusually high, but if you look back at Ellen's food record, you will see nothing out of the ordinary. In fact, you may have noticed that she had no rich desserts. Fat calories have a sneaky habit of adding up.

Before You Know It

Think of your $1000 monthly credit card bill. "What?" you cry in despair. "I didn't buy anything big." You take out your calculator. A pair of $42 shoes, a gasoline charge of $9, a TV repair bill for $59, and on and on. Nothing over $60. But it all adds up to a whopping $1000. Fat calories work the same way. A 42-fat-calorie glass of 2% milk, a 9-fat-calorie cracker, a 70-fat-calorie slice of bologna. They all add up until you've bankrupted your budget.

A Food Record = An Education

Reviewing her day's food intake has been invaluable for Ellen — and quite a surprise. She no longer wonders why she is overweight or why she is always hungry. She has discovered the sources of fat in her diet. She'll no longer regard biscuits with such a friendly eye. She'll think before dumping 4 tablespoons of high-fat dressing on her salad. She'll read labels before she gobbles down food she assumes is low in fat. Ellen now knows where to cut out fat. She knows which foods she still wants to eat and how much it will cost her — fat-wise.

Ellen is amazed to see how little food she eats in terms of bulk. Fruit, vegetables, and whole-grains are noticeably missing from her diet. Looking over her food record, Ellen can already think of many places where she could have enjoyed nutritious food instead of her high-fat choices. (Read page 110 to see how Ellen turned her meal plan around.)

Ellen's Baseline Food Record

TIME	FOOD	AMOUNT	TOTAL CALORIES	FAT CALORIES
8:15 A.M.	Blueberry muffin	1 large	400	**140**
	Coffee	1 cup	0	**0**
	Half-and-half	1 tbsp	20	**15**
10:30 A.M.	Glazed doughnut	1 large	240	**130**
	Coffee	1 cup	0	**0**
	Half-and-half	1 tbsp	20	**15**
Noon	Mixed salad			
	lettuce	2 cups	20	**0**
	tomato	½	12	**0**
	cucumber	¼	10	**0**
	carrot	¼	8	**0**
	Russian dressing	4 tbsp	308	**280**
	Sunflower seeds	1 tbsp	50	**39**
	Biscuit	1	231	**108**
	Butter	1 pat (tsp)	36	**36**
	Diet cola	8 oz	0	**0**
3 P.M.	Oodles of Noodles	3 oz	400	**140**
7 P.M.	Chicken Fettucini			
	(Weight Watchers)	1 meal	280	**80**
	Iceberg lettuce	¼ head	20	**0**
	Fat-free dressing			
	(ranch)	4 tbsp	60	**0**
	Vanilla yogurt with			
	chocolate fudge			
	crunch	6 oz	230	**45**
9–11 P.M.	Oil-roasted salted			
	peanuts	¾ cup	630	**482**

Total Calories: **2975**

Total Fat Calories: **1510**

Ellen's Fat Budget: **315**

YOUR TURN

Here's Looking at You, Kid

After seeing how Ellen's food intake adds up, are you curious to know how many fat calories you ate yesterday? Last weekend? By how much did you exceed your Fat Budget?

The Past Helps Determine the Future

Perhaps you don't even want to think about the past. You want to begin afresh and discard your old eating habits. And you want to get started NOW. Fine. But do you really know your old habits? Before you opened this book, you didn't know your Fat Budget or the number of fat calories in foods. You just ate. You chose certain foods. Some foods you ate without thought. You probably knew that some foods were fattening, but you didn't know how fattening. You might have even avoided some low-fat foods because you thought they would make you gain weight.

To make changes that will last, you need to know what to change. It is helpful to evaluate the foods you are eating to discover the sources of fat in your diet. For invaluable insight, keep a baseline record for 3 days — 2 weekdays and 1 weekend day. Write down *everything* you eat — honestly.

Even if you want to start making changes NOW and are too impatient to keep a baseline record, you need to start keeping track of everything you eat.

You will find a step-by-step guide to keeping a food record in Appendix A, page 448. You may want to purchase an inexpensive *Choose to Lose* Passbook and refills to help you keep track of your food intake. (See the order form on the last page of this book.)

People Who Keep Track Lose Weight

Food records are the ticket to weight loss success. Keeping food records will give you insight and understanding about your eating habits and will empower you to take control. You may think you eat a low-fat diet (Ellen certainly thought she did), but to lose weight you must know *exactly* what you are eating. You learn which foods are making you fat so you can make changes. You discover the high-fat foods you can't live without, the ones you can eat less of or less often, and the ones you can eliminate altogether. You know how many fat calories you have eaten so you can save for splurges. You learn if your diet is balanced, if it is filled with enough fruits, vegetables, whole-grains, and nonfat dairy for good health. How do you know if you don't write everything down?

Your Body Knows the Truth. Your records must be accurate and honest. Compulsive dieters have been known to be expert at fooling themselves. As the Nobel laureate physicist Richard Feynman so wisely advised when referring to another subject, the pitfalls of scientific investigation, "You must not fool yourself, and you are the easiest person to fool."

You Are What You Eat

To determine why they were overweight, participants in a diet study wrote down everything they ate. Their records showed that their diets were perfect — very low in fat — yet they weren't losing weight. The group was then put in a metabolic ward in a hospital where they were fed only the foods they had recorded in their food records. They all lost weight. Conclusion: You can't fool your body. The only way to know you are eating below your Fat Budget and eating enough total calories is to keep honest and accurate food records.

Keeping Track Is Only a Temporary Drag. After you get used to keeping food records, it won't even take much time. You don't eat that many foods at a meal. Just record your food as you eat. Keep a running subtotal so you know how each food you eat impacts your Fat Budget. Don't save up all your entries until the end of the day.

You won't have to keep records forever. Soon you will learn the combinations of foods you like to eat that fit within your budget and you won't have to write everything down. Of course, you will continue to refer to the Food Tables or to food labels to see how a new food can fit into your Fat Budget.

REALISTIC GOALS

Now that you have the tools to make the changes that will help you reach your fat-loss goal, you are probably feeling unconquerable. You can see the "new you" slipping into a slinky black dress or skin-tight blue jeans or you can imagine looking down and seeing your feet rather than your belly. It is important to feel optimistic and to know that you will eventually reach your goal weight, but if you start out with grandiose expectations, you will only be disappointed. If your only goal is to lose a lot of weight quickly and you don't lose it all in six weeks, you will feel like a failure and give up *Choose to Lose*. You will give up just when your body is starting to make real changes.

One Step at a Time

Make your goals small, realistic, and doable. Don't think "Fifty pounds thinner," think "Today I will eat two vegetables with dinner." Don't think, "Size twelve pants," think "This week I'll walk for thirty minutes every day at lunchtime." By meeting small goals, you will more easily reach your large goals. You might want to sit down the night before and list your goals for the day. Keep the Success Triangle in your mind's eye and attack each goal. For example, you might make a list like the following:

1. Low-fat diet:
   Bring lunch. Make a sandwich of last night's *Chili Non Carne* and heat it in the office microwave. Add carrot sticks, an apple, and a peach.
2. Adequate intake of nutritious food:
   Shop after work and buy enough vegetables to have two vegetables for dinner each night this week and enough fruit for several fruit a day.
3. Aerobic exercise:
   Walk dog thirty minutes after dinner.

Choose to Lose is not a quick fix. It is a way of eating for life and a lifelong commitment. Allow yourself only one grandiose goal — to reduce your risks of many diseases because you are eating a healthy diet. Relax, take a day at a time, and enjoy your new lifestyle of great eating, good health, and more energy.

Read On

As you begin to record what you eat, you are going to become keenly aware of the fat in food. Read the next chapter to learn "Where's the Fat?" You're in for a lot of surprises.

Remember:

1. Use the Food Tables to determine the fat calories of the foods you eat.
2. A baseline food record will help you discover the sources of fat in your diet.
3. Analyze your food record for high-fat foods.
4. Ellen was surprised to discover how much fat she consumed, especially considering how little food she ate.
5. Repeat to yourself: **I MUST EAT TO LOSE. I MUST EAT TO LOSE. I MUST EAT TO LOSE. OF COURSE, I MUST EAT NUTRITIOUS, LOW-FAT FOODS TO LOSE.**

4. Where's the Fat?

"Finally a new way of looking at food, and understanding the 'hidden fats' that many people don't realize they are ingesting."

Connie Giliberto, APO, AE

THE POWER of *Choose to Lose* is knowing your Fat Budget and the number of fat calories in foods. Before you start keeping your food record, here's a chapter devoted totally to foods, literally from soup to nuts, even including fast foods and frozen dinners — and the fat they contain.

This chapter asks the question, "Where's the Fat?" The answer is simple. EVERYWHERE! As a result, the percentage of Americans who are overweight has grown to epic proportions. The first National Health and Nutrition Examination Survey (NHANES) conducted between 1971 and 1974 found that 28.8 million American adults were obese (20 percent above their desirable weight) and, of these, 8.4 million were severely obese (40 percent above their desirable weight). Only five years later the second NHANES survey found that 34 million American adults were obese and, of these, 11 million were severely obese. In 1980, 26 percent of adults were obese. And it is getting worse and worse. The third NHANES survey conducted from 1988 to 1991 showed that 32 percent of men and 36 percent of women are obese.

Fat . . . Fatter . . . Fattest

Why are we such a fat nation? Over the last eighty years our eating habits have been changing — most dramatically since the 1950s. Our total caloric intake is slightly lower than it was in 1910, but our intake of fat is vastly higher. Fat intake is currently 40 percent of calories versus 27 percent in 1910.

Fast . . . Faster . . . Fattest

Just look at our supermarkets. The old-time grocery store stocked primarily fresh produce, meats, dairy products, and a few shelves of staples — flour, bread, sugar, coffee, and tea. Today these foods have been pushed to the outer walls. The ever-expanding inner rows of shelves and freezer cabinets are chock full of high-fat convenience foods.

What's Our Hurry?

We no longer cook. We pop a frozen dinner into our microwave or buy a prepared dish from the gourmet section of our grocery store. We feel too rushed to buy and prepare fresh vegetables. In fact, french fries and ketchup are the only vegetables many people ever eat and Froot Loops and fruit roll-ups are the only fruits.

Fast Foods Growing Fast

We eat out more often — but where? At high-fat fast-food restaurants. While rare in the fifties, fast-food restaurants are the only food service available in many areas today. If you travel on toll roads and interstates across the country, don't look for family-style restaurants. Fast-food chains have taken their place. And with the change, low-fat food choices have gone the way of the horse and buggy.

TV-Time Temptation

We are even victims within our homes. Every TV show is accompanied by a bombardment of ads for luscious, mouth-watering high-fat convenience foods and snacks. It's not only the visual onslaught — melted cheese enfolding a big, juicy hamburger; sweet, creamy chocolate swirling smoothly around a gooey nougat center; and cheese joyfully bubbling atop a pizza crust — but we have to suffer the psychological impact. People eating high-fat foods have so much fun. If you want to be one of the gang, eat the way we do.

You *Can* Resist

Yes, TV ads and fast-food restaurants and convenience foods may try to lure you into their fatty grips, but once you know where the fat lurks, you will have the power to resist their grasp. Read the rest of this chapter to discover how much fat is in the foods you eat. Use these new discoveries to make the choices that will lead directly to thinness.

Where's the Fat?

Fat is everywhere. Some is visible, like the strip of fat on a sirloin steak. But much is hidden, like the fat marbled throughout the steak and the fat added to processed frozen dinners. We Americans eat entirely too much of it. And there you are in the midst of it. To root it out of your diet you must know where it exists. You must dispel old notions. Do you consider beef a high-protein food or a high-fat food? Do you view whole milk and cheese as calcium-rich and wholesome rather than fat-laden? Do you consider skinny, little dried-out crackers good diet snacks or high-fat foods? The following discussion should start you down the road to a new, lean body.

NOTE: You may be disheartened to discover that fat lurks in so many of the foods you love, but don't lose hope. You'll learn how often and in what amounts you can comfortably fit them into your Fat Budget. True, you won't be eating your favorite high-fat foods in as large quantities or as often as before, but is this so bad? You won't just inhale that piece of apple pie, you'll *really* taste it. You will also learn to like foods you once scoffed at — vegetables and fruit, for example. Just relax. You're going to love being thin and eating healthfully. And, in just a few pages, you'll find a whole chapter devoted to great weight loss food choices you once thought were forbidden fruit.

RED MEATS

Beef: A Dieter's Undoing   (pages 354–55, Food Tables)

If you think of beef as a high-protein food that builds bulging biceps and triceps, revise your thinking. Beef is a high-fat food that creates bulging hips, tummies, and thighs. Removing the layer of fat that hugs the edge of a piece of beef will not eliminate all the fat. Invisible fat is marbled throughout. The better the quality of beef (the higher the grade), the more fat it contains. Even meats that appear to be lean contain a lot of fat. For instance, braised flank steak trimmed of fat has 35 fat calories *per ounce*. That's 140 fat calories per 4 ounces. The leanest beef is broiled top round trimmed of fat, which has 16 fat calories per ounce.

Take a look at the Meats category of the Food Tables for an eye opener. The entries are listed in 1-ounce portion size for easy comparison. Of course, no one eats just 1 ounce of meat. Be sure to multiply the fat calories by the number of ounces you eat. For instance, braised shortribs have 107 calories of fat per ounce. If you eat 4 ounces of shortribs, multiple 4 × 107 for a total of 428 fat calories. How does 428 fat calories fit into your Fat Budget?

Visions of Hamburger

The image of a big, juicy hamburger often ravages the subconscious of dieters. Until that need is satisfied, the dieter can think of nothing else, often stuffing herself or himself with everything else around to satisfy that craving. Good news: You *can* fit the hamburger into your Fat Budget. (For the leanest* hamburger meat you can buy, ask the butcher to trim the fat off a round steak and grind it.) But it won't be often.

If You'd Trade Your Right Arm for a Hamburger

If nothing but a large, 100 percent regular ground beef hamburger will satisfy you, save fat calories for your splurge by keeping your fat intake extra-low for a few days. Remember: Saving for a splurge is a better policy than paying back for it later. When you splurge without prepayment too often, you're off *Choose to Lose*. (Read about splurging in Chapter 10.)

Dieter's Plate: Guaranteed to Put on Weight

Now that you know about the fat in beef, you will scorn the diet plate offered in thousands of American restaurants. The "Diet Special" features a hamburger (without the bun), whole-milk cottage cheese, and a canned peach half. The star of the dieter's special contains 58 fat calories per ounce or about 348 fat calories per 6-ounce patty. (Aren't you glad they spared you the 18 fat calories for the bun?)

---

*Don't get taken in when a meat package boasts "Lean!" According to the Food and Drug Administration's guidelines, a meat may be described as lean if it contains less than 90 fat calories for 100 grams (about 3½ ounces). You won't remain lean very long if you eat meat that meets that requirement.

Veal: Expensive and Fattening   (pages 359–60, Food Tables)

Veal may be pale in color like chicken and turkey breast, but that is where the similarity ends. Veal is not diet food. Braised veal breast contains 54 fat calories per ounce or 216 fat calories for 4 ounces. Veal cutlet — before it becomes breaded and fried veal cutlet or even sautéed — has 27 fat calories per ounce or 108 calories per 4 ounces. Try turkey cutlets instead (2 fat calories per ounce). Pound them thin and your guests will think they are eating veal scaloppine. (Try *Turkey with Capers* (page 235), and from *Eater's Choice, Turkey Scaloppine Limone* and *Turkey Scaloppine Marsala*.

	FAT CALORIES	
	1 OUNCE	4 OUNCES
Turkey cutlet, braised	2	8
Veal cutlet, braised	27	108
Veal breast, braised	54	216

Lamb: Not Just the Wool Keeps It Warm
(pages 356–57, Food Tables)

Lamb is also a poor choice for a dieter. It should come as no surprise that a 4-ounce rib lamb chop has 360 calories of fat. You can see it. Ground lamb is no substitute for ground beef. Four ounces of ground lamb has 320 fat calories. The best lamb choice is roasted leg of lamb trimmed of fat (20 fat calories per ounce or 80 fat calories for a 4-ounce serving) or a broiled loin lamb chop trimmed of fat (19 fat calories per ounce or 76 fat calories for a 4-ounce chop).

	FAT CALORIES	
	1 OUNCE	4 OUNCES
Loin lamb chop (trimmed)	19	76
Leg of lamb (trimmed)	20	80
Ground lamb, broiled	80	320
Rib lamb chop	90	360

But remember, if a lamb chop would make you incredibly happy, just make room for it in your budget — but rarely.

Pork: You Are What You Eat (pages 357–59, Food Tables)

It may be called the other white meat by the people who sell it, but except for roasted lean pork tenderloin at 12 fat calories per ounce (48 fat calories per 4 ounces), all pork products are high in fat. Fat calories for pork products average around 65 fat calories per ounce (260 per 4 ounces). Spareribs, raw, contain 77 fat calories per ounce (308 per 4 ounces) and pan-fried loin blade has 94 fat calories per ounce (376 for 4 ounces). Your favorite roasted ham is 53 fat calories per ounce (212 per 4 ounces). It is not surprising that one skinny (ha!) strip of bacon has 28 fat calories. But would you kill for a B.L.T. sandwich? Make it with one strip of bacon. You'll get the taste without all the fat.

	FAT CALORIES	
	1 OUNCE	4 OUNCES
Pork tenderloin (lean, roasted)	12	48
Ham	53	212
Other pork products (average)	65	260
Spareribs	77	308
Pork, loin, blade, pan-fried	94	376
	PER STRIP	4 STRIPS
Bacon	28	112

Fitting It In

Although beef, veal, lamb, and pork are all high-fat foods, you can make room for them in your budget. If you want to eat an occasional (a *very* occasional) steak or chop, reduce the fat calories by trimming off the visible fat before you broil or grill it. Marinate less fatty cuts of meat to make them tender. Instead of choosing a thick steak or roast as the centerpiece of your meal, choose dishes in which small amounts of meat are added to vegetables, rice, or pasta.

Be sure to check the Meats (beef, lamb, pork, veal, & game), Fast Foods, Frozen and Microwave Foods, and Sausages and Luncheon Meats sections of the Food Tables to familiarize yourself with the fat contents of meat products not mentioned in this chapter.

POULTRY

Chicken: Basically Great . . .   (pages 363–67, Food Tables)

White meat chicken without skin, properly prepared, trounces beef, veal, pork, and lamb in the low-fat marathon. A roasted chicken breast without skin has only 13 fat calories. Chicken has the potential to be part of an infinite number of low-fat, delicious recipes. Try *Lemon Chicken* (page 230) or *Chicken with Rice, Tomatoes, and Artichokes* (page 233) and, in *Eater's Choice, Kung Pao Chicken with Broccoli* and *Pineapple Chicken* for delectable proof.

Dark meat is fattier than light meat. A roasted drumstick without skin has 22 fat calories. But one drumstick isn't much of a meal. A thigh without skin has 51 fat calories. A roasted thigh isn't all that much to eat, either. However, if you moderate the amount, dark meat chicken can fit into your Fat Budget.

. . . But Easily Ruined

White meat chicken cooked without skin is a low-fat food. Chicken *with* the skin has a fat content approaching or even surpassing that of many cuts of beef. A roasted chicken breast without skin has 13 fat calories. The same breast with skin has 69 fat calories. Take that breast with skin, dip it in flour, and fry it, and the fat calories rise to 78. Batter-dip and fry it and the calories climb to 166. Eat it extra-crispy or spicy at a KFC fast-food restaurant and the breast becomes, at 216 fat calories, almost seventeen times as fattening as the original bare skinless breast.

PREPARATION OF A CHICKEN BREAST	FAT CALORIES
Roasted without skin	13
Roasted with skin, then skin removed	28
Roasted *with* skin	69
Fried *with* skin, flour-coated	78
Fried *with* skin, batter-dipped	166
KFC Extra Crispy	216

Choose to Lose tip: Always remove the skin from chicken *before* cooking or the fat from the skin will be absorbed by the meat. If you remove the skin *after* you cook the chicken breast, your chicken breast will have accumulated 15 extra fat calories for a total of 28 fat calories. To reduce the fat even more, flour and bake skinless chicken breasts in a shallow baking pan without fat. Cooking on a cast-iron griddle or barbecue grill without fat also helps to reduce fat without impairing taste.

Turkey: Dieter's Pick (pages 369–70, Food Tables)

One ounce of unadulterated turkey breast without skin has a mere 2 fat calories. Five ounces has only 10 fat calories. That means you can eat a lot of white meat turkey without remorse. The white meat of deep-basted Butterball turkeys is not quite as fat-free. Each ounce contains 10 fat calories. This is not a lot of fat, but it can accumulate particularly with added gravy or mayonnaise. If you add the skin, Butterball turkey white meat is 17.5 fat calories per ounce (70 fat calories for 4 ounces!). Be sure to keep track of the fat-containing sauces and gravies you add to your turkey.

Dark meat without skin is higher in fat than white meat turkey even with skin. Unadulterated dark meat turkey contains 6 fat calories per ounce. That's 30 fat calories for 5 ounces. A whole leg roasted without skin is 76 fat calories. If you moderate your use of gravy, dark meat turkey doesn't have to overload your Fat Budget. Read labels. Dark meat from deep-basted Butterball turkeys contains 26 fat calories per ounce. Even without dressings and gravies this can add up quickly to a lot of fat calories.

| | FAT CALORIES | |
TURKEY	1 OUNCE	4 OUNCES
White meat turkey		
without skin	2	8
(Butterball) without skin	10	40
(Butterball) with skin	17.5	70
Dark meat turkey		
without skin	6	24
(Butterball) without skin	26	104
Ground turkey		
(93% fat free)	18	72
(frozen)	36	144

Ground Turkey: Deceptive Advertising

Ground turkey seems to be the answer to a weight-watching hamburger lover's dreams. Because turkey is so low in fat, we assume that ground turkey is also low. Not necessarily. The ground turkey you buy is often loaded with turkey skin and fat. To ensure that your ground turkey is low in fat, grind your own raw turkey breast or cutlets in a food processor or meat grinder or have your butcher do it.

Duck: Super Splurge   (page 367, Food Tables)

Have you ever seen a duck frolicking in icy water in fifteen-degree weather? The duck is padded with fat to keep it warm and afloat. Eating duck is a sure way to increase your padding and sink your Fat Budget. Half a duck with skin contains 975 fat calories — without a sauce. Has duck à l'orange lost some of its appeal? Duck without skin has 29 fat calories per ounce. Perhaps your Fat Budget can handle a pancake or two of Peking Duck (without the skin).

Be sure to check the Poultry, Fast Foods, Frozen and Microwave Foods, and Sausages and Luncheon Meats sections of the Food Tables to familiarize yourself with the fat in poultry and poultry products not mentioned in this chapter.

SEAFOOD   (pages 312–21, Food Tables)

Just plain, unadulterated fish is an excellent choice for a dieter. Two calories of fat per ounce for raw cod, dolphin, haddock, lobster, pollock, and scallops; 3 for grouper, pike, snapper, sole, and sunfish; and 4 for flounder, monkfish, perch, rockfish, and shrimp leave plenty of room in your Fat Budget for more choices later.

A few fish are high in fat and warrant caution. Watch these fat calories per ounce: sablefish 39, Pacific herring 35; Atlantic mackerel 35; chinook salmon 27; Atlantic herring 23; sockeye salmon 22; butterfish 20; Pacific mackerel 20; orange roughy 20. Check the Food Tables for the values of the fish you wish to eat.

Orange roughy! Salmon! You don't have to eliminate any of these wonderful fish from your diet — just keep track of their fat calories and fit them in.

	FAT CALORIES	
SEAFOOD	1 OUNCE	4 OUNCES
Cod, dolphin fish, haddock, lobster, pollock, scallops	2	8
Grouper, pike, snapper, sole, sunfish	3	12
Flounder, monkfish, ocean perch, rockfish, shrimp	4	16
Tuna, canned, water-packed	4.5	18
Butterfish, orange roughy, Pacific mackerel	20	80
Sockeye salmon	22	88
Atlantic herring	23	92
Chinook salmon	27	108
Atlantic mackerel, Pacific herring	35	140
Sablefish	39	156

Of course, no matter how lean a fish is, when you bread and deep-fry it, or drown it in a cream sauce or butter, it is no longer a good diet choice. Bake, broil, poach, or grill fish with little or no fat or cover it with low-fat sauces to create delectable, guilt-free dishes.

Choose to Lose tip: Choose canned tuna packed in water. A whole can of undrained tuna packed in water has 30 calories of fat or 4.5 fat calories per ounce. A whole can of undrained tuna packed in (soy) oil has 297 calories of fat or 45 fat calories per ounce. Oil-packed tuna has ten times as much fat as water-packed.

You will find the fat calories of fish listed in the Fish and Shellfish, Fast Foods, and Frozen and Microwave Foods sections of the Food Tables.

SAUSAGES AND LUNCHEON MEATS

A Poor Choice   (pages 380–85, Food Tables)

Beware of sausages and luncheon meats. They are crammed with fat (in addition to being filled with dangerous additives and excessive amounts of salt). A 3-ounce link of bratwurst has 198 calories of fat; a 2.4-ounce smoked link sausage has 194. A 2-ounce all-beef frankfurter contains 150 fat calories. Even a 2-ounce chicken frank contains 100 fat calories. The 5 little pepperoni slices atop your piece of pizza take a 50-fat-calorie bite out of your Fat Budget.

The Cold Facts about Cold Cuts

A thin slice of bologna has 70 calories of fat. Slide two slices of bologna (140 fat calories) between two slices of bread (18 fat calories) slathered with a tablespoon of mayonnaise (99 fat calories) and you have created a sandwich worth about 257 fat calories. Doesn't sound like diet food.

Check out the figures in the box that follows. Don't get carried away. *Remember these numbers are for only one slice.*

You will also find a slew of low-fat cold cuts in the luncheon meats section of the supermarket. They range from about 2 fat calories (smoked turkey) to 6 fat calories (cooked ham) for a ¾-ounce slice. This isn't much fat and it isn't much meat. Remember to multiply the fat calories by the number of slices you eat.

If you use the cold cuts that have less fat (read the labels) and make your sandwiches less thick, you can easily fit cold cuts into your budget. However, you might want to eat cold cuts less often. The cancer-causing nitrites and blood pressure–raising sodium won't make you fat, but they may shorten your life.

LUNCHEON MEATS	AMOUNT	FAT CALORIES
Turkey bologna	1 slice (28g)	35
Ham	1 slice (28g)	35
Chicken bologna	1 slice (28g)	60
Salami	1 slice (28g)	65
Beef bologna	1 slice (28g)	70
Pork and beef bologna	1 slice (28g)	70
Liverwurst	1 slice (28g)	80
Pork and turkey bologna	1 slice (38g)	100

Sliced Turkey Breast: A Deli Delight

The only luncheon meat you can eat with abandon is fresh roasted turkey breast that you roast yourself (2 fat calories per ounce). You can also find turkey breast at many grocery store deli counters for about 8 fat calories per ounce. However, if you are buying packaged turkey breast, read the label. Some turkey cold cuts have so much added fat, they approach or even exceed some beef or pork cold cuts.

Wurst Is Worst

For those of you whose default dinner selection is hot dogs, take a look at the figures in the next box. Will you still rely on hot dogs to feed picky eaters (definition of *picky eaters:* those who are not hungry because they have been snacking all day) when you know you are stuffing 150 fat calories into their mouths? When you didn't plan for dinner, will you still boil up 150 calories of fat and nitrites? We hope not. Don't let the words *turkey* and *chicken* fool you into buying poultry dogs. They are generally less fat-filled than beef hot dogs, but 70 to 100 fat calories is a hefty amount of fat for so little food.

Even really low-fat hot dogs such as Jennie-O Extra Lean at 20 fat calories for a 1.6 ounce frankfurter or Healthy Choice Low Fat Frank at 15 fat calories for a 1.8 ounce frank are best saved for rare occasions. Although a lot of fat has been removed, the excessive sodium, unhealthy preservatives, and high-fat taste remain. If you continue to subject yourself to a high-fat taste, albeit from a low-fat food, you will never lose your craving for high-fat foods.

And then, there are sausages. Don't even think of knockwurst, kielbasa, or pork sausage. Even turkey sausage touted as 90 percent fat-free is 81 fat calories for a 3-ounce link.

FRANKS AND SAUSAGES	AMOUNT	FAT CALORIES
Turkey polska kielbasa	1 inch (28g)	27
Polska kielbasa	1 inch (28g)	75
Frankfurter		
turkey	1 frank (57g)	70
chicken	1 frank (56g)	100
beef	1 frank (57g)	150
Cheese dog	1 frank (45g)	120
Beef knockwurst	1 link (85g)	210
Smoked link pork sausage	1 link (85g)	230

Fat-Free?

"90% fat-free!" "93% fat-free!" "87% fat-free!" Do these percentages imply a low-fat product? The problem lies not with the accuracy of the percentages printed so large and colorfully on the package. The problem is that these percentages are misleading because they don't tell you what you need to know. If a package says "87% fat-free," it means that 13 percent of the *weight* of the meat is fat. However, what you need to know is how many calories of fat you will be consuming when you eat the slice of turkey bologna or ham.

For a more complete discussion of hype on labels see page 128. For more illuminating cold cut fat values, take a look at the Sausages and Luncheon Meats section of the Food Tables.

FROZEN MEALS

Gain Time and Weight

There has been an explosion in the food industry, which is capitalizing on our changing society. Fast-food restaurants, microwave dinners, and a seemingly endless proliferation of convenience foods have been developed for people who don't take time for food preparation. However, what you gain in convenience you often sacrifice in taste, health, and your weight.

The price is also steep in terms of dollars. For that little box called dinner, you are paying at least five times what it would cost you if you were to purchase the ingredients separately and make the dish yourself.

Be Label-Wise: A Survival Skill

Learning how to read a food label is mandatory if you want to eat convenience foods. The food label tells it all. The package may advertise a low-fat entree such as fish, turkey, or chicken, but you need to know more. The package may claim "25% less fat," but you need to know more.

You need to know exactly how much fat the food processors have added to that dinner to make it palatable. And it is often a lot. Be sure to read Chapter 8 for more information on deciphering food labels.

Ruining a Good Thing   (pages 321–38, Food Tables)

We'd be wealthy if we had a dollar for every time we've been told, "I don't understand why I'm fat. All I eat is fish and chicken." As you will see, preparation makes all the difference.

Most fish are naturally very low in fat. Here's what happens when food companies process fish into a frozen meal. Gorton turns a 1-ounce flounder fillet (3 fat calories) into Crispy Flounder (190 fat calories) and 1 ounce of pollock (3 fat calories) into two crunchy breaded fish fillets (150 fat calories). Mrs. Paul transforms 2 ounces of crab meat (2 fat calories) into a deviled crab cake (180 fat calories). And Van de Kamp's processes less than an ounce of shrimp (4 fat calories) into breaded whole shrimps (90 calories of fat). That's some kind of magic.

	FAT CALORIES	
FISH	UNADULTERATED	PROCESSED
Crab (1-ounce)	2	80
Shrimp (1-ounce)	4	90
Pollock (1-ounce)	3	150
Flounder (1-ounce)	3	190

Abracadabra! Watch the food processors transform a low-fat chicken breast (13 fat calories) into a high-fat food:

CHICKEN	FAT CALORIES
Chicken breast without skin	13
Stouffer's Baked Chicken Breast (homestyle)	110
Banquet Chicken Nugget meal	190
Budget Gourmet Chicken & Egg Noodles	210
Stouffer's Chicken Pot Pie	300

Even a turkey would be horrified to see how its lean flesh (2 fat calories per ounce for white meat; 6 fat calories per ounce for dark meat) can be turned into high-fat frozen turkey dishes.

TURKEY	FAT CALORIES
Turkey breast without skin (1 oz)	2
Swanson Turkey Dinner	70
Stouffer's Turkey Tetrazzini	170
Banquet Turkey Pot Pie	180

Lunch Express

Not only does the frozen food industry expect you to be too busy to prepare dinner, but it's banking on the fact that you haven't the time or the inclination to fix lunch either. It has introduced a whole line of "express" lunches that you can take to work and zap in your office microwave. If you jump onto the lunch express, you may save five minutes of home preparation, but express fat will also speedily nestle into your fat stores. Check out the following chart if you need inspiration for bringing your own bag lunch to work.

LUNCH EXPRESS	FAT CALORIES
Lean Cuisine Chicken Fettucini	60
Lean Cuisine Broccoli & Cheddar Cheese Sauce over Baked Potato	80
Stouffer's Cheese Ravioli	100
Stouffer's Chicken Alfredo	150
Stouffer's Fettucini Primavera	220
Stouffer's Fettucini Alfredo	240

Take a look at the **FROZEN, MICROWAVE, AND REFRIGERATED FOODS** section of the Food Tables for a true shock.

EATER BEWARE: The food industry is adding a tremendous amount of gratuitous fat to its frozen dinners — and to you, if you eat them.

Diet (?) Frozen Dinners

Don't assume that "diet" frozen dinners are low in fat. Although hype such as "Lite!" and "Low-fat!" may be used only if a product meets low-fat criteria — less than 27 fat calories per serving — names implying healthy or a good diet choice such as Lean Cuisine, Weight Watchers, and Healthy Choice may still be used even if the product is neither. Read the label! The dishes below would take a large chunk out of anyone's Fat Budget and provide a modest amount of food. Why not make your own "diet" dinners?

DINNER	FAT CALORIES
Healthy Choice Beef Burrito Ranchero	70
Lean Cuisine Swedish Meatballs	80
Weight Watchers Grilled Salisbury Steak	80

Reduced Fat Means Reduced Food

Truly low-fat dinners are proliferating at an astounding rate. Weight Watchers Smart Ones all contain less than 9 calories of fat. Many Healthy Choice dinners have 20 to 45 fat calories each. If you read labels carefully, you can find a variety of frozen dinners that are low in fat. However, be advised that low-fat dinners may be low-fat because they are almost meat-free (many contain about ½ to 1 ounce of meat) and thus eating only one dinner leaves you hungry. (See page 124 to find out how to determine the amount of meat in a frozen dinner.) Eating modest amounts of meat is fine (and even healthy) but not if you need to consume another low-fat dinner to fill you up (45 + 45 = 90 fat calories) or you binge on high-fat snacks because the frozen dinner has left your stomach feeling empty and your psyche feeling unsatisfied.

A Box Does Not a Dinner Make

If you decide to buy commercial dinners, be sure to enhance them with fresh vegetables. Steam broccoli, carrots, cauliflower, or zucchini in a vegetable steamer. Bake a plain or sweet potato. Boil a pot of rice. Don't cheat yourself out of the vitamins, minerals, and fiber that you need to maintain your good health. Remember, this is an eating diet. You need lots of complex carbohydrates to make those fat calories vaporize.

PREPARED PASTA, NOT SO FASTA
(pages 351–53, Food Tables)

You probably jumped for joy when you found that pasta could and should be included in your eating plan. But, whoa, not just *any* pasta.

For no strain on your Fat Budget, boil up your own pasta and top it with a low-fat sauce such as *Spaghetti Sauce à la Sicilia* (page 246) at 14 fat calories a serving or make *Asparagus Pasta* (page 247) at 26 fat calories a serving.

PASTA	AMOUNT	FAT CALORIES
Lipton Rotini Primavera	1 cup	100
Cup of Noodles, beef	1 cup	110
Kraft Macaroni & Cheese Dinner	1 cup	170
Contadina Fettucine with Pasta Sauce	1 cup	300

FAST FOODS

Fast Foods = Fat Foods   (pages 285–308, Food Tables)

A person who wants to stay thin and healthy should avoid fast-food restaurants like the plague. Fast-food restaurants are a plague. Hundreds of thousands of Americans will die from fat-related, or should we say fast-food-related, diseases (heart disease and breast, colon, and prostate cancers). What is happening in Japan proves a vivid illustration of the effect of fast food on health. In the past few years since fast food has come to Japan (a country in which both fast-food restaurants and heart disease were virtually nonexistent), heart disease has increased fivefold and obesity has become a problem. Here are some figures that help explain why:

FAST FOOD	FAT CALORIES
McDonald's Big Mac	234
Dairy Queen Super Hot Dog with Cheese	306
Arby's buttermilk ranch dressing (1 packet)	347
Jack-in-the-Box Supreme Crescent	360
Jack-in-the-Box Supreme Nachos	360
Roy Rogers Egg and Biscuit Platter with Sausage	369
Denny's catfish entree	432
Dairy Queen Triple Hamburger with Cheese	450
Burger King Double Whopper	477
KFC Extra Crispy drumstick & thigh	483
Denny's French toast (2 slices)	504
Burger King Double Whopper with Cheese	549
Wendy's Triple Cheeseburger	612
Hardee's Big Country Breakfast Sausage	630

Baked potato, chicken, pasta salad, fish — what happens to all those good, low-fat foods when a fast-food restaurant gets hold of them?

FAST FOOD	FAT CALORIES
Roy Rogers **Coleslaw** (½ cup)	63
Burger King **Chef Salad**	81
McDonald's Filet-O-**Fish**	162
Jack-in-the-Box **Pasta Seafood Salad**	198
Jack-in-the-Box **Onion** Rings	207
Wendy's **Baked Potato** with cheese	216
Arby's **Chicken** Salad Croissant	324
Arby's **Baked Potato,** deluxe	328
Dairy Queen **Chicken** Sandwich	369
Long John Silver's **Seafood** Platter or Clam dinner	522
Long John Silver's **Fish** dinner, fried (3 pieces)	630

Slim Pickin's

There are no "no-no"s in *Choose to Lose.* You can eat even the highest-fat fast foods if you can fit them into your budget. But is a Wendy's Triple Cheeseburger (612 fat calories) or a Kentucky Fried Chicken Extra Crispy drumstick and thigh (483 fat calories) worth all those fat calories? Fast-food restaurants offer you such poor choices, you will do yourself a favor by staying away.

FAST FOOD	FAT CALORIES
Roy Rogers Baked Potato, plain	0
Wendy's Baked Potato	18
Kentucky Fried Chicken Corn on the Cob	27
Burger King Chunky Chicken Salad	36
Dairy Queen Chocolate Sundae (small)	36
Chick-Fil-A Chargrilled Chicken Deluxe Sandwich	44
Arby's Light Roast Turkey Deluxe Sandwich	54
Carl's Jr. Charbroiler BBQ Chicken Sandwich	54

However, if you have been knocked on the head, tied up, and dragged to a fast-food restaurant, here are a few choices that won't totally decimate your Fat Budget.

You might try the salad bar, but beware of its major pitfalls — salad dressings and toppings. (See the discussion of Salad Dressing, page 39, and **SALAD BAR** Items, Food Tables, pages 376–77).

PIZZA (pages 285–308, Food Tables)

Eating pizza is a national pastime. You don't even have to go to a restaurant to eat it. Call up your local pizzeria and within minutes, a steaming-hot pizza arrives at your door. It's so convenient. What a quick and easy way to add hundreds of fat calories to your fat bank. A Pizza Hut Personal Pan pepperoni pizza has 261 fat calories; 2 slices of Domino's 12-inch deluxe pizza contain 207 fat calories (but who eats 2 slices?). Jody Goodman-Block, a registered dietitian in New York City, estimates that a slice of pizza may contain as much as 245 fat calories. Is it a wonder that so many Americans are obese?

It is possible, however, to survive a pizza party with your Fat Budget intact. Order pizza without the cheese. Have the pizza chef add fresh mushrooms, onions, tomatoes, green peppers — whatever vegetables are available. Insist that no oil be drizzled over the pizza before it is baked. The result will taste delicious (not like cheese pizza, but still good) and will have far fewer fat calories. To estimate the fat calories for cheeseless pizza, you can assume the crust has about 18 fat calories a slice (it's about 9 fat calories per ounce). Ask if the tomato sauce contains any oil: The pizzeria staff may be able to tell you. If they say yes or if they don't know, count the tomato sauce as about 15 fat calories per slice.

RESTAURANT FOOD: CHINESE (page 373, Food Tables)

We have grown up with the misconception that Chinese restaurants are a dieter's haven. All those vegetables and rice — what could be healthier? Lots. Although homemade Chinese dishes have the potential to be relatively low in fat, most Chinese restaurant food is astronomically high. Not only do many Chinese restaurants fry and deep-fry ingredients in large amounts of oil (generally corn or cottonseed oil), they often blanch them in oil (pass meat or vegetables through hot or warm oil before stir-frying) first. In addition, oil is sometimes added after the dish is cooked to make it shiny. Check out the fat calories in the box below. Does Chinese restaurant food still seem so enticing?

It may be possible to eat like a low-fat king at Chinese restaurants if you specifically order the meat and vegetables in a dish steamed rather than sautéed and then mixed with the sauce. The food is equally as delectable as when cooked with tons of oil. The only drawback is that you don't really know if your low-fat request has been taken seriously or if the management is trying to please you by saying the dishes are oil-free. This problem always occurs when you eat out, because you are not in the kitchen yourself controlling the ingredients.

For a larger listing of Chinese dishes, look in the Restaurant Food section of the Food Tables.

CHINESE RESTAURANT DISH	AMOUNT	FAT CALORIES
Egg roll	1	103
Hunan Shrimp (not deep-fried)	1 whole dish	755
Beef with vegetables	1 whole dish	1068
Chicken with Cashews	1 whole dish	1075
Kung Pao Chicken	1 whole dish	1134
Orange Beef	1 whole dish	1216
Chinese Barbecued Spareribs	1 whole dish	1232
Sweet and Sour Pork	1 whole dish	1509

RESTAURANT FOOD: ITALIAN   (page 374, Food Tables)

Unlike Chinese food, Italian food (in America) has never been mistaken for low-fat fare. The basic ingredients of many dishes are cheese, oil, or meat. Fettuccine Alfredo, for example, is a combination of cheese, butter, cream, and pasta. Traditional lasagna is a combination of cheese, meat sauce, and pasta. (It is easy to see why pasta developed such a bad reputation considering the company it often keeps.) You know these dishes are high in fat, but would you believe 873 fat calories in a serving of fettuccine Alfredo? 558 fat calories in a serving of eggplant Parmigiana? The best choice at an Italian restaurant is the spaghetti with tomato sauce at 153 fat calories or the linguine with red clam sauce at 207 fat calories a serving. Neither are great buys. Is it becoming clearer why Americans who eat out every meal have trouble staying lean?

ITALIAN RESTAURANT DISH	AMOUNT	FAT CALORIES
Spaghetti with tomato sauce	3.5 cups	153
Linguine with red clam sauce	3 cups	207
Spaghetti with meat sauce	3 cups	225
Linguine with white clam sauce	3 cups	261
Spaghetti with meatballs	3.5 cups	351
Spaghetti with sausage	2.5 cups	351
Veal Parmigiana	1.5 cups	396
Lasagna	2 cups	477
Eggplant Parmigiana	2.5 cups	558
Fettuccine Alfredo	2.5 cups	873

Sources: Nutrition Action Healthletter; Center for Science in the Public Interest; Lancaster Laboratories

MILK AND MILK PRODUCTS

Milk: A High-Fat Food   (pages 283–84, Food Tables)

It seems un-American to regard whole milk as anything but wholesome and pure. However, whole milk should be viewed as a high-fat and thus a fattening and unhealthy food. One glass of whole milk (8 fl oz) contains 73 calories of fat. If your Fat Budget is 280, a glass of whole milk at each meal and one at bedtime would shoot your entire day's fat quota. That is not to say that all milk products are high in fat. We are fortunate to live in an age in which we can buy low-fat and nonfat milk products that are truly delicious.

Shift to Skim Milk

If you currently drink whole milk and find the thought of drinking skim milk disgusting, first switch to 2% milk. You probably think 2% milk is truly low-fat. Two percent — it's barely above zero. But a glass of 2% milk contains 42 calories of fat. How can a drink that is 2% fat contain so many fat calories? Remember the 93% fat-free cold cuts? The 2% refers to the percentage of the weight of the milk that is fat, not the percentage of the total calories that are fat. If the milk producers called this milk 35% fat milk (42 fat calories ÷ 121 total calories = 35%), would you rush to buy it?

At 42 fat calories a glass, 2% milk is a better choice than whole milk at 73 fat calories a glass, but it's still pretty high. After you get used to 2% milk, try 1% milk for a while. You'll find it tastes pretty similar, and you'll be down to 23 calories of fat per glass. **Skim milk has only 4 fat calories and more calcium than whole milk** — so go for it!

Choose to Lose tip: One of our Choosers to Lose told us how she moved her husband from 2% to skim milk without his being any the wiser. When the half gallon of 2% milk became half full, she filled it up with 1% milk. The taste was almost the same. Her husband didn't notice any difference. When he had finished half of the combination milk, she again filled the carton up with 1% milk. No negative response. Eventually he was drinking pure 1% milk without complaint (or knowledge). And then she repeated the dilution method using skim milk. Try it yourself.

MILK	AMOUNT	FAT CALORIES
Nonfat skim milk	8 fl oz	4
1% milk	8 fl oz	23
2% milk	8 fl oz	42
Whole milk	8 fl oz	73

Butter: A Spread That Increases Your Spread
(page 281, Food Tables)

Butter is 100 percent fat. A teaspoon contains 33 calories of fat; a tablespoon, 100. Each time you lift your knife to slather butter over a roll or piece of toast you are preparing to make a large dent in your Fat Budget. Keep track. Measure a specific amount — a half teaspoon (17 fat calories) or a teaspoon (33 fat calories) — and then spread. Try eating the bread with jelly or apple butter or even plain.

Butter adds fat calories even when you can't see it — when you eat baked goods, cream sauces, casseroles, and vegetables. Avoid foods containing unknown amounts of butter. Whatever the amount, it's more than you need to stay thin.

You may have heard that margarine is a better choice than butter because margarine has so much less saturated fat (18 sat-fat calories per tablespoon) than butter (65 sat-fat calories per tablespoon). Saturated fat contributes to raising your blood cholesterol and thus your risk for heart disease*. However, **both margarine and butter are 100 percent fat and both have about 100 calories of fat per tablespoon.** In addition, it is now known that the trans fats** in margarines make them behave like saturated fats in the body. So, although margarine has a heart-healthy reputation, it is just as fattening as butter, almost as heart-risky, and should be limited.

Cream   (page 283, Food Tables)

It hardly seems necessary to advise dieters that cream is full of fat. But do you know exactly how fat-laden it really is? It is necessary to keep a watchful eye on cream, for it sneaks into meals and wreaks havoc on diet goals. Cream in coffee can devastate your Fat Budget. One tablespoon of light table cream has 26 calories of fat. If you drink 4 cups of coffee a day, that adds up to 104 fat calories and you haven't eaten anything of substance. Half-and-half is better, but not great. One tablespoon of half-and-half has 15 fat calories. Half-and-half for your four cups of coffee quickly adds up to 60 fat calories.

However, if you want to use cream or half-and-half, why not drink less coffee? Or better still, use whole milk at 5 fat calories per tablespoon, 2% at 3, or skim milk at 0. Best yet, drink your coffee black.

WARNING: Some nondairy creamers may be almost as fattening as cream. One tablespoon of a powdered nondairy creamer, such as Coffee-mate, has 15 fat calories; a frozen nondairy creamer, such as Coffee Rich, or a flavored powdered or liquid nondairy creamer, such as Coffee-mate French Vanilla, has 19 fat calories per tablespoon. Four cups of coffee and you have accumulated almost 80 fat calories of nondairy creamer. Are they worth it?

Cream in Soups and Sauces: Riches to Avoid. Cream in soups can ruin your whole day. A bowl of cream of mushroom soup has about 155 calories of fat; New England clam chowder about 80, vichyssoise 210. These may be low estimates. When eating out, be sure to ask

---

*See *Eater's Choice,* Fourth edition, pages 39–40, for a discussion of saturated fat.
**See *Eater's Choice,* Fourth edition, pages 80–82, for a fuller discussion of trans fats.

whether a soup contains cream, and if it does, then choose another appetizer or figure out how to budget it in.

And cream sauces! The half cup of curry cream sauce the chef ladles over your chicken costs you 250 fat calories, the cheesy cream sauce 170. If you want cream sauces to be included in your Fat Budget, insist that they be served on the side. Then you can determine how many spoonfuls (at 30 fat calories each) you want. But remember. Don't fool yourself. Spoonfuls quickly become cups.

Whipped Cream: For Your Eyes Only. Whipped cream looks and tastes so light and airy it is hard to believe its fat content is so high. But it is. The two-tablespoon dollop that perks up your pumpkin pie has 52 fat calories. The little cloud that nestles atop your ice cream sundae may have more than 350 calories of fat. Whipped cream is not a diet food. Whipped cream splurges should be saved for very, very, *very* special occasions.

Cheese: Be Aware and BEWARE   (pages 281–83, Food Tables)

If you have been a cheese nibbler, your nibbling days are numbered. Snacking on cheese is a fattening habit because most of what makes cheese cheese is fat. One ounce of Cheddar has 85 calories of fat; 1 ounce of Gruyère has 83. One ounce of Camembert cheese has 73; 1 ounce of Gouda has 70. Those chunks of Roquefort cheese in your salad dressing add 78 calories of fat to your greens (and to your thighs). If cheese is not one of your great loves, for the sake of your body, leave cheese off your shopping list. And, if it is, buy a small amount and fit it into your Fat Budget with great care. You will appreciate every bite.

"Lo" and "Lite": Read the Label. Low-calorie and nonfat cheeses abound. Before nonfat cheeses hit the scene, most Lite-line brand cheeses had 18 fat calories per ounce. Now they have 36 or 45. While this may be half the fat of the cheese they are imitating, it still can add up to a lot of fat. Two slices may equal 72 or 90 fat calories. Be careful and read labels. If you really love cheese, you might want to skip the filled cheese imitations and budget in a small piece of the real stuff very occasionally.

Mozzarella Loses Its Reputation. Mozzarella and Parmesan cheese have gained the reputation of being low in fat. However, 1 ounce of whole milk mozzarella has 55 fat calories and 1 ounce of part skim milk mozzarella has 41. One ounce of Parmesan cheese has 77 fat calories. When you bite into that slice of pizza oozing with mozzarella and Parmesan, think about all those fat calories being deducted from your budget and added to your hulk. For delicious, low-fat pizzas, try *Focaccia* (page 244) — a cross between pizza and bread — or other pizza and calzone recipes from *Eater's Choice.*

Cottage Cheese: Not Always a Great Diet Food. Americans think of cottage cheese as the quintessential diet food. And low-fat cottage cheese really is. However, not all cottage cheeses will help you lose weight. That half-cup scoop of whole milk cottage cheese on the "diet plate" has 43 fat calories. Two percent cottage cheese is a better choice at 20 fat calories per half cup. One percent is even better at a mere 10 fat calories per half cup. Mix cut-up fruit with your one percent fat cottage cheese or scoop cottage cheese on half a cantaloupe for two super, low-fat lunches.

Yogurt: The Good and the Bad   (pages 284–85, Food Tables)

Before you gorge yourself on any brand of yogurt, read the label. Some yogurts contain cream and whole milk. Stonyfield Farm yogurts contain 63 fat calories per 8-ounce container. Whitney's 100% Natural yogurts contain 45 fat calories per three-quarter-cup serving (it looks smaller because it is smaller). Even low-fat yogurts may contain 25–40 fat calories. These yogurts are hardly worth the fat calories, especially since nonfat flavored yogurts taste so creamy and good. Nonfat flavored and unflavored yogurts have 0 fat calories per serving.

Beware of the low or nonfat yogurts with toppings. The reason Astro vanilla low-fat yogurt with chocolate fudge crunch topping tastes like a high-fat treat is because it is. This is how it adds up: a half cup of low-fat yogurt + a quarter cup of chocolate fudge crunch = a 45-fat-calorie special.

Cooking with "Cream"   (pages 283–84, Food Tables)

It is possible to make delicious dishes by substituting nonfat yogurt, buttermilk, condensed skim milk, or skim milk in recipes that call for cream, sour cream, or whole milk. The divinely delicious *Deep-Dish Pear Pie* (*Eater's Choice*) made with nonfat yogurt has 368 fewer fat calories than *Deep-Dish Pear Pie* made with one cup of sour cream. *Cantaloupe*

Dieters: Don't Give Up Dairy Products

You are embarking on a new way of eating that will keep you slim and healthy for the rest of your life. Your goal is to lose weight but not by giving up nutritious foods. For you to succeed, your diet must be well balanced. And that means eating dairy products — nonfat and low-fat dairy products.

Dairy products supply your body with calcium (skim milk has more calcium than whole milk) to keep your bones and teeth strong. Females, especially teenagers and younger, need calcium to prevent osteoporosis in old age. Children need calcium for strong bones and teeth and to grow. Fill your diet with nonfat and low-fat dairy products — nonfat yogurts, low-fat cottage cheese, skim milk, buttermilk*. Cook with nonfat yogurt, buttermilk, and skim milk. Save high-fat dairy products for splurges.

Soup (page 220) is equally as scrumptious made with buttermilk (0–36 fat calories) as it would be with cream (396 fat calories). *Potato Salad* (page 250) made with nonfat yogurt instead of sour cream saves 184 fat calories.

For a more detailed discussion of cooking with low-fat ingredients, see "Silent Substitutions," in Chapter 9.

Egg: A Fat Surprise   (page 285, Food Tables)

Before you fix yourself a four-egg omelet for a light "diet" dinner, be aware that each egg yolk contains 50 calories of fat. A four-egg omelet contains 200 fat calories. Make your omelet with one egg and three egg whites (0 fat calories) for a similar-tasting but less-fat-filled dish.

FATS

Mayonnaise   (page 311, Food Tables)

One hundred percent of the calories in mayonnaise comes from fat. One tablespoon of regular mayonnaise has 100 fat calories. At 30–45

---

*Check the nutrition label on your buttermilk carton. Fat calories of buttermilk range from 0 to 36 per cup. Nine fat calories is common.

Fat Facts

Saturated fat
Monounsaturated fat
+ Polyunsaturated fat
Total Fat

Total fat is the sum of three types of fat: saturated, monounsaturated, and polyunsaturated fat. While all three types of fat are fattening, each has a different effect on your heart-health.

Saturated fat raises your LDL-cholesterol (bad cholesterol) and your risk of heart disease. Saturated fat is found predominantly in animal fats (beef fat, veal fat, lamb fat, lard or pork fat, chicken fat, turkey fat, and butterfat) and the following vegetable fats: coconut oil, palm kernel oil, palm oil, cocoa butter, and hydrogenated vegetable oil. If you think these vegetable fats are rare, check out the labels on convenience and snack foods. Saturated fat is easily recognizable because it is solid at room temperature.

Monounsaturated fat lowers your LDL-cholesterol and your risk of heart disease. An excellent source of monounsaturated fat is olive oil. It is considered the healthiest oil because it lowers LDL-cholesterol without lowering HDL-cholesterol (good cholesterol). It also prevents oxidation of LDL-cholesterol (see *Eater's Choice* for a fuller discussion of diet, cholesterol, and heart disease). But be warned. Olive oil has 119 fat calories per tablespoon.

Polyunsaturated fat lowers LDL-cholesterol but may also lower your HDL-cholesterol. The major sources of polyunsaturated fat are vegetable oils such as soy, corn, cottonseed, and safflower. Because consumption of large quantities of polyunsaturated fats have been implicated in the development of certain cancers in animals, we recommend limiting your use of polyunsaturated oil and using olive oil instead (we use it even in baking breads and pie crusts). In addition, when vegetable oils are hydrogenated or partially hydrogenated, they become trans fats, which act like saturated fats in the body.

CAUTION: Most fats and oils contain about 100–120 calories of fat per tablespoon. For both dieters and the health-conscious, fats and oils should be limited in the diet.

fat calories per tablespoon, reduced-calorie mayonnaises are better, but may still represent a good percentage of your Fat Budget. Nonfat mayonnaise is a boon to mayonnaise lovers, but be careful. When you dump a cup of fat-free mayo into your potato salad, you are nurturing your high-fat taste. Use fat-free mayonnaise carefully.

Eating Out: Mayonnaise Salad Sandwiches. Although tuna, shrimp, and chicken are basically low-fat meats, when they are mixed with mayonnaise and made into salads, they lose their low-fat label. If you can't avoid ordering a meat salad sandwich, insist that no additional mayonnaise be spread on the bread. Turkey breast meat is a better choice — with mustard. If you must have mayonnaise on a sandwich, ask the sandwich maker to use no more than a teaspoonful — just enough to moisten the bread. For added taste, sprinkle on hot peppers.

Salad Dressings   (pages 310–12, Food Tables)

Most salad dressings are loaded with fat calories. One tablespoon of French, Caesar, or Italian dressing has about 70 fat calories, 1 tablespoon of honey Dijon has 60. The salad dressings you get in a salad bar or restaurant are almost always high in fat. At a Burger King salad bar, the packet of Paul Newman's Own olive oil and vinegar dressing contains 297 fat calories. Ask to have your dressing served on the side (or if serving yourself, find a small bowl or cup and pour in some dressing) so you can regulate the amount you use. Keep track of how much dressing you put on your salad. Measure by tablespoonfuls (or soup spoons in a restaurant) so that you don't use up your day's Fat Budget before you get to the main course. Better yet, use the fork method (page 40) and get the taste of the dressing without the fat calories.

Low-Fat and Fat-Free Dressings: Dieters' Refuge. Good news! Many low-calorie and fat-free dressings are truly low or nonfat. Read the label. Or make your own low-fat dressings. Try substituting nonfat yogurt in salad dressing recipes that call for sour cream.

DESSERTS

No dieter has to be told that desserts can cause a Fat Budget blowout. But what's the fun of living, after all, if you can never have a dessert? The beauty of *Choose to Lose* is that it allows you to eat dessert as long as you can fit it into your Fat Budget. Just eat under your budget for several days to save up enough fat calories for a big splurge. (See "Splurging" in Chapter 10.) But use caution. Desserts are not going to make you thin.

Cakes: Sweet Temptation (pages 402–6, Food Tables)

Think very carefully before that piece of cheesecake (at least 160 fat calories), carrot cake with cream cheese frosting (190 fat calories), or glazed doughnut (130 fat calories) passes between your lips. Check the Food Tables for the fat calories of your favorites. Try eating a sliver of cake. Eat it very slowly. Savor every bite.

For *very special* occasions you might also try baking other scrumptious desserts — *Key Lime Pie* (page 267) at 36 fat calories per slice or *Tante Nancy's Apple Crumb Cake* (page 266) at 60 fat calories per slice, or from *Eater's Choice* such delights as *Divine Buttermilk Pound Cake* at 66 fat calories per slice or *Strawberry Tart* at 35 fat calories per slice. While not especially low in fat, many have fewer than half the fat calories of their commercial counterparts. But before you bake a different *Eater's Choice* dessert for each day of the week, remember "reduced" fat does not mean "little" fat, and eating these desserts too often will not help you lose weight.

For really low, low-fat and divine desserts, try *Chocolate Oatmeal Cookies* (page 272) at 4 fat calories a cookie, *Cheesecake* (page 265) at 8–16 fat calories per slice, *Meringue Shells with Fresh Strawberries and Warm Raspberry Sauce* (page 273) at 0 fat calories, *Glazed Cinnamon Buns* (page 269) at 15 fat calories each, and *Cocoa Angel Food Cake* (page 264) at 0 fat calories.

Cookies: Who's Counting? (pages 409–18, Food Tables)

Now that you are so fat-savvy, would you be surprised to learn that one small Fudge Covered Oreo cookie has 50 fat calories, one Pecan Sandie has 45, and one Chips Ahoy! Chunky chocolate chip cookie has 40. Would you be shocked to find that one Peanut Butter & Jelly Sandwich cookie has 60 fat calories? Even one tiny animal cracker has 5 fat calories.

Generally small, cookies don't look fat-packed. But commercially baked cookies range in fat calories from a low of 0 fat calories for Nabisco Fat-Free Fig Newtons to a high of 70 for one Pepperidge Farm Chocolate Chunk Pecan cookie.

Read food labels to find the fat calories of your favorites. The problem with cookies is that they are addictive and additive. One (18–70 fat calories) tastes so good, why not have two? or three? or ten (180–700 fat calories)? If you know that you are a cookie monster, leave temptation in the store and keep your home and office cookie jars filled with fruit.

For a discussion of nonfat cookie abuse, see Chapter 5, page 100.

Frozen Desserts   (pages 419–26, Food Tables)

Rich Ice Cream: Poor Choice. The moment you bite into a Dove Bar or let a spoonful of Häagen-Dazs or Ben & Jerry's settle in your mouth, you know. Rich ice cream is full of fat: 260 to 440 fat calories per cup. All ice cream is not that high in fat, but it is definitely not diet food. A cup of ordinary vanilla ice cream has about 160 fat calories. Read the label. Of course, you can have half a cup or a quarter of a cup or a tablespoon or two. But don't bring a gallon of ice cream into the house "for the kids" if you know that you are the kid who'll be eating the ice cream.

Light Ice Cream: Better Choice. For those who want an alternative to the megafat varieties, there are some "light" ice creams and ice milks that will not totally decimate your Fat Budget when eaten in small amounts and with thought. Be careful to read the labels to find the flavor with the lowest number of fat calories. They range from 20 fat calories for a half cup of any Healthy Choice Ice Cream to 45 fat calories for a half cup of Edy's Grand Light French Silk Ice Cream. Be aware that although lower than most ice creams, these "light" or "low-fat" varieties still have enough fat calories to demand extra vigilance. And who eats just the half cup serving size? At 90 fat calories, one cup of Hood Light Chocolate Chip is hardly a light treat.

Frozen Yogurt: Sometimes the Best Bet. If you are an ice cream purist, no other frozen confection may satisfy you. However, a delicious, low-fat alternative does exist: frozen yogurt. Many frozen yogurts are quite low in fat. A typical small serving (5 fluid ounces) of Colombo low-fat frozen yogurt has 23 fat calories; for the same amount ICBIY has 32 fat calories and TCBY has 34.

But don't equate "frozen yogurt" with "fat-free" or "low-fat." Not all frozen yogurts are low-fat. Before you order the super-large size in three different flavors, be sure you ask the server the number of fat calories per serving and the serving size. If he doesn't know, find another yogurt parlor. Even if he does know, don't eat a frozen yogurt at every meal. Recent studies have shown that low-fat and even fat-free frozen yogurts may have more fat calories than advertised.

In the Freezer Case: You also need to check the labels of the frozen yogurt you find in the freezer cases of your grocery store. Many are truly low or nonfat. But some of the gourmet flavors rival ice cream for fat calories. Colombo Shoppe Style White Chocolate Almond has 140 fat calories per cup. The TCBY Vanilla Crunch Yog-A-Bar contains 110 fat calories.

The Best Fat Buy: Nonfat Frozen Yogurt. The greatest treat is nonfat frozen yogurt, which has 0 calories of fat and is truly delectable. But a caution: Although the basic frozen yogurt may be almost fat-free, the

FROZEN DESSERT	AMOUNT	FAT CALORIES
Frozen Yogurt		
Nonfat frozen yogurt	1 cup	0
Colombo low-fat (soft serve)	1 cup	36
ICBIY and TCBY low-fat	1 cup	72
Colombo White Chocolate Almond	1 cup	140
Ice Cream		
Healthy Choice Low-Fat Ice Cream	1 cup	40
Mattus Low-Fat Ice Cream	1 cup	54
Breyers Light	1 cup	70
Chocolate, Vanilla & Strawberry		
Edy's Grand Light Ice Cream	1 cup	70–90
Hood Light Chocolate Chocolate	1 cup	90
Chip		
Dove Bar	1 bar (78g)	150
Good Humor Candy Center Crunch	1 bar	170
Häagen-Dazs Exträas Iced	1 bar (96g)	220
Cappuccino		
Ben & Jerry's Vanilla Ice Cream	1 cup	300
Häagen-Dazs Butter Pecan Ice Cream	1 cup	440
Sherbet		
Sherbet, orange	1 cup	30
Häagen-Dazs Raspberry Sorbet &	1 cup	160
Cream		

almonds, Oreo cookie pieces, peanuts, M&M's, and coconut you load on top are not. Eat your frozen yogurt plain or with fruit toppings. Again, don't eat it for breakfast, lunch, and dinner because the fat content may be greater than 0, and the calories, whatever they contain, are empty.

Candy Packs a Fat Wallop   (pages 406–9, Food Tables)

A candy bar may be small in size, but it's gigantic in its fat-calorie count. A 1.5-ounce Mr. Goodbar has 160 fat calories. A 1.5-ounce Kit Kat has 110 fat calories. Four Hershey's Kisses have 55 calories of fat. When the taste is gone, much too quickly, all you have left is fat deposits on your frame and a few extra cavities in your mouth. However, if never eating candy would cause you deep remorse, budget candy into your diet . . . *carefully.*

Although candy has no redeeming nutritional value, some candy has little or no fat. Gumdrops, most hard candies, jelly beans, and marshmallows have no fat, so you can enjoy a few with no guilt. They are also devoid of any vitamins, minerals, or fiber, so you don't want to become a jelly bean junkie or marshmallow maniac.

SNACKS   (pages 386–98, Food Tables)

The problem with snacks is not just their high fat content. The problem with snacks is also that they are addictive. You can't eat just one — one peanut or one cracker or one potato chip. Or even two. Or even three. Try fifty.

Sitting in front of the television set or among a group of friends, the snacker reaches into a bowl of nuts, crackers, chips, over and over and over: bowl to mouth, bowl to mouth. She barely tastes what she is eating, much less thinks about it. Dieters must be thinkers. Here are some truths about snacks.

Popcorn

Homemade Air-Popped Popcorn: The Best Buy. We start with popcorn because it has the potential to be one of the greatest snacks of all time. Popcorn that you pop in an air popper has no fat. It is chock full of fiber — half insoluble (important for effective bowel function and reducing risk of colon cancer) and half soluble (helps a little bit to lower blood cholesterol and risk of heart disease). It is a perfect snack. It fills you up and satisfies that hand-to-mouth craving at no punishment to your Fat Budget. Air-popped popcorn may taste a bit like bumpy cardboard at first, but in a short time you'll develop a yen for it. And, because it contains no fat, you can eat as much as you want.

Homemade Popcorn Popped in Oil: Not Such a Great Buy. The dietary benefits of popcorn diminish when other popping methods are used because it takes a lot of fat to pop popcorn. Each cup of popcorn prepared in a saucepan with sunflower or corn oil contains about 25 fat calories. That's 1 cup. Who eats 1 cup of popcorn? (To help put 1 cup into perspective, note that the smallest container of popcorn you can buy at a movie theater holds 5 cups and the largest bucket holds 20 cups.) And then, if you flavor it with melted butter or margarine, add 100 fat calories per tablespoon. And who uses just one tablespoon of butter or margarine?

Commercial Air-Popped Popcorn: The Pits. It's a cruel world out there. The food industry has perfected deception to its highest level. And we are the victims, unless we fight back by reading labels. The newest treachery in the food industry's bag of tricks is commercially packaged air-popped popcorn. Wow, how healthy. Ha! Read the label. Bachman's All Natural (another catchword for healthy) Air-Popped Popcorn has 100 fat calories for 1 ounce — 2¾ cups. The first ingredient is popcorn, the second is partially hydrogenated vegetable oil. Bachman took a perfect dieter's food and coated it with a highly fattening and heart-risky fat. How sad.

Microwave Popcorn: No Buy. Microwave popcorns do not save you money, time, or fat calories. Microwave popcorn costs about $3.65 a pound (versus 49 cents a pound for plain popcorn kernels), takes 4½ minutes to make (versus 3 for air-popped), and ranges from 6 to 30 fat calories per cup (versus 0 fat calories for plain air-popped popcorn). Look at the next box for a comparison of 12 cups of popcorn (the amount of air-popped popcorn we each eat every day) prepared in a variety of ways and packaged by different food producers.

Movie Popcorn: BYO. Beware of movie popcorn. It is almost always prepared in coconut oil, the most saturated (heart-risky) oil there is. Don't even consider buying buttered popcorn unless you want to wipe out your Fat Budget totally for a few days. Bring your own air-popped

POPCORN	12 CUPS	
	COST	FAT CALORIES
Homemade air-popped	$ .10	0
Boston Lite	$ .99	150
Weight Watchers Butter Toffee	$8.28	300
Orville Redenbacher's Butter Light	$2.27	336
Bachman's Air-Popped	$1.73	436
Smartfood Cheddar Cheese	$2.72	617

popcorn. If the usher questions you, tell him you're following doctor's orders.

Movie Popcorn

AMOUNT	SIZE	Popped in Coconut Oil		Popped in Coconut Oil with "Butter"		Popped in Canola Shortening	
		CALORIES		CALORIES		CALORIES	
		TOTAL	FAT	TOTAL	FAT	TOTAL	FAT
5 cups	Small (A); Kids (C)	300	180	472	333		
7 cups	Small (C, U)	398	243	632	450		
	Small (A)					361	198
11 cups	Medium (A)	647	387	910	639	627	342
16 cups	Medium (C, U)	901	540	1221	873		
	Large (A)					850	468
20 cups	Large (A, C, U)	1161	693	1642	1134		

A = AMC*; C = Cineplex Odeon; U = United Artists
*Some AMC theaters use canola shortening while others use coconut oil.

Sources: Nutrition Action Healthletter; Center for Science in the Public Interest; SGS Control Services, Inc.

Nuts to Nuts   (pages 360–63, Food Tables)

Nuts make a delicious snack, add zest to entrees and desserts, possess delectable taste and crunch, and (sigh) are brimming with fat. They range from cashews at 118 fat calories per ounce to macadamia nuts at 196 fat calories per ounce. Considering that an ounce of nuts isn't many, it turns out to be a lot of fat calories. And they are habit-forming. You might want to save nuts for cooking and then, when a recipe calls for a half cup of peanuts (323 fat calories), use only a quarter cup (161 fat calories) or 3 tablespoons (121 fat calories). If having nuts around for any reason demands more self-control than you are able to muster, leave them on the shelf in the store.

Nuts to Coconut. When the soda jerk asks you if you want your dish of nonfat frozen yogurt covered with shredded coconut, you might offer him a lecture on nutrition. There are two reasons to avoid coconut: first, coconut is a high-sat-fat food—almost 100 percent of the fat is saturated. (Saturated fat raises blood cholesterol, which raises your risk for heart disease.) Coconut is what scientists feed rats (which are quite resistant to heart disease) to give them heart disease. Second, and of most importance to the new thin you, coconut is incredibly high in fat calories. One cup of shredded coconut has 241 fat calories. One half cup of coconut cream has 375 fat calories. One half cup of coconut milk has 258 fat calories. A little dab will undo you.

Nuts to Seeds. Seeds represent another sneaky fat carrier. They are so small and seem so healthy, but just a few handfuls can deplete your whole Fat Budget. Whole pumpkin seeds contain 50 fat calories per ounce. One tablespoon of sesame seeds contains 39 fat calories. Shelled sunflower seeds contain 127 fat calories per ounce, 39 fat calories per tablespoon. The little package (1⅛ ounces) of shelled sunflower seeds you pick up at the grocery store checkout line has 152 fat calories. And they are covered with salt so you want to eat more and more. If you love to nibble on sunflower seeds, apportion yourself 1 tablespoon and consider that a hefty treat.

For a real education, check the Nuts and Seeds section of the Food Tables.

Trail Mix. Trail Mix (mixed nuts, seeds, and dried fruit) conjures up the aura of outdoor vitality and good health. Out on the trail, hiking up a mountain, forging a stream (or perhaps, sitting in your den watching TV), you gobble up handfuls of this tasty mix. STOP. Consider the contents — almonds (132 fat calories per ounce), cashews (118 fat calories per ounce), peanuts (126 fat calories per ounce), sunflower seeds (127 fat calories per ounce), flaked coconut (82 fat calories per ounce), dried fruit (0 to 13 fat calories per ounce). This "healthy" snack food could contain anywhere from 60 to 80 fat calories per quarter cup.

Just Say No to Chips   (pages 386–87, Food Tables)

If you are like most normal human beings, you will find it impossible to keep from eating potato chips if they are in your house. Since 1 ounce of potato chips has 80 to 90 fat calories, you might want to avoid bringing temptation home from the store. If you have an uncontrollable urge to eat potato chips, buy the smallest deli bag (80 fat calories). It may be worth that big chunk out of your Fat Budget every once in a while.

Any chips — Fritos, Chee-tos, nachos, etc., etc. — should be eaten with considerable thought. Chips are basically fat stiffened with a bit of vegetable. In fact, the first ingredient of Durkee's French Fried Onions is partially hydrogenated soy oil. The second is onions!* And the fat calories show it. A small can (6 ounces) contains 702 fat calories. A 3-ounce deli bag of Fritos corn chips contains 270 fat calories. Snack chips are truly addictive and can be consumed by the hundreds and thousands. The last one always invites another. Our strong recommendation is to leave temptation out of the house by not bringing chips in. No one needs them.

New Chips in Town. As if potato chips, cheese twists, and corn chips weren't bad enough, bagel chips and pita chips were invented to add even more temptation to an already gigantic selection. At first glance, you may even have thought that bagel chips and pita chips were healthy and low in fat.** Ha! Three-fourths of an ounce — a whiff and it's gone — costs 36 fat calories. More likely you'll eat the whole bag for 288 fat calories.

If you are swayed to buy carrot chips or sweet potato chips for a healthy snack, read the package label, shake your head in disgust, and buy the vegetables instead. Twenty Hain's Carrot Chips contain 81 fat calories, as do 28 of Terra's Sweet Potato Chips.

Crackers   (pages 387–92, Food Tables)

Until the FDA required it, almost no cracker package sported a food label. What were they hiding? FAT. Crackers are a high-fat food and like potato chips and peanuts, crackers are consumed in great numbers with nary a thought. They are little but they add up. One cracker may

---

*Ingredients on a food label are listed in descending order by weight.
**A truly low-fat bagel chips recipe may be found in *Eater's Choice*.

have only 9 calories of fat, but ten have 90, and it is very easy to eat ten crackers. Dieters must pay attention. The best policy is to avoid the cracker section of your grocery store. But if you must have crackers, keep track of every one you eat. Perhaps, as a treat have two crackers a day. You know yourself. Will the box of crackers be so tempting that you will eventually weaken and gobble them all up? If so, leave the crackers in the store.

Fat-Free. Low-fat and fat-free crackers are making their way onto the grocery shelves. A popular brand is SnackWell's (beware: many of their *reduced* fat crackers contain enough fat to worry about). Devonsheer's Melba toast and Melba Rounds and Wasa's Crispbreads have 0 calories of fat and lots of crunch. Eat them plain or with jelly. Nonfat crackers covered with cheese, cream cheese, or some other high-fat spread are no longer diet food. See page 100 for a discussion of fat-free cracker abuse.

THE GOOD NEWS

Dry your tears. You can still fit any of these fat-laden foods into your Fat Budget. But now that you know how to choose carefully and wisely, you might ask yourself some questions. Why eat a can of solid white tuna packed in oil at 297 fat calories when a can of solid white tuna packed in water has only 30 fat calories? Do I really want that greasy cheese smokie at 112 calories of fat? Will a bite of apple pie (about 16 fat calories) instead of a whole slice (160 fat calories) satisfy me? Refer to this chapter and to the Food Tables in the back of the book to make educated choices that will produce a streamlined and glorious you.

Coming next . . . finding out the great foods you CAN eat.

Remember:
1. Americans like to eat high-fat foods, and the foods available in supermarkets, restaurants, and everywhere cater to this high-fat taste. In order to become and stay thin and healthy in this high-fat world, you need to know not only where fat lurks but in what amounts.
2. Always judge the fat content of foods with your Fat Budget in mind.
3. Use the Food Tables to compare the fat contents of foods and to find

lower-fat alternatives to high-fat favorites. Remember to adjust total and fat calories for the actual amount of a food you eat.

a. Red meats, such as beef, veal, lamb, and most pork products, are high in fat. The higher the grade of meat, the more fat it contains.

b. Turkey and chicken with the skin removed (always remove the skin before cooking chicken), shellfish, and many fish are low in fat. But these low-fat foods are easily made into high-fat foods by the way they are prepared.

c. Most sausage and luncheon meats are extremely high in fat (in addition to containing cancer-risky nitrites and blood pressure–raising sodium).

d. Many frozen dinners and convenience foods are riddled with hidden fat. Read the food labels to see how (or if) you can fit these foods into your Fat Budget.

e. Most fast foods are loaded with fat (and sodium). Do your diet and health goals a favor and approach fast-food restaurants with extreme caution or not at all.

f. Dairy products are excellent sources of calcium, but many are high in fat. A glass of whole milk contains 73 fat calories. An ounce of Cheddar cheese contains 85 fat calories. Choose nonfat or low-fat dairy products, such as nonfat or low-fat yogurt, low-fat cottage cheese, and skim milk. Fit cheeses into your budget sparingly, and you will really enjoy them.

4. Remember that your Fat Budget is a ceiling. You should not eat above it and preferably should eat well within it. But your minimum total calories are a floor and you must eat well above this amount to ensure that you provide enough calories to fuel your physical activity, maximize your basal metabolic rate, and consume adequate amounts of vitamins, minerals, and fiber.

5. Repeat to yourself: **I MUST EAT TO LOSE. I MUST EAT TO LOSE. I MUST EAT TO LOSE. OF COURSE, I MUST EAT NUTRITIOUS, LOW-FAT FOODS TO LOSE.**

5. Eat Without Fear

"For the first time I think of what I *can* eat instead of what I *can't* eat."

Dawn Monroe, Caledon East, Ontario

THINK BACK to the science you learned in Chapter 1. The earthshaking truth is that you *must* eat to lose weight. Of course, you must eat foods that are low in fat, but you should eat LOTS of low-fat foods.

It is crucial that you eat enough calories. You figured out your minimum daily total caloric intake in Chapter 2. Remember, this is a FLOOR. It is the number of calories you need to satisfy your basal metabolic rate. Make sure that you are eating *more* than this amount. You need additional calories to provide energy for your physical activity. When you reduce fat in your diet, there is a real danger that your total caloric intake will fall too low. You must replace some of the fat you eliminate with foods rich in fiber and nutrients — whole-grains, fruits, vegetables. Keep saying to yourself over and over, "I must eat to lose."

CARBOHYDRATES GALORE

And which foods these are may surprise you.

Here's the great news. You may eat bread. You may eat potatoes. You may eat rice. You may eat spaghetti. You may put jelly on your toast. You may eat a *whole* banana and an apple and pear and orange and grapes. The USDA Food Guide Pyramid recommends that you eat *at least* 2 to 4 servings of fruits, 3 to 5 servings of vegetables, and 6 to 11 servings of grains each day to maintain your health.

Remember, carbohydrates help you to LOSE weight. This is probably still difficult for you to believe and may be even more difficult for you to implement, but the more fruits, vegetables, and whole-grains you eat and the less fat you eat, the faster you will lose.

Adding Carbohydrates to the Fire

Let's review the reasons why this miraculous statement is true. Except for the small amount stored as glycogen, carbohydrates are entirely burned to provide energy to fuel your body functions and your physical activity. Any carbohydrate eaten in excess of your needs is burned and the energy is wasted as heat. It is not converted into fat under normal conditions. By eating lots of carbohydrates (as fruits, vegetables, and whole-grains), you keep your basal metabolic rate chugging away at a higher rate.

Putting Fat into Cold Storage

In contrast, the fat that you eat is immediately added to your fat stores. It doesn't get burned up. It doesn't add fuel to the fire. It is as if you took a syringe and injected the ice cream sundae that you just ate directly into your blubbery thighs. So, while occasionally you can even eat up to 2000 calories of carbohydrates in excess of your normal intake and not gain weight, any fat you eat above your Fat Budget turns into fat on your bod.

Misguidance

Carbohydrates used to be (and remain to a great extent) the Number One Forbidden Nutrient in every diet. You were advised to eat the 2 ounces of Cheddar cheese and toss the 2 slices of bread, eat the 5-ounce lean sirloin steak and chuck the baked potato. Let's see what that means in fat calories. Keep the cheese — 144 calories of fat — and toss the bread — 18 calories of fat. Keep the steak — 295 fat calories — and chuck the potato — 0 calories. Huh? They must be kidding.

Not *Choose to Lose*. Here are some good things to eat.

STARCHES: WEIGHT-LOSS STARS

Bread: A Yes-Yes

Hey! You can eat BREAD! Consider bread diet food. A slice of commercially baked bread has 10 fat calories. (Check labels — some have more.) You can eat it for a snack. Shun open-faced sandwiches. Give your sandwich a top and a bottom. You need those calories of carbohydrate. Besides, you will feel fuller and more satisfied eating both slices of bread.

Homemade Breads: MMMMmm Good! Try baking your own bread. Bread dough is easily made in a food processor (it takes less than 5 minutes). It doesn't even take that much of your time. Although you have to make an appearance an hour after you make the dough to roll it out and put it in loaf pans and then you have to return an hour later to bake it, the bread doesn't need you to do most of the time-consuming work — rising and baking. Start the bread when you finish dinner if you're staying home for the evening and you'll have it warm for a late-night snack. Make two loaves and freeze one. A slice of *Anadama* (page 258) or any of the breads in *Eater's Choice* will enhance your diet and your life. These homemade breads are not without fat calories. On the average a slice has 15 fat calories (some have as many as 25), but homemade bread tastes so good and is so filling it is worth a small bite into your Fat Budget. Have a slice for breakfast toasted and piled high with banana slices and 1% cottage cheese. Have a slice with your fruit salad and nonfat yogurt for lunch. Even a slice or two may find a place in your budget to satisfy afternoon or evening pangs of hunger.

An aside: Choose whole-grain breads. They are healthier than white. They are rich in fiber, protein, thiamin, riboflavin, niacin, folic acid, vitamin E, iron, phosphorus, magnesium, zinc, and other trace minerals. Check labels. The first ingredient should be whole-wheat flour. Some breads labeled "wheat bread" may contain no whole-wheat. Some bread manufacturers substitute caramel coloring for whole-wheat flour.

Eat Potatoes to Avoid Looking Like One

Can you believe it? Eating potatoes will help you lose weight. Bake them, boil them, broil them. Fill them with nonfat yogurt or eat them plain. Bake *Potato Skins* (page 241). At 7 fat calories a serving (or 0 if you use no oil), you can eat them with zest. Bake an extra potato for dinner and eat it cold as a snack.

Your mouth drops open in disbelief. How can potatoes be diet food? Potatoes are almost completely free of fat. And they are a good source of vitamin C, thiamin, niacin, and iron. Sweet potatoes are also loaded with vitamin A. Screw up your courage and eat a potato or two every day. See if you don't look less and less like a potato.

Low-Fat Potato + Fat = High-Fat Potato. Of course, if you stuff your potato with a fat (butter, margarine, cheese, sour cream) or slice and fry it into french fries or slice it even thinner and fry it into potato chips, you can no longer consider potatoes diet food. French fries and potato chips are among the worst offenders on the Most Unwanted Fat list.

Pastas + Rice = Fat-Loss Success

Two more complex carbohydrates to add to your diet list — pasta and rice. Don't be shy. Pile a heap of steamed rice on your plate and top it with a low-fat chicken or vegetable dish. Fill a large bowl with spaghetti and cover it with a low-fat tomato sauce. Eat more of the pasta or rice and less of the topping.

Are you having difficulty imagining piles of rice or spaghetti on your plate? And actually eating them? Those who have always considered a quarter cup of rice or spaghetti extravagant must make an effort to regard them in a positive light. Repeat over and over: "Pasta and rice are NOT fattening. Eating pasta and rice will help me LOSE weight." You'll see.

Pasta + Cream Sauce = Weight Gain

Of course, pasta or rice are not always reducing foods. Mix in butter or margarine or cover them with high-fat sauces or cheese and you destroy their beneficial weight loss properties. Prepared pastas such as Contadina Chicken and Rosemary Ravioli (110 fat calories for 1 cup) don't even need added sauces to give your Fat Budget a nervous breakdown.

You must also be sure that the basic pasta is really nonfat. Pastas such as Oodles of Noodles and Top Ramen Noodles sound like great nonfat choices. They are not. A quick bath in sizzling hydrogenated vegetable oils has made them into high-fat no-no's.

Cereals: Breakfast of Champions

What a treat it is to eat a large bowl of cereal without feeling like a sinner. Eat cereal for breakfast and eat it for a snack. Of course, the milk should be skim and the cereal should have no more than about 9 to 18 fat calories per serving. Check the fiber listing on the box. The more the better. (Read on to learn about the importance of fiber in your diet.)

VEGGIES

No one needs to tell you that vegetables are an important part of a diet. You have probably followed diets in which the fear of turning into a rabbit was justified. But don't disparage vegetables. Not only are they fat-free, high in vitamins, minerals, and fiber, they are also just plain delicious. Eat them raw. Or cut them into matchsticks, steam them until just tender, and press garlic or grind pepper over them or sprinkle them with herbs. Create a vegetable dip by mixing Dijon mustard into nonfat yogurt. Try vegetables you have never tried before. Have you ever baked spaghetti squash? When you scrape out the cooked interior, it separates into strands, exactly like spaghetti but more nutritious and delicious. Top it with a low-fat tomato sauce. Bring home a cartful of vegetables each time you shop. Then you'll have cucumbers for Cucumber Soup, lemons for Lemon Chicken, and sweet potatoes, spinach, zucchini, carrots — a panoply of vegetables — to enhance your dinners.

FRUIT

Food of the Gods

Fruit makes a great snack, a great lunch, and a great dessert. In fact, we should emulate the Europeans and top off our meal with fruit instead of rich, high-fat desserts. In season, cantaloupe, honeydew melon, watermelon, strawberries, raspberries, peaches, nectarines, pears, plums, taste divine. Packed with vitamins, minerals, and fiber, fruit is nutritious and will put no strain on your Fat Budget. You can eat fruit until you feel like a human fruit bowl. Don't limit it (except for avocado, which has 270 fat calories). Eat a *whole* banana. Eat *two bananas!* Bring a bag of fruit to the office and dig in whenever hunger strikes.

Fattening Fruit

Of course, even fruit can be ruined. Vanilla ice cream covered with strawberries, raspberries in cream, or blackberries in sour cream may taste delicious, but they won't keep buttons from popping off your shirts. Substitute nonfat yogurt or nonfat frozen yogurt for a similar but nonfattening effect.

FIBER

By eating all these wonderful fruits and vegetables and whole-grains, not only are you getting a heaping amount of vitamins and minerals, you are also fulfilling your requirement for fiber. Fiber is essential for good health. A high-fiber diet reduces the risk of colon cancer and may reduce the risk of breast cancer. It helps prevent diverticulosis and hemorrhoids, as well as constipation. It can even lower blood glucose levels.

The chart that follows shows you the amount of fiber in a variety of foods. The Food and Drug Administration recommends eating 25 grams of fiber a day. Most Americans eat less than 10 (which may be why, along with a high-fat diet, we have such high rates of colon cancer). But don't overdo a good thing. Eating more than 50 to 60 grams of fiber a day may decrease the amount of vitamins and minerals your body absorbs.

When you are making choices, keep fiber in mind. Eat the fruit rather than just drinking the juice. Eat the skin on your potato. Choose a cereal with a high fiber content*. Eating the *Choose to Lose* way, you will automatically be eating enough fiber. See Chapter 12, "Ensuring a Balanced Diet," for guidelines on how many servings of fruit, vegetables, and whole-grains you need to eat to ensure an adequate intake of fiber.

SUGAR GUILT

Sugar guilt is intense in dieters. Intense but misguided because sugar by itself will not make you gain weight. It is the fat that accompanies the sugar that makes you fat. Think of all those wonderfully rich desserts you have been avoiding. They contain sugar *and* butter, chocolate, whipped cream, cream, or sour cream. The big *and* makes the dessert fattening.

So although you can only occasionally fit high-fat desserts into your Fat Budget, you can give yourself a daily treat by using real jelly or jam

---

*Nutrition labels of commercial foods list dietary fiber. See pages 124–25.

Table 3
Dietary Fiber in Foods

FOOD	AMOUNT	DIETARY FIBER (G)	FOOD	AMOUNT	DIETARY FIBER (G)
Vegetables, cooked			**Legumes, cooked**		
Broccoli	½ cup	2.0	Baked beans, canned	½ cup	9.8
Brussels sprouts	½ cup	3.4	Kidney beans	½ cup	7.3
Potato, baked, with skin	1 medium	3.6	Lentils, cooked	½ cup	3.7
Spinach	½ cup	2.0	**Breakfast cereals**		
Sweet potato	½ medium	1.7	All-Bran	⅓ cup	8.5
Zucchini	½ cup	1.3	Bran Chex	⅔ cup	4.6
Vegetables, raw			Bran flakes	¾ cup	5.3
Carrots	1 medium	2.3	Cornflakes	1¼ cup	0.6
Celery	1 stalk	0.6	Granola	¼ cup	3.2
Cucumber, sliced	½ cup	0.5	Oat bran, raw	⅓ cup	4.9
Lettuce, romaine	1 cup	1.0	Oatmeal, cooked	¾ cup	1.6
Mushrooms, sliced	½ cup	0.5	Raisin bran	¾ cup	4.8
Spinach	1 cup	1.5	**Breads, grains, and pasta**		
Tomato	1 medium	1.6	Bagel	1	1.2
Fruits			French bread	1 slice	0.8
Apple, with skin	1 medium	3.0	Pumpernickel bread	1 slice	1.9
Banana	1 medium	1.8	Rice, brown, cooked	½ cup	1.7
Blueberries	½ cup	1.7	Spaghetti, cooked	½ cup	1.1
Cantaloupe	¼	1.1	Whole-wheat bread	1 slice	1.9
Figs, dried	2	3.5	**Snack foods**		
Orange	1 medium	3.1	Popcorn, air-popped	1 cup	0.9
Peach, with skin	1	1.4			
Pear, with skin	1 medium	4.3			
Prunes	3	1.8			
Raisins, seedless	¼ cup	1.9			
Strawberries	1 cup	3.9			

Pennington, J.A.T. *Bowes and Church's Food Value of Portions Commonly Used.* 15th ed. Philadelphia, Pa.: J.B. Lippincott Co., 1989.

on your English muffin without a twinge of conscience. (In fact, you should use jelly and forget about the margarine or butter.) You can suck an occasional peppermint, jelly bean, or hard candy without guilt.

Sweet Treat

No, you should not binge on sugar, either. Sugar is just a lot of empty calories containing no vitamins, minerals, or fiber. If you are diabetic or have high triglycerides, you should avoid sugar. Otherwise, treating yourself to an occasional hard candy may give you a lift. (Be sure to check labels for ingredients; some hard candy, such as butterscotch, is made with heart-risky, fattening oils.) If you ordinarily skimp on maple syrup on French toast, pouring a little more of the maple syrup and eating a lot less of the French toast will do both your psyche and chassis a lot of good. A cup of vanilla nonfat yogurt may have about 120 calories of sugar, but since it has 0 calories of fat — eat away.

Alcohol — NOT a Fat-Free Panacea

Although alcohol has no fat, its consumption should be limited for other reasons. Not only are alcohol calories empty — they provide no nutritional benefits — drinking too much alcohol can wreak havoc on your health. In addition, alcohol can weaken your inhibitions and you may end up eating more fat than a sober you would have allowed. Limit alcoholic beverages to a maximum of 1 to 2 drinks a day.

SNACKS

Popcorn

Air-popped popcorn — that is, TRUE air-popped popcorn that you pop yourself (as opposed to commercial packaged brands, which may add 100 calories of fat per ounce) — has no fat. If you ate the same amount of air-popped popcorn with no added fat which fills the large container of coconut oil–popped movie theater popcorn — 20 cups — you would not gain weight. (However, your jaws might never work again.)

Pretzels

Bravo, Snyder's of Hanover. Pretzels can make a great diet snack if eaten in moderation. (We eat a few for dessert.) Some, such as Snyder's of Hanover Sour Dough Pretzels, are fat-free. Many are very low in fat. Ten two-inch pretzel sticks may have only 9 fat calories. However, before you invest in a warehouse of pretzel tins, note that most brands are heavily encrusted with salt (sodium raises blood pressure in some people and causes fluid retention) and, as your aim is to eat primarily nutritious (not processed) foods, you don't want to go hog-wild on even the lowest sodium nonfat pretzels.

Tsk, Tsk, Snyder's of Hanover. Don't take it for granted that all pretzels are low- or nonfat. A small handful (1 ounce) of Snyder's of Hanover Cheddar Cheese-Flavored pretzel pieces has 63 fat calories. Their Honey Mustard and Buttermilk Ranch pretzel pieces contain 45 fat calories an ounce. Rold Gold Honey Mustard Pretzel Bits go for 70 fat calories an ounce. Even some ordinary-looking pretzels are made with significant amounts of fat. Read the labels.

Self-Control

You are following *Choose to Lose* because you want to lose weight and eat healthfully. Keep this in mind at all times. Eating an entire box of pretzels or a whole bag of hard sucking candies because they have little or no fat is misusing the *Choose to Lose* system and will not lead to weight loss.

Yogurt: Too Good to Be True

Nonfat flavored yogurts (0 to 9 fat calories per 8-ounce container) are truly a treat. Choose coffee, lemon, vanilla, and a variety of fruit flavors. Even if you don't think you like yogurt, check these out. They make good snacks and desserts. Try the Roland Lippoldt special for a nonfat dessert delicacy: mix apple sauce and nonfat plain yogurt and top with a sprinkle of pumpkin pie spice; add a cut-up apple for extra crunch.

CHOICE MEATS

Chicken: Infinite Variety

Chicken can be prepared in umpteen million delicious ways without harming your diet. Choose the breast. It's the part lowest in fat. Always remove the skin *before* you cook it. Steam, bake, broil, or stew to minimize added fat. Use spices for interest. Substitute nonfat yogurt, skim milk, or buttermilk for cream, sour cream, or whole milk to create tasty, low-fat dishes.

Turkey without Skin: Low-Fat Treat

White turkey meat has only 2 calories of fat per ounce. You can't do much better than that. For a low-fat treat, fill a whole-wheat pita or French bread baguette to overflowing with turkey breast meat and dress it with mustard, tomato, lettuce, and hot peppers. Try Ron's most favorite lunch in all the world — Ted Mummery's Turkey Barbecue (page 255) in a whole-wheat pita. Throw cooked turkey into low-fat sauces. Roast a big tom and you'll have turkey leftovers to freeze and use for weeks.

Seafood: Lean Cuisine

Many fish are irresistibly lean and delicious — 2 calories of fat per ounce for raw cod, dolphin fish, haddock, lobster, pike, pollock, and scallops; 3 for grouper, snapper, and sunfish; and 4 for flounder, monkfish, perch, rockfish, shrimp, and sole. Just bake it, grill it, poach it, or broil it. Skewer it with vegetables. Cover it with low-fat sauces. Eat away.

WARNING: Chicken, turkey, and fish can be exceedingly fattening if prepared incorrectly. Read the Chicken, Turkey, and Seafood sections in Chapter 4, "Where's the Fat?," to learn how easily these low-fat meats can be pumped up with fat.

Treat Yourself: Turn Chicken, Turkey, and Seafood into *Choose to Lose* and *Eater's Choice* Entrees

Nancy Goor loves to eat. She's not wild about cooking. She does it because she loves to eat so much. Most of the recipes she has created in *Choose to Lose* and *Eater's Choice* are quick and easy to prepare because she doesn't want to spend her life cooking. She has other things to do and she knows you do, too. If you want to lose weight, you (or someone in your household) has to cook. You need to be satisfied. You need to eat full dinners. It is not enough to eat only a baked sweet potato and three carrot sticks for dinner. How long will you stay on a low-fat diet if you eat so little? But if you eat them with *Vegetable Soup with Spinach, Potatoes, Rice, and Corn* (page 225) and *East Indian Chicken* (page 230) and *Curried Whipped Potatoes* (page 241), you will be full and content. Eating lots of delicious, low-fat food is the secret to staying thin.

Healthy Food Can Be Delicious. How does *Chili Non Carne* (page 245) sound? *Barley Vegetable Soup* (page 220)? *Sweet Potatoes with Oranges, Apples, and Sweet Wine* (page 242)? All will easily find room in your Fat Budget. REALLY! Read Chapter 9, "Cooking Low-Fat and Delicious," to learn how to reduce the fat in your favorite recipes. When you start changing your eating habits and eat wonderful low-fat foods, you will find life worth living. Not only will your fat melt away, your whole life will be richer. You'll see.

DON'T FORGET: THIS IS A HEALTHY WAY TO EAT . . .

. . . Not a License to Overdo

Now that you are feeling free as a bird, here is a warning. You need not count carbohydrates, but you must use sense. Don't gobble up a whole loaf of bread. One slice of bread has only 9 calories of fat. But try multiplying 9 calories of fat times 17 slices of bread — 153 fat calories are no longer inconsequential.

Don't eat a food without paying attention just because you think it is a carbohydrate. The oat bran muffins you greedily devour without guilt or thought may contain anywhere from 75 to 250 fat calories each. Think first! Don't make assumptions. Always check the Food Tables or food labels.

Watch Simple Sugars

Choose to Lose allows you to eat jelly on your bagel or pop a Life Saver into your mouth. But don't abuse the system by consuming a can of hard candy and two six-packs of soda. Eating too much simple sugar will do nothing for your health and could push out nutritious foods you should be eating instead. Don't deprive yourself, just use sense.

FAT-FREE FOOD ABUSE

Free May Cost You

When many new Choosers to Lose find out that calories don't count, they race to their supermarket. They whiz by the produce department and slide into the baked goods section, where they pile their baskets full of fat-free and low-fat goodies. They think they are following *Choose to Lose* by keeping their calorie count high with loaves of nonfat cakes and boxes full of fat-free cookies and zero-fat crackers. WRONG! Choosers to Lose need to eat lots of food but not just *any* food. They need to eat nutritious foods like fruits, vegetables, whole-grains, nonfat dairy, low-fat poultry, and fish. A nonfat cookie or two after dinner, a fat-free pretzel or two with lunch, is a treat. But when your menu consists of mainly ersatz nonfat food instead of nutritious food, not only do you deprive yourself of necessary vitamins, minerals, and fiber for good health because you are forcing out nutritious foods, but you will find it difficult to lose weight.

We said that *only* if you eat more than 2000 calories of pure carbohydrates in addition to your normal diet for five or six days will it turn to fat. But accumulating a mighty number of calories is not so difficult when you ersatz-load. Eat 10 slices (they're minuscule) of an Entenmann's Banana Crunch Cake and you will have consumed very little fat, but a hefty 900 total calories. Add 10 slices of an Entenmann's Cinnamon Apple Twist — not hard to do — and you will have consumed another 900 total calories. Add 2 cups of Sealtest Free frozen dessert — no fat, but 400 total calories. Get the picture? Those extra empty carbohydrate calories slide right down the ol' gullet.

And then there is the problem of whether food labeled fat-free is truly fat-free. In its May 1994 issue, *New York* magazine had a variety of low- and nonfat foods sold in local food shops analyzed for their fat content. A tofu cheesecake billed as fat-free contained 221 fat calories; a fat-free, sugar-free diet corn muffin, 204. Tasti D-lite Frozen (peanut butter*) dessert claimed less than 9 fat calories per small serving, when in truth an 8.9 fluid ounce serving contained 58 fat calories. If you are not losing weight even though you are eating a perfect diet, you might be a victim of false labeling.

---

*Beware of peanut butter nonfat yogurt. Although the basic yogurt may contain little or no fat, the peanut oil added for flavor is not required to be fat-free.

To avoid a fat-free overload and to be successful in your quest to be lean and healthy, follow the recommendations of the Food Guide Pyramid (see page 170). It is almost impossible to eat enough high-fiber fruit, vegetables, and whole-grains to exceed the 2000-calorie carbohydrate overflow limit. Your jaw would be too tired to open ever again and you would be too full to look kindly on even a kernel of popcorn.

Nonfat High-Fat Taste. The reason the American food supply is so high in fat is because Americans have developed a fat tooth. Even the nonfat and low-fat foods are doctored to appeal to our high-fat taste. Look at the low-fat frozen dinners — Fettuccini Alfredo, Lasagna Florentine, Veal Patty Parmigiana, pizza. They almost all include cheese or cream. An abundance of nonfat cheeses, nonfat cream cheeses, nonfat sour creams, and nonfat mayonnaises allows us to continue our high-fat taste without the fat calories. But will these substitutes help you achieve your long-term fat-loss goals? The most successful Choosers to Lose are those who use the Fat Budget to wean themselves from fatty foods and replace them with high-fiber, nutritious foods. While there is nothing harmful about spreading a tablespoon of fat-free cream cheese on your bagel or pouring a few tablespoons of nonfat dressing on your salad, those who overdo their use of creamy and cheesy-tasting low-fat and nonfat ersatz foods are less likely to be successful because they never give up the taste and craving for fatty foods. If you are a nonfat fat addict, you must ask yourself, when you are no longer keeping track of what you eat, will you slip back to your old high-fat habits because you never really let them go?

Scientific experiments have shown that it takes about 12 weeks to change to a low-fat, tasty taste *if* you don't keep subjecting yourself to your old high-fat tastes. Give yourself a chance to let the change take place.

RECAP

This may sound like our chorus, but it is soooo important, we will say it again. You need to eat a lot of calories to lose weight — calories from nutrient-dense foods, not empty calories from ersatz nonfat foods. Your minimum total caloric intake is a floor. Eat away!

Coming Next . . .

Read the next chapter to get the scoop on making *Choose to Lose* work for you.

Remember:

1. You must eat foods rich in carbohydrates to lose weight.
2. Carbohydrates are burned and not stored as fat.
3. Some low-fat and nonfat foods you will want to eat in abundance are potatoes, bread, rice, pasta, fruit, vegetables, and low- and non-fat dairy products. Be sure to keep track of any fat you add to them.
4. Chicken and turkey without skin and most seafood are naturally low in fat and can be prepared in a large variety of delicious low-fat dishes. But they can become very fattening if prepared incorrectly.
5. While allowing you to eat within your Fat Budget, ersatz nonfat processed foods have the following drawbacks when eaten in large amounts:
   a. they have no vitamins, minerals, or fiber;
   b. they crowd out more nutritious foods;
   c. they can cause carbohydrate overload and be stored as fat;
   d. they perpetuate a high-fat taste and make the switch to a low-fat cuisine more difficult.
6. Repeat to yourself: **I MUST EAT TO LOSE. I MUST EAT TO LOSE. I MUST EAT TO LOSE. OF COURSE, I MUST EAT NUTRITIOUS, LOW-FAT FOODS TO LOSE.**

6. Putting *Choose to Lose* to Work for You

"I kept track of everything I ate for the first 100 days, and that got me really into KNOWING what I was eating — all the time. It was great — and it worked and works. Thanks."

Joanne Ferguson, Baltimore, Maryland

"This is not like struggling with a diet but is becoming more and more a permanent part of our lifestyle."

Mildred Clark, Mentor, Ohio

ARMED with your own Fat Budget, insight into the sources of fat in foods, and a desire to be as light as a feather, you are ready to . . . begin making changes!

SLASHING THE FAT

Take Your Time

But, whoa! Don't expect to revamp your entire eating repertoire today and lose 25 pounds tomorrow. (Ah, were it so easy.) You have been eating the way you have been eating for a long time. Changes made too quickly are rarely permanent, and you want to be permanently slim. Take a few weeks to work into your new eating plan. You'll even lose during this time because you will be making changes — enduring changes.

Cut to the Bone

For those of you who want to cut your fat intake to budget level immediately and know that you can stick to these big changes, disregard the last paragraph. Each to his or her own style.

Collect Data

To analyze and change your eating habits, you need to know what they are. If you haven't done it already, order yourself a Choose to Lose Passbook (see the ad at the back of the book) or make your own and read Appendix A: "The Nitty-Gritty of How to Keep a Food Record." Keep a three-day (two weekdays and one weekend day) baseline food record. It will be extremely helpful to have this information in hand as you read on.

Paring Down by Stages

One approach to making gradual changes is to focus your attention on the worst culprits. Can you eat these foods less often, in smaller amounts, or eliminate them entirely? Go for the worst first. Make changes in stages. Don't go from whole milk to skim; go from whole milk to 2% milk (the taste is very similar). Then go from 2% milk to 1% milk (the taste is close); then from 1% milk to nonfat skim milk. You made it.

Choices and Changes

First, you want to target your high-fat food choices. Make four lists:

1. high-fat foods you can eat in smaller amounts;
2. high-fat foods you can eat less often;
3. high-fat foods you can eliminate entirely;
4. high-fat foods you can replace with low-fat substitutes.

Study this list and use it to analyze your food records. Perhaps you find that margarine, cheeseburgers, potato chips, and waffles made with whole milk are your high-fat downfall. (If you can pinpoint just a few offenders, you are lucky. For most people no one item is making them fat — fat is riddled throughout their diet.)

Choose Smaller Amounts. You decide that margarine is a high-fat food that you are willing to eat in smaller amounts. Check the Fats and Oils section of the Food Tables. The tablespoon and a half of margarine (150 fat calories) you use to butter your bagel inflicts major damage on your Fat Budget. Although not insignificant fat-calorie-wise, 1 teaspoon (30 fat calories) would still give you the taste and texture of margarine, but would make only a minor wound. (Best, of course, would be to use jelly and no margarine.)

Choose Less Often. Your food records show that you ate three cheeseburgers in a three-day period. According to the Meats, Dairy Products and Eggs, and Grain Products sections of the Food Tables (and your food diary), a cheeseburger has 286 fat calories (4 ounces of lean hamburger = 188 fat calories, 1 ounce of American cheese = 80, a hamburger roll = 18). Realizing that you are not that crazy about cheeseburgers — certainly not at that price — you choose to cook them rarely and instead fix low-fat dishes that are just as simple and quick to prepare.

Choose Not at All. How do you want to treat your third high-fat booby trap, potato chips? You look at the Food Tables under Snacks. Eliminating potato chips at 50 fat calories for a mere 10 chips (and who eats only 10 potato chips?) is a change you can make with no pain.

Choose Low-Fat Alternatives. You love making waffles Sunday morning. Light streaming through the kitchen window, the aroma of coffee filling the air, maple syrup flowing over a pile of light brown crispy waffles — a scene to warm the heart. Why start such a beautiful day with a dent in your Fat Budget? Why not replace the ¾ cup of sour cream (276 fat calories) and ¾ cup of whole milk (55 fat calories) with 1½ cups of nonfat buttermilk (0 fat calories)? Why not replace the half cup of melted butter (800 fat calories) with 1 tablespoon of olive oil (119 fat calories) or no fat at all (0 fat calories)? The waffles will still be incredible.

Use the Food Tables to find alternatives. For example, if you normally fry up a rasher of bacon for breakfast, check the Meat (Pork) section in the Food Tables for a lower-fat substitute. You'll find that for about one-third fewer fat calories, you'll get four times more Canadian bacon.

A DAY TO BE RECKONED WITH

It's amazing how total calories and fat calories accumulate while you're not paying attention. Without even eating much food, Ellen has accumulated 1510 fat calories (Chapter 3). Ellen needs to look over her meal plan and pinpoint the worst culprits. Knowing the bad news, she can then make the changes that will bring her fat intake in line with her Fat Budget.

Let's look at Ellen's baseline food record (pretend it's one day of your food record) on page 108 of this chapter. Start with breakfast. Which is the biggest fat offender? The large blueberry muffin contributes 140 calories of fat. She could have had a bowl of Wheat Chex (10 fat calories) with ¾ cup of skim milk (3 fat calories) and half a banana worth of banana slices (2½ fat calories), a slice of whole-wheat toast (9 fat calories) with fancy preserves (0 fat calories), and a half cup of 1% cottage cheese (15 fat calories) mixed together with slices of the remaining banana (2½ fat calories) for a total of 42 fat calories instead.

Chuck the glazed doughnut at 130 fat calories. What about toasting a bagel in the office microwave (10 fat calories)? How about a carton of flavored nonfat yogurt (0 fat calories)? How about a peach, apple, orange, or pear? Her snack would then cost 10 fat calories — a saving of 120 fat calories.

The 280 fat calories of Russian dressing can easily be reduced to 0 fat calories with a nonfat dressing or about 35 using the fork method (see page 40). The 108-fat-calorie biscuit with butter (36 fat calories) could be replaced with an English muffin with jelly at 9 fat calories. But what kind of lunch is a dinky salad and biscuit, anyway? Instead of submitting herself to fast-food temptation, she could bring a sandwich of sliced deli turkey breast (8 fat calories per oz) with mustard, sliced tomato, sprouts, and hot peppers on multi-grain bread (a total of 34 fat calories). Or bring a few pieces of last night's *Chinese Chicken* (13 fat calories) and eat it cold. Add carrots and an orange and top it off with a dish of nonfat frozen yogurt (0 fat calories). Ellen's diet cola can be replaced with a healthy drink — skim milk or orange juice. Instead of spending 463 fat calories for a few boring bitefuls, she will be spending at most 35 fat calories for a full, satisfying lunch.

Ellen called her snack fiasco "oodles of ignorance." Never again will she consume 140 fat calories without knowing exactly how much fat she is eating. She will choose the optimal way to spend her fat calories. Instead of eating Oodles of Noodles, Ellen might have had a carton of strawberry or peach nonfat yogurt (0 fat calories) or a pear.

For dinner Ellen spent 80 fat calories for the Chicken Fettucini dish. Why waste 80 fat calories on such a skimpy meal — a cup of mostly white sauce? She doesn't have to punish herself this way. Try this scenario on for size. Before she goes to work or the night before, Ellen takes five minutes to make *Cucumber Soup* (0 fat calories or 10 fat calories with the walnut garnish). When she returns home at the end of the day, the soup is chilled and ready to eat. Then she starts the rice (0 fat calories) so it will be cooking while she whips up *Turkey Mexique*

(23 fat calories). Steaming the zucchini (0 fat calories) takes her 3 minutes. She cuts up a tomato and half a cucumber and drizzles a tablespoon of nonfat dressing over them. Voilà — a 33-fat-calorie feast! Ellen could even include one of her yogurts with a crunchy topping for dessert (although she's probably too full to enjoy it) if she makes a low-fat substitution for her evening snack extravagance.

At 482 fat calories, the cup of peanuts was a blunder of earthshaking proportions. However, Ellen has no reason ever to repeat this mistake. The solution is simple. If nuts are your weakness, don't keep them in the house. Ellen could have enjoyed 6 cups of air-popped popcorn with 0 fat calories, loads of soluble and insoluble fiber, and lots of crunch.

With all these changes she has brought her fat intake down to 148 — way below her Fat Budget of 315. When she switches to 2% or 1% milk instead of half-and-half, her fat intake will come down 30 more fat calories.

No Pain. Making these changes didn't hurt Ellen a bit. You'll notice that the modified menu is filled with much more food — more interesting tastes, more bulk, a more balanced and healthier combination of foods.

First Cut. In your first round of fat modification you may not be able to make as many changes as Ellen has. If so, start slowly. For example, if giving up a blueberry muffin would make you cry, you might eat it today and substitute an English muffin or whole-wheat toast with jam tomorrow. If you can't imagine eating a baked potato plain, cut the 3 tablespoons of sour cream you normally eat in half. Next time, you can reduce the amount even more or try nonfat yogurt or a nonfat sour cream substitute. When you feel ready, perhaps in a few days, try to modify more of your high-fat choices.

Try a Little Harder. Next round, take another look at your food record to see if there are other foods you wouldn't mind eating less often or in smaller amounts or eliminating entirely. Do you need half-and-half in your coffee? Why not give 1% milk a chance? Try replacing the high-fat yogurt combo (45 fat calories) with nonfat flavored yogurt with no topping. Mix in some raisins and apple pieces and make your own crunch.

Table 4. Ellen's Food Record

Baseline			Replacement Meal Plan		
	CALORIES			**CALORIES**	
FOOD ITEM	**TOTAL**	**FAT**	**FOOD ITEM**	**TOTAL**	**FAT**
Breakfast			*Breakfast*		
1 large blueberry			1 bowl Wheat Chex	190	10
muffin	400	140	¾ cup skim milk	65	3
			1 banana	105	5
			1 slice whole-wheat toast	70	9
			1½ tsp jelly	27	0
			½ cup 1% cottage cheese	82	10
1 cup coffee	0	0	1 cup coffee	0	0
1 tbsp half-and-half	20	15	1 tbsp half-and-half	20	15
Snack			*Snack*		
1 large glazed doughnut	240	130	1 bagel	300	10
			1 tbsp fat-free cream		
			cheese	25	0
1 cup coffee	0	0	1 cup coffee	0	0
1 tbsp half-and-half	20	15	1 tbsp half-and-half	20	15
Lunch			*Lunch*		
2 cups mixed salad	20	0	1 turkey sandwich		
½ tomato	12	0	2 oz sliced turkey		
¼ cucumber	10	0	breast	76	16
¼ carrot	8	0	tomato slice	4	0
4 tbsp Russian dressing	308	280	2 slices multi-grain		
			bread	140	18
1 tbsp sunflower seeds	50	39	1 carrot	31	0
			1 orange	60	0
Biscuit	231	108	8 oz skim milk	86	4
1 pat butter	36	36	5 oz nonfat frozen		
1 diet cola	0	0	yogurt	100	0
Snack			*Snack*		
Oodles of Noodles (3 oz)	400	140	8 oz nonfat yogurt	190	0
Dinner			*Dinner*		
Chicken Fettucini			1 cup *Cucumber Soup*	78	10
(Weight Watchers)	280	80	*Turkey Mexique*	153	23
			¾ cup white rice	168	0
¼ head iceberg lettuce	20	0	1 cup zucchini	36	0
4 tbsp fat-free dressing	60	0	1 tbsp nonfat dressing	15	0
6 oz vanilla yogurt with			1 tomato, sliced	24	0
crunch	230	45	½ cucumber	20	0
Snack			*Snack*		
¾ cup peanuts	630	482	6 cups air-popped		
			popcorn	180	0
Total:	2975	1510		2265	148

The *Word*

Always keep in mind that you are trying to lose weight, and the less fat you eat, *without feeling like a martyr,* the faster you will lose. You can easily fit many wonderful low-fat foods into your budget. You just have no room for greasy, ugly high-fat foods.

Treat this time of transition as an adventure. Explore new foods, new tastes, new textures — experiment.

ADDING BACK CARBS

Ellen analyzed her food record to find the biggest fat donors so she could make better choices. She can't stop there (and neither can you). It is equally important that she review her day's intake to see if she is satisfying her Minimum Basic Nutritional Requirements (MBNR). According to the Department of Agriculture Food Guide Pyramid (see page 170), you must eat a minimum of 2 to 3 servings* of fruit, 3 to 5 servings of vegetables, 6 to 11 servings of grains, and 2 to 3 servings of dairy every day to maintain your health and to ensure that you are eating a nutritious diet.

IMPORTANT: The beauty of this recommendation is that when you combine it with eating a low-fat diet, you get the perfect prescription for weight loss.

A BIG TIP: The easiest way to reach and maintain your goal weight is to:

• eat below your Fat Budget.
• eat a lot of total calories — more than the minimum total caloric intake you used to determine your Fat Budget.
• **make sure these calories include foods to satisfy your Minimum Basic Nutritional Requirements.**
• exercise aerobically every day.

Soon people who don't even know you will comment on how great you look.

---

*See page 174 for definitions of what constitutes a serving.

Check Out the MBNR Rating of Ellen's Baseline Food Record

Fruit: 2–3 Servings. Ellen: 0 servings. One quick glance shows you that Ellen is in the hole concerning fruit. She is supposed to eat at least 2 servings and she has eaten none.

Vegetables: 3–5 Servings. Ellen: 2 servings. Although lettuce has little nutritional value, she can count her 2 cups of lettuce as 1 serving, and the tomato, carrots, and cucumber add up to another. She is short 1 serving of vegetables.

Grains: 6–11 Servings. Ellen: 0 servings. Grains are a tricky category. The idea is to eat nutritious whole-grains, not a little flour holding together a lot of fat. Use this rule of thumb: If a food is about 20 percent fat or more, do not count it as a grain. By this criterion, Ellen ate no grains.

Dairy: 2–3 Servings. Ellen: 1 serving. Ellen's 6-ounce vanilla yogurt fulfills one of her dairy requirements.

Ellen's Replacement Meal Plan Gets an A⁺

Ellen has easily met the nutritional requirements in her new meal plan. Her choices are filled with vitamins, minerals, and fiber. By fulfilling these recommendations, she will be so stuffed at the end of the day she won't have room to pig out on empty and/or fat calories.

Look over her new meal plan yourself and see how she satisfies each requirement.

Did you make the following analysis?

Fruit: 2–3 Servings. Ellen: 2 servings. Ellen ate a banana at breakfast and an orange at lunch. She should have included an apple with her afternoon snack.

Vegetables: 3–5 Servings. Ellen: 4 servings. The carrot, cup of sliced zucchini, cucumber half, and tomato each count as 1 serving.

Grains: 6–11 Servings. Ellen: 9 servings. Except for the bagel and white rice, all of Ellen's grains are whole-grains. Her bowl of Wheat

Chex, slice of whole-wheat toast, and ¾ cup of rice each count as 1 grain. Her bagel, 2 slices of multi-grain bread, and 6 cups of air-popped popcorn each count as 2 servings. Popcorn is really a vegetable, but it is counted as a grain. 3 cups = 1 serving.

Dairy: 2–3 Servings. Ellen: 3¾ servings. Ellen's 1¾ cups of skim milk, the ½ cup of cottage cheese, and the 8 ounces of nonfat yogurt fulfill her dairy requirement. The fat-free cream cheese contributes no dairy to her diet. Her frozen yogurt (even nonfat) does not fulfill a dairy requirement because the amount of dairy in frozen desserts is often negligible. Again, the idea is to satisfy your MBNR with nutrient-dense foods, not with processed, ersatz fluff.

For more on eating a balanced diet, see Chapter 12.

Educated Choices

We gave you our modification of Ellen's meal plan, but you could have modified it in an infinite number of different ways to suit your taste. It is your choice. But now, when you make choices, you will think before you choose. The quarter cup of butter you pour over your popcorn will scream 400 FAT CALORIES! You'll pause before you bite into the 65 fat calories of a Reese's peanut butter cup. You'll think vitamins, minerals, and fiber when you choose whole-wheat toast over white bread.

Don't worry. You'll still be able to enjoy and love food. You'll just be able to make more informed choices. When you do choose that hot apple turnover with vanilla ice cream after a month of low-fat desserts, you'll love every bite. You'll even taste every bite. Or, perhaps, you'll take a bite and push it away because it isn't worth 350 fat calories.

Remember:
1. Gradual changes are more likely to be lasting.
2. Four ways to reduce your fat intake:
   a. Choose some high-fat foods in smaller amounts.
   b. Choose some high-fat foods less often.
   c. Eliminate some high-fat foods entirely.
   d. Replace some high-fat foods with low-fat alternatives.
3. Use the Food Tables to choose lower-fat alternatives.
4. Be sure you are meeting your daily minimum basic nutritional requirements:
   a. 2–4 servings of fruit

    b. 3–5 servings of vegetables
    c. 6–11 servings of grains
    d. 2–3 servings of dairy
5. Satisfying your MBNR ensures an adequate supply of vitamins, minerals, and fiber and will keep you full and happy.
6. Repeat to yourself: **I MUST EAT TO LOSE. I MUST EAT TO LOSE. I MUST EAT TO LOSE. OF COURSE, I MUST EAT NUTRITIOUS, LOW-FAT FOODS TO LOSE.**

7. Taking the Show on the Road: Planning Your Meals

"By counting fat calories, I find I can eat so much more than on other diets. I never go to bed hungry. We all know diets do not work but lifestyle changes do and *Choose to Lose* makes this possible and relatively simple."

Pam Vasquez, Minneapolis, Minnesota

"*Choose to Lose* taught me there is nothing I can't have. I just need to plan for it."

Rhonda Carothers, Bremen, Indiana

Moving Right Along

You are ready to make wise choices for the rest of your life. You have a Fat Budget so you know how much fat you should eat each day. You have targeted your high-fat favorites so you know how often and in what amounts you plan to fit them in. Now for the actual meal planning.

To Plan or Not to Plan?

If planning is impractical or not in your nature, you can keep a running total of the fat you eat each day as you eat it. Before you consume any food, however, you must look it up in the Food Tables or read the food label to determine how many fat calories it adds to the fat you have already accumulated. For example, if your Fat Budget is 315 and you have already consumed 220 fat calories by mid-afternoon, you better think twice before you accept that 170-fat-calorie cheese Danish your secretary just brought you. Toast up the 10-fat-calorie blueberry bagel you brought from home instead and enhance it with 0-fat raspberry preserves.

113

Or you can plan your meals for the day or week and add up your fat calories in advance. Planning ahead gives you the opportunity to make choices before you eat. "Hmm," you say, "I'll spend _____ fat calories on _____ and _____ fat calories on _____. Better still, if I eat _____ instead of _____, I'd have _____ fat calories left for dessert." Advance planning also makes grocery shopping more efficient and ensures you will have plenty of low-fat and nonfat foods on hand.

When you plan ahead, you can save up fat calories for splurges (see Chapter 10). If some great food emergency arises (your mother-in-law bakes your very favorite chocolate cheesecake as a special treat *just for you*), you can deduct those added fat calories from your budget and compensate for the splurge by eating less the next day. Of course, your Fat Budget has just so much room for emergencies. Too much borrowing from tomorrow's Fat Budget and you're off *Choose to Lose.*

Benefits of Keeping Track

You may think adding up fat calories will take all the fun out of eating. However, you probably eat a limited number of foods and dishes, so sooner than you think you will know their fat values as well as you know the telephone numbers of your family and friends.

You may feel that you can lose weight without keeping a record of the foods you eat. While just knowing your Fat Budget and the fat calories in foods will help you make educated choices, if you don't keep track of the foods you eat, you may be consuming more fat than you realize. It is very easy to overeat fat calories when you are not keeping track.

Another Plug for the Handy, Inexpensive Choose to Lose Passbook:

To help you record your fat intake, you may want to use the order form at the end of the book to order the handy *Choose to Lose* Passbook (checkbook size), which includes abbreviated Food Tables and a balance book for keeping a two-week record of the total fat calories you consume.

EATING WELL WITHIN BUDGET

Here are some suggestions for easing into your new eating pattern:

Making Changes: Breakfast

A low-fat breakfast can be nourishing and delicious. Some quick and easy choices are: hot cereal (0 to 25 fat calories per ½ cup of dry); cold cereal (generally 0 to 20 fat calories per ounce; check the label) with skim milk (4 fat calories per cup) and banana (5 fat calories); whole-wheat toast (9 per slice) with jelly (0); 1% cottage cheese (15 fat calories per ½ cup); nonfat yogurt (less than 9 fat calories per cup); fruit or juice (0 fat calories). Take a few minutes to eat at home. (That doesn't mean slipping a 60-fat-calorie toaster pastry into your toaster or heating a 230-fat-calorie Great Starts breakfast in your microwave oven.) You narrow your choices (but not your waist) when you pick up breakfast at a snack shop or coffee shop.

Skipping Meals: A Dieter's Undoing

Do you nobly skip breakfast and/or lunch to save calories? Don't. Skipping a meal makes you only hungrier for the next meal or snack. So hungry, in fact, you may eat twice the fat calories you saved by not eating. Missing a meal may even depress your basal metabolic rate so that everything you eat later is burned more slowly. You need carbohydrates to stoke your fat-burning fires. No breakfast or lunch makes for an empty furnace. An empty furnace (depleted glycogen reserves) leads to fatigue. Glycogen reserves are the source of fuel for your immediate energy needs. Functioning with your glycogen reserves depleted is like running your car on empty. No wonder you feel like a limp rag when you haven't eaten breakfast or lunch.

Making Changes: Lunch

Brown-bag it. Leftovers make great (and quick) lunches. Make a sandwich or two of last night's *Blackened Chicken* (page 232) or *Bar-B-Que Chicken* breast (page 231). Use mustard instead of mayonnaise and add tomatoes and lettuce. Cook up a batch of *Pawtucket Chili* (*Eater's Choice*) or *Ted Mummery's Turkey Barbecue* (page 255) and store it in the refrigerator. Each day, heat a little and spoon it into a pita or two. (At work, heat the whole sandwich in the microwave.) Mix 1% cottage cheese or nonfat yogurt with cut-up fruit. Pack a nonfat flavored yogurt, fruit, carrot, and celery sticks. Add air-popped popcorn for a crunchy, filling "dessert."

If you have to buy lunch, select a sandwich shop where you can order turkey (with mustard or a teaspoon or less of mayonnaise) rather than a fast-food restaurant where your options are limited. A fancier restaurant might offer grilled chicken breast for lunch. If the only chicken breast on the menu is breaded and deep-fried, ask that it be grilled (without the skin and with no fat) instead. If the menu offers Cajun steak, have the grilled chicken cooked with Cajun sauce. Ask for a baked potato, plain, instead of french fries. Have a chef's salad, but hold the cheese and ham. Ask for the dressing (preferably low-fat) on the side so that you control the amount you use. Cold shrimp, although expensive, have almost no fat and can be dipped fat-free into cocktail sauce (not tartar sauce, which is made with mayonnaise). If you're forced to have a higher-fat-than-you-want lunch, keep track of the fat so you can balance it with low-fat dinner choices.

Be Salad-Bar-Wise

Salad bars offer a tempting array of greens and sliced vegetables, fresh fruits, and . . . high-fat salads. Red potatoes in sour cream dressing, bacon pieces lurking in apple salad, mayonnaise salad with a bit of cabbage mixed in, cold-cut strips marinated in oil — each one is overflowing with fat calories. A little bit of this and a little bit of that adds up to triple your Fat Budget for the day. Unless you eat only the fruit or vegetables with little or no dressing, salad bars are not a buy for the diet-conscious. Check out the Salad Bar items listed in the Food Tables (pages 376–77) for a real shock.

Making Changes: Dinner

For Starters. Stay home for dinner and give your diet goals a boost. Start dinner with soup. Soup is a wonderful invention for weight watchers. It cheers the soul as it fills you up. With a low-fat soup as a filling first course, you are less tempted to gorge yourself on the higher-fat main course or dessert. If you have regal tastes, you'll love *Sour Cherry Soup* (page 224) or *Ginger Squash Soup* (page 223). To soothe the spirit, prepare *Vegetable Soup with Spinach, Potatoes, Rice, and Corn* (page 225), and in *Eater's Choice, Avgolemono Soup, Mushroom Soup,* and *Vegetable Soup Provençal.*

For equally wonderful results, substitute nonfat yogurt, buttermilk, skim milk, or evaporated skim milk in soup recipes that call for sour cream, cream, or whole milk. A tasty example is *Zucchini Soup* (page 226). Make large batches of soup and freeze them in small containers for future pleasure.

Spice Up the Main Course

Delectable dishes can be made without cream, butter, or cheese. Beef doesn't have to be eaten in a slab. Foods can taste good without being drowned in oil.

Rethink your preferences and retrain your palate. Modify favorite recipes by reducing the fat. Make "cream" sauces with skim milk, nonfat yogurt, or buttermilk. To reduce fat and add texture and flavor, cut a small piece of meat into bite-size pieces and mix it with masses of vegetables. Pile on the pasta or rice so you'll need less meat.

Give up the rich, bland, fattening dishes you eat too much of because they are so unfulfilling. Use spices instead of fat to create savory dishes. Spicy doesn't necessarily mean "hot." Spicy means tasty. Spices satisfy your palate and you. It's easy to eat well on a low-fat diet. Does *Chicken Paprikash* (*Eater's Choice*) or *Asparagus Pasta* (page 247) sound like diet food? With 28 or fewer fat calories each, they slip easily into anyone's Fat Budget.

Fitting In Your Favorites . . .

Don't forget: The reason you have a Fat Budget is so that you can occasionally splurge on a thick steak or cherry cheesecake. You really should splurge occasionally, because if you don't you will feel as if you are on a *DIET* and your commitment will be temporary. The big surprise is that what you now consider the most delectable treat in the world may revolt you in a couple of months. Your tastes are going to change and you won't crave the high-fat foods you once did.

. . . But Not Too Often

If you are fitting in too many high-fat foods, you will be denying your taste buds a chance to change. A Chooser to Lose told us that she once considered McDonald's french fries ambrosia to the gods. After a few months following *Choose to Lose*, she couldn't even look at those greasy yellow sticks. If she had included french fries in her daily meal plan, she never would have lost her taste and craving for them. Eating a low-fat diet would have been a struggle for her instead of simply a way of life.

A Balanced Diet

Once you see the cost of many foods, you are going to find that eating below your Fat Budget is a cinch. However, it is extremely important that you do not just cut out fat. You must replace some of the fat you eliminate with complex carbohydrates (fruits, vegetables, and whole-grains) and low-fat or nonfat dairy products. Your body needs all the vitamins, minerals, and fibers that these foods provide. You need to eat lots of complex carbohydrates to keep up your basal metabolic rate to burn fat. (See Chapter 12, "Ensuring a Balanced Diet.")

You need to eat real, full meals. If you are eating a baked potato and broccoli and calling it dinner, your days as a Chooser to Lose are numbered. You need to be satisfied. Eat the baked potato and broccoli, but eat it with *Tortilla Soup* (page 224), *Broiled Ginger Fish* (page 236), steamed rice, and *Cucumber Salad* (page 249).

Eat, Eat, My Darling

When you reduce the fat in your diet, you will also reduce the total calories. For many of you, this dual reduction will bring your total caloric intake below a healthy and fat-reducing level. You must make an effort to eat more. (Did you ever think you would be urged to eat more?) Eat more fruits, vegetables, and whole-grains, that is. Eat a lot.

A Chooser to Lose told us that, without telling her husband, she started cooking *Eater's Choice* recipes to reduce fat in their diet. He was delighted with the new dishes and ate with gusto. After several months he came to her visibly distressed. "Dear," he began, "I think I have cancer. I have never eaten so much and I keep losing weight." Can you imagine the anguish he felt? She calmly explained that he had become an unwitting Chooser to Lose. Don't be distressed if *you* are eating more than ever and losing weight. Celebrate.

And in the Next Chapter . . .

Practical advice to fit *Choose to Lose* into your life.

Remember:
1. Budget your fat intake by keeping a running total for each day or planning ahead for a day or a week.
2. Keep track of your fat intake so that you know you are truly eating under your Fat Budget.
3. Be sure your total caloric intake is well above your minimum daily total caloric intake (Table 2) to ensure that you:
   a. maximize your BMR;
   b. consume an adequate supply of vitamins, minerals, and fiber;
   c. have maximum energy and stamina.
4. Repeat to yourself: **I MUST EAT TO LOSE. I MUST EAT TO LOSE. I MUST EAT TO LOSE. OF COURSE, I MUST EAT NUTRITIOUS, LOW-FAT FOODS TO LOSE.**

8. Decoding Food Labels

"I didn't realize how important label reading was until I went grocery shopping the next time after reading your book. I found myself putting back things after taking them off the shelf just because I finally knew what the number of grams of fat really meant. . . . Your book has also opened up a dimension in my taste buds and I really seem to enjoy food more now than ever before, without the added butter or other fats."

Diana Firey, Sand Springs, Oklahoma

TODAY everyone is in a hurry. No time to shop. No time to cook. No time to eat. No time to sit down and enjoy a meal. If you want to succeed in your quest for long-term good health and a lean body, you need to shift your priorities. You will have to take time both to shop, to cook, and to eat. Here's some advice to make shopping and low-fat cooking as easy as pie (low-fat pie, of course).

SMART SHOPPING

The only *real* way to control your diet is to cook from scratch. Only when you have added all the ingredients yourself can you be certain your meals will be nutritious and low in fat. However, we realize that many of you feel harassed and pressed for time and may occasionally (let us hope, *very* occasionally) resort to zapping a frozen dinner in your microwave. There are some commercial products that even the cook-it-from-scratch cook will need to buy. To know exactly what is hiding behind the carefully crafted hyperbole, you need to acquire the shopper's most important survival skill: understanding how to read a food label.

120

THE ART OF READING FOOD LABELS

"25% LESS FAT!" "50% LESS FAT!" "95% FAT-FREE!" "NATURAL!" "CHOLESTEROL-FREE!" "SMART CHOICE" "HEALTHY CHOICE" "WHOLESOME CHOICE!" Are the products as healthy and wholesome as their names and claims imply? The answer to this question is easy to discover. Forget the hype. Look beyond the bright lettering on the packages. The truth can be found in the nutrition label.

In the following section we will show you how to become a label-reading expert. Before you read on, please select a can or package from your kitchen or pantry so that you can examine the label.

Ingredient List

Find the list of ingredients on the container you chose. Although ingredient lists do not give you quantitative information, they may give you facts that influence your choice. Do you want a product with lard as its main ingredient? Find the ingredient list on your package. What ingredient is listed first? The ingredients are always listed in descending order by weight.

TOMATO SOUP

INGREDIENTS: TOMATOES (WATER, TOMATO PASTE), HIGH-FRUCTOSE CORN SYRUP, WHEAT FLOUR, SALT, VEGETABLE OIL (CORN, COTTONSEED OR PARTIALLY HYDROGENATED SOYBEAN OIL), SPICE EXTRACT, VITAMIN C (ASCORBIC ACID) AND CITRIC ACID.

The ingredient list for this tomato soup tells you that tomatoes account for more weight than any other ingredient. On second glance you see that the first ingredient isn't *really* tomatoes. It's water and tomato paste. Now you know there is more water and tomato paste than any other ingredient. Unfortunately, since the actual weights of the ingredients are not provided, you have no way of knowing if these two ingredients comprise 50 percent of the soup or 40 percent or 10 percent.

Read on and you will see that high-fructose corn syrup is the ingredient second in weight, wheat flour is the third, and so on.

Notice that the listing for vegetable oil is a choice among corn, cottonseed, or partially hydrogenated soybean oil. Manufacturers typically list a variety of oils and they generally choose whichever is cheapest at the time. Of course, you have no idea which oil was used. But the choice of oil (fat) makes a big difference to your arteries. (See page 77 for discussion of the health effects of saturated, monosaturated, and polyunsaturated fats.)`

What does the ingredient list on the package *you* chose tell you?

Nutrition Facts Box

Thanks to the Food and Drug Administration's new food label regulations, every food package has a shiny, new easy-to-read label. The format is standardized so that every product must include the same nutrition information.

In many ways the new nutrition labels are a great improvement. Calories from fat are boldly listed near the top. Saturated fat is also listed (albeit in grams, not calories). Fiber is an important new category. These are the pluses. The minuses concern the Daily Value and % Daily Value concepts, which we will discuss later.

Dissecting a Food Label

We are going to analyze food labels from top to bottom so you will understand what every part means. However, because you are a Chooser to Lose and have a Fat Budget, most of the numbers and percentages on the label need not concern you.

The only two numbers you really need to know are the calories from fat and the serving size. With this information you can determine the number of fat calories for the amount of food you want to eat. Then you can decide if you want to fit the food into your Fat Budget.

Let's dissect the Weight Watchers Chicken Fettucini label. All of the information — calories, calories from fat, total fat, and cholesterol — is for one serving of food. The serving size is listed at the top of the Nutrition Facts box.

First, find the information that is most important to you:

Calories from Fat: 80

At the top right of the Nutrition Facts box you can see the listing of calories from fat. Calories from fat! A boon for us Choosers to Lose.

Chicken Fettucini

Nutrition Facts
Serving Size: 1 meal (233g)
Servings Per Container: 1

Amount Per Serving

Calories 280 Calories from Fat 80	
	% Daily Value*
Total Fat 9g	**14%**
Saturated Fat 3g	**15%**
Cholesterol 40mg	**13%**
Sodium 590mg	**25%**
Total Carbohydrate 25g	**8%**
Dietary Fiber 2g	**8%**
Sugars 5g	
Protein 22g	

Vitamin A 4%	•	Vitamin C 0%
Calcium 20%	•	Iron 10%

*Percent Daily Values are based on a 2,000 calorie diet. Your daily values may be higher or lower depending on your calorie needs:

	Calories:	2,000	2,500
Total Fat	Less than	65g	80g
Saturated Fat	Less than	20g	25g
Cholesterol	Less than	300mg	300mg
Sodium	Less than	2,400mg	2,400mg
Total Carbohydrate		300g	375g
Dietary Fiber		25g	30g

Calories per gram:
Fat 9   Carbohydrates 4   Protein 4

Potato Chips

Nutrition Facts
Serving Size 1 oz. (28g/about 20 chips)
Servings Per Container: 4

Amount Per Serving

Calories 150 Calories from Fat 80	
	% Daily Values*
Total Fat 9g	**14%**
Saturated Fat 2g	**10%**
Cholesterol 0mg	**0%**
Sodium 95mg	**4%**
Potassium 370mg	**11%**
Total Carbohydrate 14g	**5%**
Dietary Fiber 1g	**4%**
Sugars less than 1g	
Protein 2g	**4%**

Now you know exactly how much fat you are getting. No more multiplying grams of fat by 9. This bantam-weight meal contains 80 fat calories for 1 serving (**Total Fat 9g** is a listing you can ignore because since it is rounded to the nearest gram, it gives you less specific and accurate data than the Calories from Fat information.)

Serving Size: 1 meal (233g)

Look under the heading "Nutrition Facts" for the serving size. In this case, the serving size is one meal or the whole package. Thus, one serving of this "diet" meal costs 80 fat calories. That's a lot of fat for a little convenience. How does this dish fit into your Fat Budget?

Serving Size Smarts

Many people read the "calories from fat" and then they stop reading — but they don't stop eating. The food label tells you the calories from fat for *each* serving. But you don't necessarily eat only 1 serving. The serving may also be smaller than you expect. Ignoring the serving size can have calamitous consequences.

In the old, pre–*Choose to Lose* days, you might have grabbed this bag of potato chips off the shelf and swallowed it whole. Perhaps you would have known enough to look at the fat calories listed on the nutrition label first: 80. This is where most people terminate their label review. They figure the whole bag of chips contains 80 fat calories and tear into it. If you have a Fat Budget, you know that 80 is a heap of fat calories, but that is nothing compared with the true number of fat calories in this bag. You must *always* look at the serving size. The serving size for these potato chips is 1 ounce or 20 chips. Twenty thin little greasy chips cost 80 fat calories. The whole bag contains 4 servings or 4 × 80 = 320 fat calories. How does this fit into your Fat Budget? Or vice versa?

If you want your suits to drop three sizes and your cholesterol level to fall 50 points, always take note of serving size and the number of servings you are eating or you may seriously underestimate the amount of fat you are consuming.

Making Sense of the Rest of the Label

Take a look at the Fettucini label on page 123. These listings may also be of interest to you:

Saturated Fat: 3g. Everyone who is interested in a healthy diet, and especially people with elevated blood cholesterol, should limit their intake of saturated fat. Read page 77 about saturated fat (for *everything* you need to know about saturated fat, also read *Eater's Choice*). To determine the calories of saturated fat, multiply the grams by 9. There are 9 calories per gram of saturated fat (3 grams × 9 calories per gram = 27 sat-fat calories). To help put the 3 grams or 27 sat-fat calories into perspective, a sedentary female who wants to weigh 140 pounds has a Sat-Fat Budget of 176.

Cholesterol: 40 mg. This number is useful, not because you should be concerned with cholesterol (dietary cholesterol has a very minor effect on raising blood cholesterol) but because the cholesterol content can help you determine the amount of meat in a product. For example, this product lists 40 milligrams of cholesterol. Since 1 ounce of chicken contains about 24 milligrams of cholesterol,* this meal contains about 1½ ounces of chicken (the Parmesan cheese accounts for some cholesterol). Although it is healthier to eat less meat, you might be a bit annoyed that you paid so much for so little food. Now do you understand why eating these frozen dinners leaves you hungry?

Dietary Fiber: 2g. Because the FDA considered dietary fiber an essential element of a healthy diet, it was added to the new nutrition

---

*All meats (beef, veal, lamb), poultry, and seafood (except for shrimp at 43 milligrams per ounce) contain 18 to 28 milligrams of cholesterol per ounce.

labels. What a great addition. With a diet of fast foods, frozen dinners, and convenience foods, Americans eat too little fiber (the current average American intake is 10 grams), and it shows in our massive health problems. (See page 94 for discussion of the benefits of consuming dietary fiber.)

You're in luck. By following *Choose to Lose* and eating a diet high in vegetables, fruit, and whole-grains, you will be eating a high-fiber diet. (To be sure you are meeting your minimum daily nutritional requirements and thus getting adequate fiber, see page 94.) The FDA recommends eating 25 to 30 grams of fiber a day (more than 50 or 60 grams may decrease the amount of vitamins and minerals your body absorbs). By listing dietary fiber, the new food labels help you choose higher-fiber foods.

Special K Cereal

Nutrition Facts
Serving Size 1 Cup (31g/1.1 oz.)
Servings per Container 6

Amount Per Serving	Cereal	Cereal with ½ Cup Vitamins A & D Skim Milk
Calories	110	150
Fat Calories	0	0

	% Daily Value **	
Total Fat 0g*	0 %	0 %
Saturated Fat 0g	0 %	0 %
Cholesterol 0mg	0 %	0 %
Sodium 250mg	11 %	13 %
Potassium 60mg	2 %	7 %
Total Carbohydrate 22g	7 %	9 %
Dietary Fiber 1g	3 %	3 %
Sugars 3g		
Other Carbohydrate 18g		

All-Bran Cereal

Nutrition Facts
Serving Size 1/2 cup (31g/1.1 oz.)
Servings per Container 13

Amount Per Serving	Cereal	Cereal with ½ Cup Vitamins A & D Skim Milk
Calories	80	120
Calories from Fat	10	10

	% Daily Value **	
Total Fat 1.0g*	2 %	2 %
Saturated Fat 0g	0 %	0 %
Cholesterol 0mg	0 %	0 %
Sodium 280mg	12 %	14 %
Potassium 350mg	10 %	16 %
Total Carbohydrate 23g	8 %	10 %
Dietary Fiber 10g	40 %	40 %
Insoluble Fiber 9g		
Sugars 5g		
Other Carbohydrate 8g		
Protein 4g		

A good way to use dietary fiber information is to comparison-shop at the cereal aisle in your grocery store. Look at the amount of dietary fiber in the Kellogg's Special K at the left. Compare it with the dietary fiber in the Kellogg's All-Bran at the right. At 1 gram per serving, the Special K is almost fiber-free. At 10 grams per serving, the All-Bran cereal meets almost half your daily fiber needs. Before you choke down a spoonful of a high-fiber cereal as if it were medicine, remember that you can get lots of fiber in other foods. But if a cereal tastes good and also contains 10 grams of dietary fiber per serving, why not choose it over another favorite that has only 1 gram?

Daily Value: Universal Nutrition Budget

Woe to the people who have no *Choose to Lose* Fat Budget. The Food and Drug Administration (FDA) was worried that most Americans had no way of judging food labels to make healthy food choices. After many months of hearings and debate, they came up with a solution. Give all Americans a nutrition budget — they called it a Daily Value (DV) — for fat, saturated fat, cholesterol, sodium, total carbohydrate, and dietary fiber. Look in the circled area of the Pepperidge Farm Bread Crisps label. These Daily Values are based on a 2000-calorie diet for everyone, regardless of sex, weight, shape, or size. Those who think this basic caloric intake is too small can choose the 2500-calorie diet listed in the last column on the right. You can see that the DV for cholesterol is less than 300 milligrams, the DV of sodium is less than 2400 milligrams, and so on.

Bread Crisps

Low Cholesterol
Nutrition Facts
Serving Size 1 oz. (28g / about 1/6 of package)
Servings Per Container About 6

Amount Per Serving

Calories 140   Calories from Fat 50

	% Daily Value*
Total Fat 6g	9%
Saturated Fat 1g	4%
Polyunsaturated 1g	
Monounsaturated 2g	
Cholesterol 5mg	2%
Sodium 180mg	8%
Total Carbohydrate 18g	6%
Dietary Fiber Less than 1g	2%
Sugars Less than 1g	
Protein 4g	

Vitamin A 0%	•	Vitamin C 0%	
Calcium 0%	•	Iron 4%	
Thiamine 10%	•	Riboflavin 4%	
Niacin 8%			

* Percent Daily Values are based on a 2,000 calorie diet. Your daily values may be higher or lower depending on your calorie needs:

		Calories:	2,000	2,500
Total Fat	Less than		65g	80g
Sat. Fat	Less than		20g	25g
Cholesterol	Less than		300mg	300mg
Sodium	Less than		2,400mg	2,400mg
Total Carbohydrate			300g	375g
Dietary Fiber			25g	30g

Calories per gram:
Fat 9 • Carbohydrate 4 • Protein 4

Daily Value Total Fat: Ticket to Weight Gain. The Daily Value for Total Fat is the only one that is truly off the mark. The others are reasonable. At 180 sat-fat calories, the DV for saturated fat is actually low for most people and that's healthy. But at 30 percent of 2000 total calories, the DV for total fat is so huge (65 grams or 585 fat calories) that anyone using it is bound to gain weight. This DV of 585 fat calories is supposed to fit your needs whether you are a man or a woman, 4 feet 10 inches or 6 feet 7 inches tall, or your goal weight is 105 pounds or 195. How does 585 fat calories compare with your Fat Budget?

% Daily Value: Complicating a Simple System

Choosers to Lose have always found reading labels a snap because they have their own personal Fat Budget by which to judge the fat content of any food. But because everyone else had no way of judging

Bread Crisps

	% Daily Value*
Total Fat 6g	**9%**
Saturated Fat 1g	4%
Polyunsaturated 1g	
Monounsaturated 2g	
Cholesterol 5mg	**2%**
Sodium 180mg	**8%**
Total Carbohydrate 18g	**6%**
Dietary Fiber Less than 1g	2%

if 10 grams was a lot of fat, the FDA invented % Daily Value (% DV). This turns out to be the most confusing part of the nutrition label.

In case you are curious, this is how it works. Look at the Daily Value section of the bread crisps label. Nutrients and the amount of each nutrient contained in the product are listed on the left. On the right is a list of percentages. Each of these percentages represents the percentage of the Daily Value for that nutrient which is contained in 1 serving of this product. Clear as mud?

A specific example will make it clearer. Let's take total fat. The label lists Total Fat 6g . . . . 9%. This means that 1 serving of these bread crisps contains 6 grams of fat or 54 fat calories*, and 54 fat calories represents 9 percent of the DV for fat (9 percent of 585 fat calories). What are you supposed to do with this information? If you didn't have a Fat Budget, you might say, "Nine percent? That's not much," and finish off the whole bag, which contains 6 servings for a total of 300 fat calories. Would you realize that *each* serving was 9 percent of your Daily Value and that if you eat 2 servings, you would be eating 18 percent of your DV? Would you keep track each day of all the percentages of all the commercial food you eat until you reach 100 percent and then stop eating? Most likely, you would mistakenly think that the 9 percent represents the percentage of fat in the food and eagerly gobble up the entire package of crisps.

Choose to Lose: Getting Straight to the Facts

Not only is the % DV unnecessarily complicated and thus extremely confusing, it is misleading too. How should an educated Chooser to Lose analyze this bread crisp label (above)? First, look at the calories from fat: 50 fat calories per serving. Next, look at the serving size.

The bread crisps label tells us that the serving size is 1 ounce (28 grams) or about one-sixth of the package. Unless you open the package, you really don't know what 1 ounce means in terms of these bread crisps. You do know that one ounce is a picayune amount of food. The

---

*There are 9 calories per gram of fat. So 6 grams × 9 calories per gram of fat = 54 fat calories. These bread crisps actually contain 50 calories of fat per serving.

label says there are 6 servings in the package. You can eyeball the bag and try to estimate what one-sixth of the package might contain. It turns out to be 7 tiny, tiny crackers, which is very, very, very little for all that fat. If you eat 14 crackers (not difficult to do) you are eating 2 servings or 2 × 50 fat calories = 100 fat calories. Compared to a DV of 585, even 100 fat calories doesn't seem so high, but compare it to your Fat Budget and you'll appreciate the cost.

CONSUMER BEWARE!

The food industry has you pegged. They know that you and millions like you want to buy products that will help you in your quest for a perfect body. They count on your not being knowledgeable enough to read nutrition labels so you can evaluate their claims. Watch out for the following traps.

The Health Connection

The FDA regulations on food labeling have greatly restricted the misleading and deceptive practices so common in the past. But the rules still allow a considerable amount of duplicity and confusion to slip through.

You need to be ever vigilant. Always be suspicious of hype that implies a product is healthy or weight-reducing. Never devour the contents of a package that screams, "I am healthy," "I will help you lose weight," until you read the nutrition label. For a real-life example, take a look at the popcorn packaging and label on the next page.

All-Natural Fat. Although the food processor does not claim outright that this popcorn is healthy and a good choice for weight loss, he has designed his package so you will leap to this conclusion on your own. His choice of words is perfect. Read "All Natural," but think "healthy." Read "Air Popped," but think "fat-free." But, if like Sergeant Friday, you just want the facts, ma'am, just the facts, read the label. The label tells the true story.

Calories from Fat: 100; Serving Size: 2¾ cups. Wow! 100 fat calories for a mere 2¾ cups of popcorn (about 2 handfuls). This popcorn may contain no unhealthy additives, but the fat content negates any chance it has of being a healthy choice. And how did fat-free air-popped popcorn accumulate 100 fat calories, anyway? Look at the list of ingredients. Popcorn, vegetable oil (corn and/or sunflower and/or partially

Air-popped Popcorn

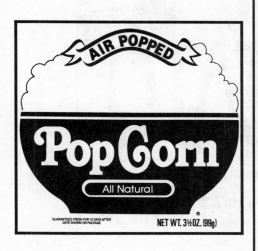

Nutrition Facts
Serving Size 2 3/4 cups (30g)
Servings Per Container about 3

Amount Per Serving	
Calories 170 Calories from Fat 100	
	%Daily Value*
Total Fat 11g	16%
Saturated Fat 1g	7%
Cholesterol 0mg	0%
Sodium 240mg	10%
Total Carbohydrates 15g	5%
Dietary Fiber 6g	23%
Sugars 0g	
Protein 2g	

Vitamin A 0%	•	Vitamin C 0%
Calcium 0%	•	Iron 2%

* Percent Daily Values are based on a 2,000 calorie diet. Your daily values may be higher or lower depending on your calorie needs:

	Calories	2,000	2,500
Total Fat	Less than	65g	80g
Sat Fat	Less than	20g	25g
Cholesterol	Less than	300mg	300mg
Sodium	Less than	2,400mg	2,400mg
Total Carbohydrate		300g	375g
Dietary Fiber		25g	30g

Calories per gram:
Fat 9 - Carbohydrate 4 - Protein 4

INGREDIENTS: POPCORN, VEGETABLE OIL (CORN AND/OR SUNFLOWER AND/OR PARTIALLY HYDROGENATED SOYBEAN AND/OR PARTIALLY HYDROGENATED COTTONSEED), SALT AND ANNATTO COLORING.

hydrogenated soybean and/or partially hydrogenated cottonseed). Vegetable oil? That's pure fat. The manufacturers took fat-free popcorn, air-popped it so they could claim "Air Popped"! and then covered it with 100 fat calories of vegetable oil.

% Fat-Free: Noninformation. 95% fat-free! 88% fat-free! 97% fat-free! The food manufacturers who use % fat-free claims are not lying. They are just giving you an irrelevant fact — that fat accounts for a small percentage of the *weight* of a product. (In most foods, much of the weight is water, so even a glass of whole milk, which has 73 fat calories, is only 4 percent fat by weight.) You assume they are telling you the percentage of calories coming from fat and conclude the product is low-fat and you can eat it in unlimited quantities. Wrong.

For an example, take a 4-ounce bag of 95% FAT-FREE, LOW CAL

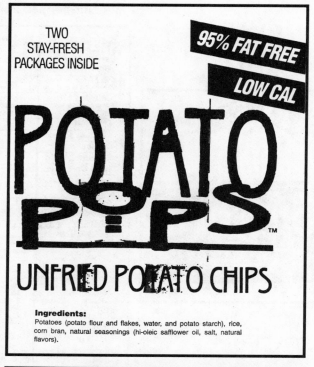

TWO
STAY-FRESH
PACKAGES INSIDE

95% FAT FREE

LOW CAL

POTATO
POPS™

UNFRIED POTATO CHIPS

Ingredients:
Potatoes (potato flour and flakes, water, and potato starch), rice, corn bran, natural seasonings (hi-oleic safflower oil, salt, natural flavors).

Nutrition Facts	Amount/serving	% DV*	Amount/serving	% DV*
Serving size 1/2 oz. (14g)	**Total Fat** 1g	**2%**	**Total Carb.** 11g	**4%**
Servings Per Package 8	Sat.Fat 0g	**0%**	Fiber 1g	**4%**
Calories 50	**Cholest.** 0mg	**0%**	Sugars 0g	
Fat Cal. 9	**Sodium** 165mg	**7%**	**Protein** 1g	
*Percent Daily Values (DV) are based on a 2,000 calorie diet.	Vitamin A 0% • Vitamin C 8% • Calcium 0% • Iron 4%			

Potato Pops UNFRIED POTATO CHIPS. Sounds like a great choice. You might as well eat the whole small bag. Whoa! Look at the nutrition label. The claim "95% fat-free" is based on the fact that the weight of the fat — 1 gram — is 5 percent of the weight of the Potato Pops — 14 grams per serving. Actually, 1 gram is 7 percent — not 5 percent — of 14 grams. The producers should have claimed "93% fat-free," but let's not quibble; the information is useless, anyway.

If the manufacturer had based his claim on total calories as you probably assumed, he would have called this snack "82% fat-free." (9 fat calories ÷ 50 total calories = 18%; 100% − 18% = 82%). But "82% fat-free" doesn't look so enticing. This is also extraneous information

Peanut Butter

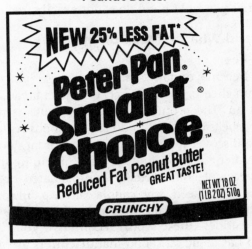

NEW 25% LESS FAT*

Peter Pan®

Smart Choice™

Reduced Fat Peanut Butter GREAT TASTE!

NET WT 18 OZ
(1 LB 2 OZ) 510g

CRUNCHY

Nutrition Facts
Serv. Size 2 Tbsp (36g), Servings about 14

Amount/serving – % Daily Value**

Calories 190   Calories from Fat 110

Total Fat 12g - **18**%, (Sat. Fat 2g - **10**%),
Cholest. 0mg - **0**%, **Sodium** 140mg - **6**%,
Total Carb. 15g - **5**%, (Fiber 1g - **5**%),
(Sugars 6g), **Protein** 8g

Vit. A <2% • Vit. C <2% • Calcium <2% • Iron 4%
**Percent Daily Values are based on a 2,000 calorie diet.

*THAN REGULAR PEANUT BUTTER WHICH CONTAINS 16g FAT PER
SERVING. SMART CHOICE CONTAINS 12g FAT PER SERVING.

(see page 11). The only information that is *really* important to you is that there are 9 fat calories for a ½-ounce serving and that since you plan to eat the whole small bag you will be eating 8 servings or 8 × 9 = 72 fat calories, *not* an inconsequential amount of fat. An aside: Don't you think it is clever that the manufacturer lists safflower oil as a natural seasoning?

~~Smart Choice.~~ This peanut butter label is practically jumping off the jar it is so excited: "NEW 25% LESS FAT." This must be a SMART CHOICE. You must be smart to be choosing such a healthy, "low-fat" product. Really? Check out the label.

Calories from Fat: 110; Serving Size: 2 Tbsp (36g). Why don't we think 55 fat calories a tablespoon is such a smart choice? Yes, it is less fat than the 75 fat calories for a tablespoon of regular peanut butter, but 55 fat calories per tablespoon does not exactly make it diet food.

More Claims and What to Make of Them

1. CLAIM: Fat-free

   TRUTH: Fat-free mayonnaise, salad dressings, sour cream, cheese, cream cheese, cookies, crackers, cake, bread, butter, and on and on. The profusion of fat-free foods is mind-boggling. The label says 0 fat, but do fat-free foods really have no fat?

   To discover if a food is truly free of fat, look at the list of ingredients. If you find any fat-containing ingredient such as vegetable oil, partially hydrogenated or hydrogenated corn, cottonseed, soy, canola, olive, palm, palm kernel, or coconut oil, butterfat, cheese, beef, lard, monoglycerides or diglycerides (these words mean fats), you can assume the food has some fat. Food manufacturers are allowed to call a food fat-free if a serving contains less than half a gram or 4.5 fat calories. So, if a product labeled fat-free includes a fat-containing ingredient, it is safest to assume the food has 4.5 fat calories per serving. You may think so few fat calories seem trivial, but even few calories can add up, especially if the serving size is small. See "Fat-Free Food Abuse," page 100, for a discussion of the real problem with fat-free foods.

2. CLAIM: Cholesterol-free

   TRUTH: The average consumer translates "Cholesterol-free" to mean "heart-healthy" or "healthy." First, since dietary cholesterol has a minor effect on raising blood cholesterol, the cholesterol content of a food is of little importance. What is significant for your heart health is the amount of saturated fat and fat the food contains. Second, cholesterol-free just means that a foodstuff contains no animal products because cholesterol is found only in animal products. Every plant product, no matter how high in saturated fat, is cholesterol-free. Coconut, palm, and hydrogenated vegetable oils, which are among the most heart-risky foods around, are cholesterol-free because they are plant products.

   According to the FDA regulations, if a product claims it is cholesterol-free, it cannot be loaded with saturated fat and thus be heart-risky. Specifically it must contain no more than 18 calories of saturated fat per serving and 27 calories of fat. If the serving is small, such as 1 cookie, it must contain no more than 9 calories of sat-fat. But who eats 1 cookie? How about 5 or 6 (45 or 54 sat-fat calories)? Or, for some cookie freaks, 10 or 15 (90 or 135 sat-fat calories)? How does this fit into a Sat-Fat Budget of 176?

3. CLAIM: Low Cholesterol

TRUTH: As the claim on the top of the bread crisps label (page 126) makes clear, a product can claim it is "Low cholesterol" even if it is horrendously high in total fat. At 1 gram or 9 sat-fat calories, this snack meets the criteria for saturated fat, but at 50 fat calories per ounce or 7 piddling crackers, it is certainly not a healthy choice.

4. CLAIM: Light

TRUTH: Food producers bank on the fact that we associate the term light with low-fat. However, although a product which advertises itself as "light" must contain one-third fewer calories or half as much fat as the "regular" product, it may still not qualify as low-fat in our book. A "lite" brand of potato chips that contains 45 fat calories per ounce rather than 90 is definitely an improvement, but 45 fat calories is still a whopping amount of fat for such a small amount of food.

5. CLAIM: 2% Low-fat Milk

TRUTH: Because of a grandfather clause in the FDA regulations, 2% milk is still called low-fat, although at 45 fat calories a cup, it is hardly low-fat fare. The 2% sounds like such a low percentage of fat, but it refers to the fact that fat accounts for 2% of the *weight* of the milk. Milk is mostly water, so the percentage contributed by fat to the total weight is small. It would be more accurate to advertise this milk as 35% high-fat milk since fat contributes 45 of the total 130 calories ($45 \div 130 = 35\%$). However, neither the claim 2% fat or 35% fat tells us what we need to know — that one 8-ounce glass contains 45 fat calories, two glasses contain 90 fat calories, three glasses contain 135 fat calories, and that this is a drink our body can ill afford.

6. CLAIM: Lean

TRUTH: Consumers associate the word "lean" with low in fat. However, to qualify as "lean" a meat must contain less than 10 grams of fat (90 fat calories) per 100 grams (3½ ounces) of food. You are not going to remain very lean if you spend 90 fat calories on a mere 3½ ounces of meat; or more likely, 128 fat calories for 5 ounces of "lean" meat.

7. CLAIM: Extra-Lean

   TRUTH: Under the FDA regulations, a meat can qualify as "extra lean" if it contains less than 45 fat calories for 3½ ounces of food. This amount hardly seems extra-lean when you compare it with turkey, cod, crab, haddock, lobster, pike, pollock, and scallops that contain only 7 fat calories for 3½ ounces or skinless chicken breast, red snapper, or sole at only 11 fat calories for 3½ ounces.

Words of wisdom: Only an educated consumer can remain healthy and lean.

Coming Next:

If you love to eat (even if you don't love to cook), read the next chapter to learn how to prepare quick and easy low-fat meals.

Remember:

1. Read food labels to make wise selections.
2. The only two numbers on the food label that you need to know are:
   a. Calories from fat.
   b. Serving size.
3. Be sure to adjust the fat calories for the number of servings you eat.
4. Beware of misleading advertising claims, such as Lite! Lean! 95% fat-free! Low cholesterol! Lower in fat!
5. Repeat to yourself: **I MUST EAT TO LOSE. I MUST EAT TO LOSE. I MUST EAT TO LOSE. OF COURSE, I MUST EAT NUTRITIOUS, LOW-FAT FOODS TO LOSE.**

9. Cooking Low-Fat and Delicious

"A friend recently recommended *Choose to Lose* to me. I am absolutely delighted with it. I feel there is hope! I don't feel deprived! Ingredients are usually ones I have on hand. Most of the recipes are able to be made quickly, which fits into my busy schedule."

Barbara Karpinski, Rockville, Maryland

REALLY SMART SHOPPING

Fresh Ingredients: An Unlimited Source of Riches

Tomatoes, potatoes, green peppers, onions, garlic cloves, broccoli, bok choy, carrots, mushrooms, salmon steaks, shrimp, boneless chicken breasts, turkey cutlets, pasta, rice, chicken broth, and on and on. Think of all the wonderful dishes you can make — and eat! If your approach to grocery shopping has been hit-and-run forays into the frozen dinner freezers, throw the microwave boxes out of your cart and take time to explore the natural riches along the perimeter of the store.

Get to know the produce section. Just walking through the aisles and looking at the colors, shapes, and textures that make each fruit or vegetable unique and beautiful is a pleasure. Fill up your cart with produce. It's a capital investment. You can't take an orange for a snack if you have no oranges in the refrigerator. You can't make *Indonesian Chicken with Green Beans* (page 229) if you don't have green beans. You can't make *Carrot Soup* (page 221) if you don't have carrots and potatoes.

Be adventuresome. If your supermarket stocks a variety of produce, experiment. Try cilantro and fennel. Try bok choy and kale. Buy peppers of all colors and types — red, yellow, green, jalapeño. Even if your grocery store is not so well endowed, each week choose a vegetable and fruit you've never brought home before.

Check out the fish counter. Try a different species every week.

Make sure you have the basics in stock at home (see "Stocking Up," page 140) — foods such as flour, sugar, rice, canned tomatoes and chicken broth, molasses, onions, and potatoes in the cupboards; lemons, limes, garlic, ginger in the refrigerator; chicken breasts, turkey cutlets, corn, and peas in the freezer. Have a variety of spices on hand to enhance your dishes instead of adding fat.

The message! If you want to become lean and stay that way for a lifetime, you need to keep your kitchen jam-packed with the ingredients needed to create wonderful, low-fat and healthy dishes.

COOKING LOW-FAT

You can't help but notice how many times we have mentioned the *fantastic!* recipes in *Eater's Choice: A Food Lover's Guide to Lower Cholesterol.* We are not trying to strong-arm you into buying another book, but as you can see from our hearty endorsement, we believe you would greatly enjoy the 240 additional recipes in *Eater's Choice.* They are generally quite low in fat, delectable, and helpful for losing weight. In fact, one of the reasons we wrote *Choose to Lose* was that so many people told us they lost weight using *Eater's Choice* recipes.

You probably also have your own favorite recipes that are too high-fat to keep your Fat Budget in the black. With a few substitutions and modifications you may be able to fit them into your new eating plan.

Silent Substitutions

In most cases, the following low-fat or nonfat substitutions will greatly reduce the fat content of your recipes without diminishing the taste or texture.

WHEN THE RECIPE CALLS FOR:	SUBSTITUTE:
Cream	Nonfat yogurt, buttermilk, skim milk, evaporated skim milk
Whole milk	Skim milk
Sour cream	Nonfat yogurt, buttermilk
Veal cutlets	Turkey cutlets
Pork	White meat chicken
3 egg yolks	1 egg yolk
2 whole eggs	1 egg + 1 egg white
Ground beef	Ground turkey (without skin and fat) that you grind yourself

Hints for Quick and Easy Meal Making

Preparing dinner need not be a 3-hour endeavor. If you plan ahead, meal making can be quick and easy. Here are some hints:

- At the beginning of the week, glance through *Choose to Lose* or *Eater's Choice* or other low-fat cookbooks and choose recipes for the week. Jot down the ingredients you will need so you won't waste time when you shop. Be sure to add foods such as fruits, vegetables, and bread, which you will need for snacks, side dishes, and desserts.
- When you go to the supermarket, follow your shopping list, but if you see a food that entices you, buy it. For example, perhaps you hadn't even thought of making shrimp creole, but the shrimp look so large and appetizing, you decide to buy them for that night's dinner.
- Buy enough food so you have material to work with. Buy a variety of vegetables so you always have a vegetable or two with dinner. Make sure you keep your larder well stocked with the basics (see "Stocking Up," pages 140–42).
- Cook up several soups (double or triple the recipes) over the weekend. Freeze them in small containers (enough for one meal) to reheat and eat all through the week.
- Make enough of an entree so you can eat it for two days. Make even more so you can also freeze some to reheat for later.
- To save preparation time, flour chicken breasts and bake them (with no fat) the night before so you can use them in a recipe the next day.
- Plan so your recipes last at least two days. Alternate so you don't have to make soup and an entree the same day.

Reducing the Fat

Recipes often recommend more fat than is necessary. Another way to modify a recipe is to reduce the amount of fat you use.

- If the recipe calls for sautéing in ¼ cup oil, use 2 tablespoons of olive oil instead. If the reduced amount works, try 1 tablespoon. If a recipe calls for sautéing in 2 tablespoons of fat, use 1 teaspoon of olive oil or less, plus a splash of water, or sauté in strained chicken broth.

- DON'T dot the top of your fish or pie with margarine or butter. You may find the dish doesn't need the extra fat.
- Instead of sautéing chicken breasts in a few tablespoons of olive oil, dredge them in a mixture of flour, salt, and pepper, and then bake them in a single layer in a shallow baking pan. Add no fat. When the breasts are fully cooked, either refrigerate or freeze them for later use or cut them up and add them to the sauce you have just prepared.

Modifying a Recipe

We easily modified the high-fat recipe for Curry Soup into a tasty low-fat treat.

A Recipe: Before and After

HIGH-FAT CURRY SOUP		LOW-FAT CURRY SOUP	
INGREDIENTS	FAT CALORIES	INGREDIENTS	FAT CALORIES
¼ cup butter	400	1 tsp olive oil	40
2 medium onions		2 medium onions	
3 stalks celery		3 stalks celery	
2 tbsp flour		2 tbsp flour	
1 tbsp curry powder		1 tbsp curry powder	
2 apples		2 apples	
1 cup diced chicken (light and dark meat)	31	1 cup diced chicken (white meat)	13
2 qts chicken broth	184	2 qts chicken broth, strained	5
1 cup light cream	417	1 cup nonfat yogurt	0
Total Fat Calories	1032	Total Fat Calories	58
Makes 10 cups		*Makes 10 cups*	
Per cup of soup	**103**	Per cup of soup	**6**

This is how we did it:

- Four tablespoons of butter had more fat than necessary to sauté the onions. We reduced the fat to 1 teaspoon of olive oil and a splash of water and saved 360 fat calories. (We chose olive oil because it is a heart-healthy oil; but being heart-healthy does not make it any less fattening.)
- Instead of dark and light chicken meat, we used only white breast meat and saved 18 fat calories.

- Straining the chicken fat from the broth saved 179 fat calories.
- Replacing the cream with nonfat yogurt saved 417 fat calories.

The resulting soup tastes fine, and at 6 fat calories per cup you could easily enjoy a pint of it.

Determining Fat Calories per Serving. If you want to determine the fat calories per serving for a recipe, add up the fat calories for all the fat-containing ingredients and then divide by the number of servings. For example, in the high-fat curry soup recipe, the fat calories for all the fat-containing ingredients total 1032. To determine the fat calories per serving, you divide 1032 by the number of servings, which is 10. $1032 \div 10 = 103$ fat calories per serving.

If you want to determine the fat calories per serving after you have reduced the fat in a recipe, see Appendix B, page 457.

Cooking Tips

The following cooking tips will help you stay within your Fat Budget:

- Steam vegetables. Purchase an inexpensive metal steamer and place it in a saucepan filled with about an inch of water. Spread out the steamer and place cut-up fresh vegetables on top. Cover the saucepan and steam the vegetables until they are tender. Steamed vegetables need no fat. For added flavor, mix in some pressed garlic, vinegar, or herbs (thyme, basil, etc.).
- Sauté vegetables in 1 teaspoon of olive oil and add splashes of water to steam-cook them.
- Sauté vegetables in broth.
- Always steam or bake eggplant. When it is sautéed, it absorbs gobs of oil.
- Combine flour, salt (optional), and pepper on a plate or in a plastic bag. Flour chicken and place it in one layer in a shallow baking pan without fat and bake it at 350°F for about 20 minutes or until cooked through.
- Always remove skin *before* cooking chicken to keep the chicken from absorbing the fat from the skin. A skinless chicken breast has 13 fat calories. A chicken breast that was cooked with the skin has 28 fat calories after the skin has been removed. Eating the skin more than triples the fat calories in a chicken breast. A chicken breast with skin has 69 fat calories.

- NEVER deep-fry fish or chicken. NEVER EVER flour or bread and fry fish or chicken. Breading soaks up fat like a sponge.
- Bake, broil, grill, or poach chicken or fish. Limit the amount of fat you use. Use low-fat sauces for added taste.
- If you cook beef, lamb, pork, or veal, trim off all visible fat. Broil or bake on a rack to drain the fat. Wrap cooked meat in paper towels to remove more fat. Avoid pan-frying.

Fat-Reducing Cooking Equipment

- Cast iron makes a great nontoxic, nonstick cooking surface. You can purchase cast-iron griddles that fit over two stove burners and quickly cook chicken breasts, turkey cutlets, French toast, and pancakes with little or no added fat. Small cast-iron griddles that fit over one stove burner are also available.
- Steamer: See the preceding list of Cooking Tips.
- Clay cooker: Keeps chicken moist and tender without adding fat.
- Gravy skimmer: Removes fat from canned chicken broth.

Is Low-Fat Cooking and Eating Expensive?

No way. Replacing foods high in fat with vegetables, fruits, and whole-grains will keep you thin and your wallet fat. Convenience foods and snacks are high in fat and expensive. Frozen dinners are about five times as expensive as the raw ingredients used to prepare them. Compare the cost of a pound of potatoes with a pound of potato chips. Beef costs more than chicken or turkey. Sour cream, sweet cream, and cheeses are rich foods that impoverish both your pocketbook and your Fat Budget.

In contrast, a variety of vegetables, rice, or pasta, with small amounts of chicken or beef, keep both budget and body trim. Even if eating low-fat were more expensive — which it definitely is not — the saving in health costs and the psychological benefits of not being overweight would balance the expense.

STOCKING UP

For some of you, reducing fat will mean a big change in the foods you cook. You may wonder what foods will replace the cream in your refrigerator or the Twinkies in your cupboard. What foods should you have on hand to make cooking a snap? Here is a list of foods and spices to keep in your cupboard, your refrigerator, and your freezer.

FOODS TO KEEP ON YOUR SHELVES:

Almonds, slivered
Anchovies
Apricots, dried
Apricot jelly
Artichoke hearts in water
Baking powder
Baking soda
Barley
Beans, dried (black, pinto, etc.)
Beans, kidney, canned
Chicken broth
Chickpeas
Cocoa, unsweetened
Cornstarch
Flour, unbleached white
Flour, whole-wheat
Honey
Lentils
Molasses
Oat bran
Oatmeal (not quick)
Oil, olive
Oil, sunflower or safflower

Olives, black and green
Onions
Pastas (spaghetti, noodles, etc.)
Pineapple chunks, canned
Peaches, canned
Peanuts, unsalted
Potatoes
Prunes
Raisins
Salt
Sesame paste (tahini)
Sherry, dry
Sugar, brown
Sugar, white
Sugar, confectioners'
Tomatoes, canned
Tomato juice
Tomato paste (6 oz)
Tomato sauce (8 oz)
Vanilla
Vermouth
Vinegar
Walnuts, shelled
Yeast (if you plan to make bread)

SPICES:

Basil leaves
Caraway seeds
Cardamom, ground
Cayenne pepper
Chili powder, hot (if you like)
Chili powder, mild
Cinnamon, ground
Cinnamon sticks
Cloves, ground and whole
Coriander
Cream of tartar
Cumin, ground and seeds

Curry powder
Dillweed
Ginger, ground
Mustard seed, black
Nutmeg, whole
Oregano
Paprika
Peppercorns, black
Rosemary leaves
Sesame seeds
Tarragon
Thyme leaves
Turmeric

FOODS FROM THE ORIENTAL FOOD STORE:

Bamboo shoots, canned	Mushrooms, dried black
Bean sauce	Sesame chili oil
Black beans (fermented)	Sesame oil
Chili paste with garlic	Soy sauce and double black soy sauce
Hoisin sauce	Water chestnuts, canned

FOODS* TO KEEP IN YOUR REFRIGERATOR:

Buttermilk (for baking)	Limes
Carrots	Margarine
Celery	Mayonnaise or salad dressing
Garlic cloves	Mushrooms (always good in salads)
Ginger root (store in jar with sherry)	Mustard, Dijon
	Peppers, red or green
Lemons	Yogurt, nonfat plain

FOODS TO KEEP IN YOUR FREEZER:

Boned and skinned chicken breasts	Peas, frozen
	Turkey cutlets
Corn, frozen	Whole-wheat bread
Margarine	Whole-wheat pita bread

THESE ALL-SEASON FOODS WILL ENHANCE YOUR MEALS — KEEP SOME ON HAND:

Broccoli	Spinach
Eggplant	Squash** (acorn, butternut, etc.)
Potatoes, white or sweet**	Tomatoes
Snow peas (Chinese peapods)	Zucchini

Buy fruits in season. Apples, bananas, oranges, and pears can usually be purchased year-round. Use for baking, cooking, and snacks.

---

*These foods will stay fresh at least several weeks.
**These vegetables will keep fresh at least a week or more.

And coming next . . .

Learn how you can become the master of your fate in every eating situation.

Remember:

1. Reduce fat content of recipes.
   a. Use less fat than called for; experiment.
   b. Substitute low-fat or nonfat ingredients for their high-fat counterparts.
2. Prepare food with little or no fat.
   a. Steam, broil, grill, bake, poach, or boil rather than fry.
   b. Use cast-iron cookware, vegetable steamers, or clay cookers for low-fat cooking.
3. Repeat to yourself: **I MUST EAT TO LOSE. I MUST EAT TO LOSE. I MUST EAT TO LOSE. OF COURSE, I MUST EAT NUTRITIOUS, LOW-FAT FOODS TO LOSE.**

10. Coping in a World You Did Not Make

"We had a church picnic on Sunday. I fixed the *Choose to Lose* cucumbers and also took some bagels, no-fat cream cheese, and turkey. I also ate a bowl of cereal before I left. I chose not to have a hot dog — my ALL-TIME FAVORITE! I didn't even miss it. All I saw was the fat I would be eating. I didn't feel funny or embarrassed about bringing my own food. I felt in control for the first time in my life!"

Susan Mallams, Oak Harbor, Washington

YOUR GOALS are high. You are making all the right changes — and loving it. Soon you will find that your clothes are slipping off your bony body. You'll be so perky and alert your boss will give you a raise or if you're the boss you'll give yourself a bonus. You are beginning to prefer plain air-popped popcorn to buttered. Your life is shaping up. And so are you.

We hope this first paragraph describes you. However, the road to thinness may not be quite so smooth. Temptation abounds. Television ads assault you with visions of rich, dark chocolate flowing smoothly over clusters of peanuts, thick, juicy hamburgers glistening with fat, breaded shrimp floating in pools of butter. Birthday parties, office parties, dinner parties, threaten your resolve. Here are some tips to get you through the hard times.

SPLURGING

The beauty of *Choose to Lose* is that you can go to a party and eat what you want. You just have to plan. Say you are going out to dinner Saturday night and want to eat a 6-ounce steak (276 fat calories), a baked potato with a teaspoon of butter (34 fat calories), and a piece of cheese-

> Important. *Choose to Lose* is quantitative. You have a Fat Budget. If you weaken and eat 2 large slices of Aunt Miranda's famous whipped cream pie, just compensate by making low-fat choices for the next few days — and you know exactly how many fat calories that is. Don't say, "I've been bad," give up, and pig out for the rest of the day because you splurged. You can fit it in. You are in control.

cake (162 fat calories) for a total of 472 fat calories. WOW! Even if your budget is 268, you can afford the splurge. Here's how:

If you eat 220 fat calories each day from Sunday to Saturday you will have accumulated $268 - 220 = 48$ fat calories per day; 48 fat calories $\times$ 6 days = 288 extra fat calories to spend on Saturday. Add these to your budget $(288 + 268)$ and you have 556 fat calories for Saturday. You can enjoy your splurge and have 84 fat calories left for breakfast and lunch on Saturday. Just plan ahead.

Here are some hints for the many occasions that will arise when you haven't saved for a splurge, but don't want to decimate your budget.

AT PARTIES

It's guaranteed. Any party you attend will be overloaded with high-fat foods. In fact, at some parties the only low-fat choice will be soda water.

> ### Important Advice for Chronic Dieters
>
> Don't starve all day so that you go wild when you arrive at the table. You'll break your fat bank in a millisecond or two. If you want to save fat calories for the affair, just eat extra-low-fat all day (but eat a lot so you won't be hungry) or for several previous days. (See "Splurging" at the beginning of the chapter.)

Pre-party

Ask your host or hostess if you can bring something — hors d'oeuvres, bread, salad, vegetable, main course, dessert, and, of course, you'll make it low-fat. Most hosts will be delighted, but if one should resist, you insist. Your contribution may be all you get to eat.

Eat a light snack before the party so that blinding hunger won't cause you temporary failure of will power and result in overeating.

At the Party

The first glance may make your heart sink. How can you resist the sumptuous array of the most delectable foods you have craved for your entire life? But look again. Does the breaded shrimp look luscious or just greasy? Does the twelve-layer rum cake taste good or just look beautiful? Granted, some of the food will be delicious, but not all. Pick and choose.

Leave the Scene of the Crime Before It Becomes a Crime

When you have finished savoring a few offerings, leave the area. Don't stand around listening to the food cry, "Eat me! Eat me!" Go to a room where there's no food. Out of sight, out of mind; in sight, in mouth. (Eventually, you may not have to avoid rooms with food. I just spoke with a Chooser to Lose who said that this is the first holiday season that she was able to pass by doughnuts and cookies and cakes rather than frantically scarfing them down. She knew she could have them so she could ignore them. She ate the one piece of cake she had chosen for herself. This may happen even to you.)

Regrets to the Hostess

Before you arrive at a dinner party devise a plan of action. Be ready with an appeasing comment. "You know I adore your desserts, but I'm off sweets until I can button my slacks." Or privately before dinner (if you know the food will be full of fat): "Please give me tiny portions. I'm trying so hard to lose weight."

At Your Own Party

This is a perfect opportunity to show your friends how well they can eat low-fat. Give a dinner party and start with *Ginger-Carrot Soup* (page 222) at 4 fat calories per cup. Then serve *Shrimp Creole* (page 238) on rice for a main course at 28 fat calories per breast, steamed carrot sticks with garlic for a vegetable (0 fat calories), *Onion Flat Bread* (page 259) for 7 fat calories a slice, or made with no fat (0 fat calories per slice), and for dessert, *Key Lime Pie* (page 267), 36 fat calories. When's the party? We'll be there.

If time limitations force you to weaken and buy a high-fat dessert (better to serve fruit), be sure any leftovers leave with your guests. Stuff them into their pockets and purses if necessary. Don't leave a trace even in your garbage can because we all know that food in garbage cans can be retrieved.

AT RESTAURANTS

Eating at home makes keeping to your Fat Budget a breeze. Although you can't always be expected to eat at home, keep eating out to a minimum. Take a look at the fat calories for Restaurant Foods and Fast Foods in the Food Tables if you need a reason to dine at home. How does a serving of fettuccine Alfredo at 873 fat calories fit into your Fat Budget? Or lasagna at 477 fat calories per serving? Or a bowl of wonton soup at 108 fat calories or a dish of kung pao chicken at 1134 fat calories? Can your Fat Budget be stretched to accommodate that amount of fat every couple of days and bounce back?

> REMEMBER: If you eat out once or more a week, it is no longer a special treat that justifies splurging. Eat as you do at home — with care.

Here are some tips for eating out.

Be Choosy

If possible, *you* pick the restaurant. If others choose, you may have no options. Select a restaurant that you know serves food you can eat. Want to try some place new? Call early in the day and ask what's on the menu. If nothing suits your Fat Budget, ask if the chef can prepare something with little fat or with a low-fat sauce. Be specific.

Beforehand

Don't starve all day in preparation for dinner or you'll frantically gobble up your Fat Budget before you get through the soup and salad. Eat low-fat all day, but eat. In fact, you might want to munch on a carrot or two or even snack on a nonfat flavored yogurt an hour before you depart for the restaurant.

Ask

Don't be shy. Always ask the waiter what you want to know. It's your body, not his. Ask how the sole amandine or chicken Dijon is prepared. Is it fried? Baked? Broiled? Is it made with butter? Oil? What kind of oil? What's in the soup or the sauce? Cream? Milk? Sour cream? Ask enough questions so you can make educated choices.

Make Requests

Ask the waiter if the chef will broil, bake, poach, or grill the chicken or fish without fat. Then you can add it later in the amounts you choose. Ask if the nonfat mustard sauce that spices up the steak dish can be used on a grilled fish instead of fat. Be creative.

On the Side

Always ask to have butter, salad dressings, and sauces served on the side so that you can regulate how much you use. You'll see how quickly a few tablespoons add up to more than you need to eat.

Dip In or BYO

When you order your salad dressing on the side, keep it in the serving dish instead of pouring it over your salad. Use the fork method: Dip your fork into the dressing, then spear your salad greens or vegetables. You will get the salad dressing taste with many fewer fat calories. You might want to order your salad plain and enhance it with packets of nonfat or low-fat salad dressing you bring from home.

Give It Away

If a portion served is more than you should eat, give what you don't want to your dining partner. If you are eating alone, place the extra on a salad plate and ask the waiter to take it away. Send back the butter served with the bread. Ask for the potato plain. You can't eat what's not there.

You may feel compelled to lick your plate clean because you paid for your meal, but resist the urge. The cost to your Fat Budget is not worth the salve to your conscience.

Share

If you are dying for a taste of that sinful-looking Black Forest cake that has been haunting you from the tent-card on your table, share it with a friend, or better yet, several friends. Choose your friends wisely and you might find one who will give you a bite of everything she eats. Main dishes and appetizers can also be shared without anyone starving. Restaurants often serve single portions large enough for two.

Taste

Don't just shovel in the food, particularly a high-fat splurge. Concentrate when you eat. Don't just grab some vegetables at a salad bar and call it dinner. Make a quick, but glorious *Eater's Choice* meal and savor every bite. Eating is one of life's great pleasures.

IN AN AIRPLANE

Flying? Plan Ahead

Why waste hundreds of fat calories on mediocre airline food? If you plan ahead, you won't be forced to choose between 2 greasy sausages (140 fat calories), a greasy cheese omelet (125 fat calories), and a greasy minimuffin (40 fat calories) for breakfast or nothing to eat for three hours. Just plan ahead. Call the airline at least 24 hours before your flight and order a special meal. Explain that you are on a low-fat diet. Be as specific as they allow in making your request. Ask for a fruit plate. Ask for chicken breast without skin. You'll find that the meals you order will not only be lower in fat, they will also taste better.

AT WORK

A Fat Minefield

In the abstract, one might think that a worksite would be a safe haven from temptation, but no such luck. Boxes of big, shiny, glazed doughnuts arrive every morning like clockwork. Vending machines full of little bags of fat are ever ready in the lounge. Is there ever a day without a cake to celebrate a birthday, anniversary, the office baseball team's victory, the receipt of a big contract? Then there are the meetings, office lunches, and office parties. Although it seems an impossible job to avoid all the booby traps, you can take control of each fat mine and disarm it.

Remove the Lure. Move the doughnuts or birthday cake to another office so they won't keep yelling "Eat me!" in your ear. Bring a large bag of fruit, bagels, nonfat pretzels, to munch on during the day so you never need to invade the vending machine. Keep an air popper in your office so you can enjoy a snack of fresh air-popped popcorn every day. Help plan the refreshments for a meeting so there will be food for you to enjoy. Instead of the typical Danish, doughnuts, cookies, sweet cakes, for the morning break, make sure fruit (how about a beautiful arrangement of cut-up fruit?), English muffins, and bagels are offered. For lunch, insist that the cold cut platter include turkey breast, the bread tray not be limited to croissants, and that mustard be made available. If a birthday is going to be celebrated at a restaurant, make certain that it is a restaurant with low-fat choices. For the office party, join the planning committee to make sure a table of low-fat offerings (fruit, vegetables, low-fat dip, low-fat dishes) is included. Bring a favorite *Choose to Lose* or *Eater's Choice* recipe as a treat for yourself and the crowd. You can take control of the fat aspects of your working conditions if you make an effort — and it's worth it.

Eat! Eat! Eat!

Don't allow work to interfere with eating. *Never go without lunch!* If you know you are going to be chained to your desk through your lunch hour, be sure you have brought lunch so you have something to eat. Keep a few flavored nonfat yogurts in the office refrigerator so you can take one for your afternoon break. Remember: If you do not eat lunch or an afternoon snack, you will be hungry and tired all day. The fatigue will follow you home and wipe you out for the entire evening. The hunger-fatigue combo will make you fall off the *Choose to Lose* wagon, go berserk, and eat margarine sandwiches. Eat! Eat! Eat! Eat low-fat, vitamin-mineral-fiber-packed foods and do it all day.

AT HOME

For many, entering their front door is the beginning of their weight loss problems. This doesn't have to be. Your home is where you can take control. You can start in your kitchen.

How "Clean" Is Your House?

The amount of high-fat food that lingers in your home is an indication of how seriously you are trying to change your way of eating to lose weight. What about your hidden fat stores? Do you keep ice cream in the freezer? Do you keep crackers in the cupboards? Do caches of high-fat foods offer irresistible temptation? Get rid of it. You can't devour a gallon of ice cream if it isn't in your freezer. You can't demolish a bowl of macadamia nuts if you never buy them. Keep high-temptation foods out of your house. Splurge elsewhere. If you have accumulated a stock of high-fat goodies, give it away to neighbors. Feed it to your dog. Take a deep breath and throw it into the garbage. To be safe, throw it in your neighbor-down-the-street's garbage can.

Plenty. Instead of fixating on the high-fat food you are eliminating, pamper yourself with an abundance of delicious, nutritious low-fat food. How about starting dinner with rich, creamy, and completely fat-free *Apple-Squash Soup* (*Eater's Choice*)? Take time (and it takes very little) to marinate skinless chicken breasts in a mixture of equal amounts of mustard, molasses, and vinegar and then broil or grill them until cooked through. Or place fish fillets in a baking dish, pour in ¼ to ½ cup of vermouth or white wine, grind pepper over fish, and then cover with 2 to 4 tablespoons chopped shallots and bake until the fish flakes easily. Press a garlic clove over steamed broccoli. Sprinkle vinegar, basil, salt, and pepper over sliced tomatoes. You can create a feast in almost no time. Eat well the low-fat way and you'll find the pounds melting away.

Fixing the Problems

You can also try to eliminate the underlying causes for uncontrolled eating.

Fatigue. When you come home from work do you use what little energy you have to drag yourself to the refrigerator? Is your self-control exhausted so you binge on everything in sight?

Fatigue need not be your undoing if you take the following advice. Only have low-fat food around so if you binge the binge is benign. Don't go directly to the kitchen; go to your bedroom and take a nap. Some Choosers to Lose have told us they like to take a walk or run as soon as they return from work. This activity seems to energize them for the remainder of the evening. If you are tired because you are hungry, remember to take a low-fat snack — a piece of fruit, a nonfat yogurt, during the afternoon or before you leave work. And be sure you never, ever skip lunch.

Boredom. Many people eat because they are bored or lonely. They spend their evenings and weekends watching television. To satisfy their feeling of emptiness, they fill up on food. Of course, the food industry makes thinking about high-fat foods as easy as flicking on the TV. You can't help fantasizing about food you shouldn't eat because it pops out at you every ten minutes.

How about overcoming your boredom by taking up a hobby? It's never too late. How about photography, oil painting, or ceramics? Take an adult education course at your local high school or Y. What about square dancing or folk dancing? Join a barbershop quartet or a chess club. Work for your local politician or volunteer at your library or neighborhood hospital. Get out, meet people, get involved. You'll feel better about yourself and you won't have time to fixate on high-fat food.

Food Cues

Are you driven to eat by subconscious forces? Think about it. What makes you feel like eating besides hunger? Make a list in your mind. Do you react to the following food cues? When you sit down at your desk to work, are you immediately impelled to go to the vending machine for something to eat? When you turn on TV, do you automatically reach for a bowl of chips? When you talk on the phone, do you make forays into the refrigerator? Many people have told us that walking in their front door is the first food cue they encounter.

Solutions: Figure out your food cues and then figure out how to overcome them. If your subconscious thinks the best way to postpone working is to eat, bring a large bag of fruit to keep at the office. Nibble on bananas, apples, and oranges all day (while you work!) instead of the high-fat garbage offered in your vending machine. Don't turn on the TV, do something productive. Write your memoirs. Read. If reading makes you want to snack, make 10 cups of air-popped popcorn and munch away. If the kitchen offers too much temptation, talk on the phone in the living room.

Sabotage. When you decide to lose weight, does your boyfriend bring you a box of chocolates? Does your wife prepare your favorite strawberry pie? Does your husband take you out to dinner? Does your mother tell you you're getting too thin? Is this love? Whether your loved ones know it or not, this behavior is not without design — they want to thwart your new lifestyle changes. They may fear that a new, lean you will be attractive to others; a new, lean you may be more independent and not need them as much. They may feel threatened because they should be doing something about their own weight problem. They may just not want to find a grilled chicken breast on their plate instead of a lamb chop.

This ostensibly generous behavior is triply hard to resist. First, the gift is an irresistible treat. Of course you'd love to eat a box of Godiva chocolates or dine at a fine French restaurant. Second, a guilt trip comes along free of charge: "If you don't eat what I give you, you don't love me." Third, refusing the gift means an uncomfortable confrontation with the saboteur. But if you want to be a successful Chooser to Lose, you must resist, reject, and confront. Be strong. You can do it.

Communicate. The best way to effect a change is to communicate. Talk to the saboteurs. They may not even be aware of what they are doing. Tell them that you appreciate their thoughtfulness, but you are staying away from fat. You still love them, but at this moment losing weight and eating healthfully are the number-one priorities in your life. Tell them that you don't feel good being fat; you are ready to make changes and you need their help. They should bear with you and keep high-fat foods out of the house and be open to eating new low-fat dishes. If you are thinner and healthier, they will benefit. Ask them for their support.

If they don't get the message and continue to shower you with unwanted fat packages, get tougher. Say, "No thanks." If they brought you arsenic, would you eat it because they wanted you to? Tell them it's hard enough to change habits that you've developed and nurtured for all these years, you don't need to deal with their guilt trips, too. Ask them why they are trying to sabotage your efforts. If they still turn a deaf ear to your needs, don't give up your resolve. When you are a lean person glowing with self-confidence and good health, you will know why you were uncompromising in the pursuit of your new lifestyle.

Self-Sabotage. Does it turn out that you are your own best saboteur? Do you eat the mocha truffles your husband brought you to spare hurting his feelings, or do you just want an excuse to eat them? Do you prepare spareribs for your relatives because it is their favorite dish or because it is yours? Do you take your kids to a fast-food restaurant because it's convenient or do you want a Big Mac? Don't fool yourself. If any high-fat wind that comes along blows away your resolve, you aren't really interested in changing your lifestyle. If you *really* want to eat healthfully, you can.

People have told us that they went "off" *Choose to Lose* because their husband changed his job, their mother had dental work, their uncle Mo stubbed his toe. Impossible. *Choose to Lose* is an eating plan for life. It is not an exercise in starvation or balancing exchanges that you can follow only for a few weeks. When you follow *Choose to Lose,* you eat lots of healthy food. You reduce your fat, but you can still fit in an occasional high-fat favorite. If you go "off" *Choose to Lose,* it means you were never "on" it. In crisis situations, like having a child in the hos-

---

Psychology

The emphasis of *Choose to Lose* is not on restructuring psyches. The emphasis is on knowledge. Knowing you can eat what you want and becoming food-smart will remove a lot of psychological stumbling blocks. You may have developed feelings of inferiority and self-hate because you are overweight, but many of your deep-rooted psychological problems probably didn't cause you to become fat. Like millions of Americans, you were exposed to the American food system and didn't know the rules. Now you know the rules. You can take control and your self-esteem will grow as you shrink.

For those of you who are fat to avoid sex, fat because of self-hate, fat because of an overprotective parent or sexual abuse as a child, *Choose to Lose* will not rid you of these problems. You may find, however, that when the pounds start coming off easily and naturally without much thought, you will feel so much better about yourself, you'll be able to reach your goal — and stay at that size.

pital or moving to a new city, there is no reason to abandon *Choose to Lose*. You can still make wise choices. In fact, having control in this part of your life will help you cope with the rest of the chaos.

Boy Scouts, Move Over

The theme of this chapter is the Boy Scout's marching song: "Be Prepared." That's all it takes. Think ahead and you can face any eating situation and master it.

Remember:
1. The key to surviving every social situation is planning ahead.
2. Splurging: *Choose to Lose* allows you to splurge without guilt. By eating fewer fat calories than allowed on your Fat Budget, you can save up for special occasions.
3. Party Survival
   a. Eat a light snack before the party.
   b. Station yourself AWAY from the food.
   c. Make low-fat choices.
   d. Serve low-fat dishes at your own parties.
4. Restaurant Survival
   a. Choose a restaurant with low-fat options.
   b. Ask questions about preparation and ingredients.
   c. Specify exactly how you want your food prepared — be creative.
   d. Have sauces, dressings, gravies, toppings, and butter served on the side so you can regulate the amount you use.
   e. Eat with care (when you dine out once a week or more, it is no longer a special occasion justifying high-fat gluttony).
5. Work Survival
   a. Remove high-fat temptation from your work area.
   b. Take control in choosing restaurants, planning menus, or bringing food.
   c. Eat lunch.
   d. Have fruit, bagels, popcorn, pretzels, and other low-fat food around to snack on.
6. Home Survival
   a. Keep tempting high-fat foods out of your home.
   b. Stock up on delicious low-fat/high-carbohydrate foods.
   c. Eliminate causes for bingeing, such as fatigue, boredom, and food cues.

   d. Confront sabotage
     (1) Communicate with the saboteur.
     (2) Know thyself.
7. Repeat to yourself: **I MUST EAT TO LOSE. I MUST EAT TO LOSE. I MUST EAT TO LOSE. OF COURSE, I MUST EAT NUTRITIOUS, LOW-FAT FOODS TO LOSE.**

11. Exercise:
Is It Necessary?

"Thank you for saving my husband's life. Mike was overweight with a high triglyceride count, high cholesterol, family history of heart disease, and no exercise. A statistic waiting to happen. Your *Choose to Lose* book gave him the tools to change. He has lost 45 pounds . . . and he exercises *daily*. We eat mostly fish, legumes, grains, fruits, and vegetables. It is wonderful and *he likes it!*"

Sharon Darr, Beaverton, Oregon

EATING RIGHT + EXERCISE = PERFECTION

You're almost there. You now know how to modify your fat intake to lose weight. Soon you will be watching your clothes get baggier and baggier as you become slimmer and slimmer. To keep *you* from getting baggier and baggier as you change your eating habits, you will need to indulge in an activity you may have tried to avoid — *exercise*.

Relax. We are not proposing marathon running, Olympic swimming, 2000 pushups six times a day. We are suggesting that you walk at least 20 to 30 minutes every day. Is that so bad?

LET'S HEAR IT FOR EXERCISE

Exercise Builds and Preserves Muscle

Exercise will help you lose weight as well as benefit your health and make you feel good.

As we discussed in Chapter 1, exercise helps you lose weight because exercise builds muscle and muscle burns fat. The more muscle you have, the more fat-burning capacity you have.

If you don't exercise, the muscle is broken down and not rebuilt. The protein released from the muscle is burned instead of fat stored in the

157

adipose tissue. Exercise protects your muscle from being broken down and burned for energy. By exercising you force your body to burn fat from the fat stores instead of protein from the muscle tissue.

Exercise Raises Your Metabolic Rate

Exercise increases your metabolic rate, the rate at which you burn calories. Not only does your metabolic rate increase *while* you are exercising, there is evidence (though it is somewhat controversial) that your metabolic rate *remains elevated* for a number of hours *after* you finish exercising. If this is true, then you continue to burn off calories at an accelerated rate even after you stop exercising.

Fat but Not Overweight

If you do not exercise when you reduce your fat intake, you will lose muscle tissue instead of fat tissue. You can end up weighing less but being fatter; that is, a higher percentage of your weight is fat. "So what," you say. "As long as I weigh less, who cares what percentage is what?" You *should* care. Being fatter and having less lean body mass puts you at greater risk of regaining weight because you have less metabolically active muscle tissue to burn off the fat you eat.

Losing Pounds Doesn't Always Make You Thin

To make this concept clearer, let's look at George and Henry. Initially, George and Henry both weighed 180 pounds and both were 30 percent fat (54 pounds of body fat). They both lost 20 pounds, but because George exercised he lost 25 pounds of fat and gained 5 pounds of muscle. Sedentary Henry lost 4 pounds of fat and 16 pounds of muscle. If you subtract George's fat loss from his original body fat (54 lbs − 25 lbs = 29 pounds of fat), you will find that George is now 18 percent fat (29 lbs body fat ÷ 160 pounds total weight = 18% body fat) and considered lean. Although Henry also lost 20 pounds, his fat loss (4 lbs) is much less than George's, making his percentage of body fat considerable (54 lbs of total body fat − 4 lbs = 50 lbs of body fat ÷ 160 lb total weight = 31% body fat). Henry is fatter than when he started even though he weighs less than he did.

George and Henry may weigh the same, but George has much more metabolically active muscle and much less metabolically inactive fat. George will have an easier time maintaining his new weight.

BEFORE WEIGHT LOSS	GEORGE (EXERCISE)	HENRY (SEDENTARY)
Total weight	180 lb	180 lb
Body fat	54 lb	54 lb
Percent body fat	30%	30%
AFTER WEIGHT LOSS		
Total weight	160 lb	160 lb
Body fat lost	25 lb	4 lb
Body fat remaining	29 lb	50 lb
Percent body fat	18%	31%

This graphic illustration shows why the scale gives no meaningful information and may even mislead you into thinking you are making no progress. If you change your sedentary ways and begin to exercise, you will build new muscle. Muscle has weight. At first, the scale may show you are actually gaining weight. But this weight (new muscle) is fat-burning tissue and soon it will burn the fat away. People who weigh in daily may get discouraged and stop just as everything is beginning to work. Once again, do yourself a favor. Throw away your scale or give it to someone you wish to torture. You'll know you are losing fat when your clothes get looser and you fit into smaller sizes.

Give a Cheer for Exercise

In addition to helping you become lean, regular aerobic exercise provides the following important benefits:

- Cardiovascular fitness — helps protect you against fatal heart attacks
- Helps protect you against osteoporosis (if weight-bearing)
- Helps protect you against some forms of cancer
- Lowers blood pressure
- Helps you cope with anxiety, stress, and tension
- Relieves insomnia
- Enhances mood — makes you feel good
- Strengthens, tones, and shapes muscles
- Increases stamina

WHAT IS THIS THING CALLED EXERCISE?

There are three types of exercise that are crucial for long-term health and peak performance. These are aerobic exercise, resistance or strength training, and stretching. We will discuss resistance training and stretching at the end of the chapter, but for fat loss, you need to focus your attention on aerobic exercise.

AEROBIC EXERCISE

Aerobic exercise is repetitive and rhythmic. It includes walking, jogging, continuous aerobic dancing, biking, and swimming. It does not include lifting weights, bowling, golf, tennis, or most other competitive sports because they are start-and-stop activities.

Aerobic exercise need not be strenuous nor does it require any athletic ability. But in order to realize the maximum weight loss benefits, you should do at least 20 to 30 minutes of nonstop aerobic exercise every day.

Consult your physician before you begin an exercise program if you are over forty, have heart trouble, experience pain during or after exercise, or suffer from arthritis, dizzy spells, or any condition that would lead you to believe you should consult your physician.

Why Aerobic Exercise?

Back to the science. When you eat carbohydrates your body breaks them down into glucose, a simple sugar. Some of that glucose is burned immediately, some is stored as glycogen. When you exercise in spurts and bursts, as when you play tennis, you body burns mainly glucose for quick energy. Burning glucose has no effect on removing fat from your fat stores. In contrast, when you exercise aerobically for more than 20 minutes, your body burns mostly fat from the fat stores.

How Long Should I Exercise?

When you exercise you burn a mix of fuels. During the first 20 minutes you burn mostly carbohydrates. After 20 minutes you burn more and more fat. The longer you exercise nonstop the more fat you burn. For fat loss, it is more effective to walk for 40 minutes than to run for 15.

How Often?

If you exercise every day, you can't put it off until tomorrow because you are already exercising tomorrow. Just make exercise a normal part of your daily routine, like brushing your teeth.

How Intensely?

For fat loss, it is better to exercise longer and less intensely than intensely for a short time. When you exercise intensely you burn more glucose than fat. You can tell if you are exercising at the correct intensity if you can carry on a normal conversation without getting out of breath.

The Number-One Choice: Walking

The best, easiest, and safest exercise is plain old walking, which almost anyone can do almost anywhere. This is the least expensive and least punishing exercise. You need no special facility or special equipment except good walking shoes. The risk of injury is negligible. So go to it. Work up to 30 minutes a day. You need not walk briskly, but you should not stop and start. In other words, walking in a mall and stopping to buy a sweater doesn't count. For the greatest aerobic effect, bend your elbows at a 90-degree angle and move them straight back and forth, slightly brushing your sides as you walk.

If you are overweight, you may find that walking literally takes your breath away. Don't give up. Begin by walking for 5 minutes, slowly at first. Stop for a few moments when you get out of breath. But keep walking. And continue to walk — a little faster and a little longer each day. As you get thinner, you will find that walking will become easier.

Aerobic Dance

Many local YMCAs, hospitals, adult education programs, and spas offer aerobic dancing classes. Aerobic dancing is fun and, for some, paying for a class that meets on a schedule is a strong incentive to exercise. These classes are offered at both low-impact and high-impact levels. Even if you are not Jane Fonda, there is a class you can handle. Be sure, however, that you keep moving even when the music stops. Starting and stopping will cause your body to burn more glucose and less fat.

> Be careful. It is easy to injure yourself doing aerobic dancing.

Video Exercise

If you prefer exercising in the privacy of your home, an extensive array of exercise and aerobic workout tapes are available at your local video store and through catalogues. They range from low-impact to strenuous and are adjusted to different ages and exercise goals. Try to schedule your video exercise at the same time each day. Make it part of your routine.

Bicycling

Riding a bicycle outdoors in fair weather is a visual and emotional treat as well as excellent exercise. If your neighborhood has accessible bike paths or streets that are safe for riding, and you enjoy biking, budget half an hour of bicycling into your daily routine.

However, if the weather or terrain of your area does not encourage biking out of doors, a stationary bicycle is an excellent substitute. You can do it at any time and in any weather. For those with bad feet, bikes offer the advantage of supporting your weight as you exercise. The drawback to riding a stationary bike is that it is boring. Some exercisers overcome this problem by watching TV or reading while they bike.

Swimming

Swimming is a particularly effective exercise for those who find walking difficult. Swimmers use muscles in both the upper and lower body, but their weight is supported by the water. The disadvantage of swimming is that, as most of us do not own our own pools, we must fight kiddies for swimming lanes in the summer and endure overchlorinated indoor pools in the winter. As with any exercise, start slowly and work up to swimming 20 to 30 minutes of laps five times a week.

Jogging

We do not recommend jogging for most people. Jogging incurs a high risk of injury to backs, knees, legs, and ankles. Walking is much safer and more effective in terms of fat loss.

Trampolining

For about $20, you can buy a mini-trampoline (about 3 feet in diameter) that sits about 9 inches above the ground. Rain or shine, snow or sleet, you can jog in place in comfort with little or no risk of damaging yourself.

Exercise Equipment

We have just described the safest and easiest forms of aerobic exercise that require the least equipment and expense and can be easily incorporated into anyone's routine and budget. Of course, you can buy exercise equipment such as treadmills, stationary rowing machines, and cross-country skiing machines. All of these machines provide perfectly acceptable aerobic exercise if used properly and regularly.

Tip: Don't buy cheap exercise equipment. It won't last. It was constructed for people who like the idea of exercise but not the actual practice of it.

Combination Exercise

You may choose to swim in the summer and walk or bike in the winter or do aerobic dancing in the morning and walk in the evening. Whatever exercise or combination of exercises you choose, be sure you do some aerobic exercise every day. Soon exercise will become a part of your routine, like taking a shower or bath, and you will miss it sorely when circumstances force you to forgo it.

The BEST Exercise

As one exercise equipment salesman told us, the best exercise is the one that you will continue to do. And only you know which one that is. Experiment. Try a variety of exercises until you find the one or the combination that suits you.

But Not for Me

"Of course I know how important exercise is and I'd love to do it but . . ."

☐ I'm too busy to exercise.
☐ Exercise takes time away from my family.
☐ I get sweaty.
☐ I look funny in leotards.
☐ I get out of breath.
☐ It's too dark, too light, too cold, too wet, to exercise.
☐ My Aunty Syl is coming to town.
☐ I (fill in the blank)_____.

Have you found your favorite excuse(s) for not exercising? Here's why your excuse is no excuse:

☐ **I'm too busy to exercise.** No one is too busy to exercise. You can always fit it in. Get up 30 minutes early and ride a stationary bike or take a walk before you leave for work. Walk during your lunch hour. Take a walk before you go to bed. What do you do that is more important than exercising? Watch TV? Work overtime? Exercise is essential to your well-being, both physical and mental.

☐ **Exercise takes time from my family.** Include your family when you exercise. Take a walk after dinner with your daughter, son, husband, wife. Leave the car at home and walk your spouse to and from the bus, subway, or train. Take a bike ride with your family on the weekend. Exercise won't hurt them a bit.

☐ **I get sweaty.** Walking should not make you sweaty. If your chosen exercise causes excessive perspiration, exercise at a place where showering is possible.

☐ **I look funny in leotards.** Almost everyone looks funny in leotards. They exaggerate what you want to flatten and flatten what you want to exaggerate. Don't wear leotards. Wear comfortable shorts. If you look funny in shorts, who cares? The exercise is for you. And if you eat right and exercise, you will soon look great in shorts.

☐ **I get out of breath.** Take it easy. After all, if you haven't exercised in a long time you are probably out of shape. If you are overweight you are carrying a lot of extra pounds. Start slowly, a few minutes a day, and work up to 30 minutes of walking a day. However, you should check with your physician before you begin any exercise program.

☐ **It's too dark, too light, too cold, too wet, to exercise.** Come on! You can find a solution to any problem if you try. If the weather is bad, take a walk in a covered mall, exercise at home on a stationary bike, mini-trampoline, NordicTrack, rowing machine, or treadmill, or pop an exercise tape into your VCR and move with the beat.

☐ **My Aunty Syl is coming to town, I have a big job to finish, my son skinned his knee, it's my dentist's birthday.** You make time for what is important to you. If someone gave you a free ticket to a football game or a concert, you'd be able to fit it in. You must fit exercise in. Aerobic exercise is an essential component of good health and weight control.

TIPS TO KEEP YOU ON THE STRAIGHT AND NARROW

It is so easy to put off exercise. The following tips will help you incorporate exercise into your life and keep it there.

1. Make Exercise a Part of Your Routine

Schedule exercise at a specific time so you will really do it. Reserve 30 minutes every weekday morning for a ride on your stationary bicycle. Walk for 30 minutes every day after dinner. Work out to a videotape every morning at 7:00. Make exercise a habit. Do it even if you're not in the mood. Force yourself. You'll be glad you did.

Walking Fits in Everywhere. Incorporating walking into your schedule is probably the easiest and most practical exercise program. Make it an integral part of your lifestyle, rather than an activity grafted onto an already busy schedule. For example, walk to work or partway by getting off the bus early or parking your car 20 to 30 minutes away.

Walk on Your Lunch Break. Walk for 30 minutes at lunchtime. It's good to get out of the office and into the fresh air. You can combine the walk with errands. But remember, the exercise *must be continuous*. Walking 5 minutes to the bank and standing in line for 15 minutes doesn't count as exercise.

2. Do Exercise You Enjoy

Choose an exercise you enjoy or make the exercise you do more enjoyable. If you find a stationary bike too strenuous, walk. If you find walking boring, plug in earphones, turn on your Walkman, and listen to your favorite music or talk show. Slide in language tapes and teach yourself Italian. Watch television as you stride along your treadmill, ride your bike, or jump on your mini-trampoline.

3. Exercise with a Buddy

Exercising with another person (spouse, child, neighbor, friend) can be more fun than exercising alone. Instead of spending an hour every evening gathered around the kitchen table nibbling and chatting, spend the time taking a walk and chatting. Let it become a ritual. Exercising with a friend can also give you the added nudge you need. How can you say, "Sorry, I'd rather sleep," when Barbara comes by to drive you to the nine o'clock aerobics class?

However, if you exercise with a partner, do not use his or her absence (due to illness, other commitments) as an excuse to stop. Either find another partner or go it alone. If you know you don't have the discipline to exercise on your own, join a spa or exercise group. But do whatever it takes.

4. Wear the Best Equipment: Good Shoes

Be sure to wear comfortable shoes with good support. You need not buy $125 sneakers with bubble-filled soles and foam-layered heels especially constructed for walking on pavement in temperate climates. In fact, you might find tie-up leather shoes more comfortable for walking because they don't get as hot as sneakers. Whatever type of shoe you prefer, make sure it fits and offers support.

ADD STRENGTH OR RESISTANCE TRAINING + STRETCHING

Aerobic exercise is essential to facilitate your fat loss as well as to keep your body in good working order throughout your life. Here are two more types of exercise that will help you to remain independent, strong, and flexible as you age.

Strength or Resistance Training

As its name implies, strength training is exercise that builds up your strength by building up your muscles. Strength training involves lifting weights such as dumbbells and/or using a Nautilus or multigym equipment.

You probably are amused to imagine yourself as a muscle-bound body builder and wonder why we think this form of exercise is so important. We are not urging you to become Mr. or Ms. Universe, but many adults, especially sedentary ones, lose muscle through disuse and, as a result, when they get old they lose the strength to lift objects, to walk distances, sometimes even just to move across the room. If you want to be independent through old age, you need to start building your muscles now. You don't have to lift heavy weights or spend hours at the gym every day. In fact, you should give your muscles a rest every other day. To learn the correct way to lift weights, to avoid hurting yourself and to maximize the benefit, you need to consult a personal trainer, get guidance at a gym, fitness center, or YMCA, or read an appropriate book.

Stretching

As you age, you lose your flexibility. You get stiff and may find moving your body difficult and sometimes painful. So to keep yourself flexible and limber for your entire life, you need to stretch your muscles. This won't take much time and it will feel good. Again, you need to get professional advice or read an appropriate book so you know your stretching exercises will not hurt you and that you are getting the most for your effort.

THE MESSAGE

Daily aerobic exercise will both help you lose weight and keep it off. It will enhance your life. Start now. Schedule it in. Add strength training and stretching. You'll be glad you did — and your body and psyche will be ecstatic.

Recommended Reading

To learn more about exercise, check the reference list for Chapter 11 on pages 461–62. In particular, the books by Kenneth Cooper, M.D., are an excellent resource.

Remember:
1. Regular aerobic exercise is a necessary part of *Choose to Lose* because it:
   a. protects your muscle from being burned for energy and builds new muscle, which burns fat.

   b. maximizes the burning of stored fat.
   c. increases your metabolism.
   d. increases your energy expenditure.
   e. helps you reach and maintain your desirable and healthy body weight.
   f. improves cardiovascular fitness, reduces risk of osteoporosis (if weight-bearing) and other diseases, and enhances your sense of well-being.
2. Walking is a safe, convenient, and inexpensive form of aerobic exercise. Alternatives include bicycling, swimming, rowing, and aerobic dance.
3. Make exercise a regular part of your daily schedule.
4. Repeat to yourself: **I MUST EAT TO LOSE. I MUST EAT TO LOSE. I MUST EAT TO LOSE. OF COURSE, I MUST EAT NUTRITIOUS, LOW-FAT FOODS TO LOSE.**

12. Ensuring a Balanced Diet

"This is absolutely the best program available for *anyone* wishing to eat healthy. Weight loss is a side benefit of how one feels while on your diet."

Thomas and Pauline Going, Chesapeake, Virginia

"I feel very confident that the pounds lost will not come back since I don't feel I 'dieted' but rather 'ate healthier.'"

Mark Mandel, Erie, Pennsylvania

CHOOSE TO LOSE is not just about reducing fat in your diet. It is also about eating an abundance of nutrient-dense, delicious foods. Eating a well-balanced diet should be easy to do if you replace your excess fat calories with fruits, vegetables, whole-grains, and nonfat dairy.

THE FOOD GUIDE PYRAMID

The Food Guide Pyramid was proposed by the Department of Agriculture to replace the original four basic food groups wheel. Although both diagrams stress the importance of eating foods from all groups, the pyramid (page 170) emphasizes the importance of eating more of some foods than others. The base gives you a healthy foundation. You should consume whole-grain breads and cereals, rice, and pasta pictured in the base of the pyramid in greatest quantities, followed by vegetables and fruits. Milk products and meat may be eaten in smaller amounts, and fats, oils, and sweets (not even part of the original basic food groups) should be eaten sparingly. In general, Americans have turned this pyramid on its head and have, as a result, been totally out of balance for years.

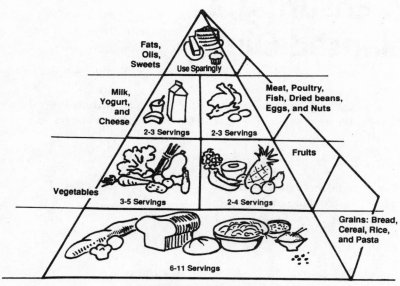

Food Guide Pyramid

Meeting the Recommendations

To maintain your health it is essential that you eat at least the minimum recommended number of servings of these foods, as illustrated on the Food Guide Pyramid (at the end of the chapter you will find a table that summarizes the recommended servings and serving sizes of foods from each group). Just meet these standards and you are set. Consuming at least 6 to 11 servings of grains, 2 to 4 servings of fruits, 3 to 5 servings of vegetables, and 2 to 3 servings of nonfat or low-fat dairy ensures that you will get enough vitamins, minerals, protein, and fiber for good health. It also means you won't be hungry. You will be too full from all these healthy, nutritious foods to have room for ersatz fat-free fluff or high-fat junk.

WHOLE-GRAIN BREADS, CEREALS, RICE, AND PASTA

For good health and weight control, you should consume 6 to 11 servings of whole-grain breads, cereals, rice, and pasta per day. (See Table 5 on page 175 for sizes of servings.)

The following whole-grain products are rich in starch, fiber, protein, thiamine, riboflavin, niacin, folic acid, vitamin E, iron, phosphorus, magnesium, zinc, and other trace minerals. Choose from:

Brown rice	Oatmeal	Whole-wheat bread
Buckwheat groats	Pumpernickel bread	and rolls
Bulgur		Whole-wheat pasta

The following enriched-grain products contain starch and protein, but thiamine, riboflavin, niacin, and iron have been added. Eat these foods less often. Whole-grain products are far more nutritious.

Bagels	French bread	Pasta
Cereal (ready-to-eat)	Noodles	Rice

VEGETABLES

Vegetables contribute vital fiber, vitamins, and minerals to your diet. They should be varied and eaten in abundance, at least 3 to 5 servings a day.

The best way to prepare vegetables is to steam them for a short time so they are tender but still crunchy (overcooking causes loss of vitamins and taste). In restaurants, beware of vegetables cooked in butter or drowned in high-fat sauces. To keep them delicious, healthy, and non-fattening, ask that vegetables be steamed with no fat and served with sauces on the side.

Dark green vegetables should be included several times a week. They are an excellent source of vitamins A and C, riboflavin, folic acid, iron, and magnesium. Choose from:

Beet greens	Chicory	Romaine lettuce
Bok choy	Endive	Spinach
Broccoli*	Escarole	Turnip greens
Chard	Kale	Watercress

Deep yellow vegetables are an excellent source of vitamin A. Choose from:

Carrots	Sweet potatoes
Pumpkin	Winter squash

---

*This cruciferous vegetable may reduce your risk of some cancers.

Other vegetables also contribute varying amounts of vitamins and minerals. Choose from:

Artichokes	Chinese cabbage	Okra
Asparagus	Cucumbers	Onions
Beets	Eggplant	Radishes
Brussels sprouts*	Green beans	Summer squash
Cabbage*	Green peppers	Tomatoes
Cauliflower*	Lettuce	Turnips*
Celery	Mushrooms	Zucchini

Starchy vegetables are rich in starch, fiber, vitamin B_6, folic acid, iron, magnesium, potassium, and phosphorus. Choose from:

Corn	Potatoes (white)
Green peas	Rutabaga*
Lima beans	Sweet potatoes (rich in vitamin A)

Dried beans and peas are excellent sources of protein, soluble fiber (known to reduce blood cholesterol levels), calcium, magnesium, phosphorus, potassium, iron, and zinc.

Choose from these dried beans and peas, which should be included as a starchy vegetable several times a week. Dried beans and peas are a healthy substitute for meat, poultry, fish, and eggs. They may be included in both the vegetable and meat food groups in the Food Guide Pyramid.

Black beans	Lentils	Split peas
Black-eyed peas	Lima beans	Other types of dried
Chickpeas	Navy beans	beans and peas
Kidney beans	Pinto beans	

FRUITS

Fruits contain vitamins, minerals, and fiber. Eat a variety — at least 2 to 4 servings of fruit daily. Have fruits available around the house instead of nuts, cookies, crackers, or candies. Bananas, oranges, pears, apples, strawberries, peaches, nectarines, cantaloupes . . . all fruits make sweet or crunchy treats. Take a bag of your favorite fruits to

---

*These cruciferous vegetables may reduce your risk of some cancers.

work: when hunger or boredom strikes, dip into the bag instead of heading for the vending machine and its high-fat temptations.

Citrus, melon, and berries are rich sources of vitamin C, other vitamins, folic acid, and minerals. Choose from:

Blueberries	Lemon	Tangerine
Cantaloupe	Orange	Watermelon
Grapefruit	Orange juice	Other citrus fruits,
Grapefruit juice	Raspberries	melons, and
Honeydew melon	Strawberries	berries
Kiwi fruit		

Other fruits are also a rich source of vitamins and minerals. Choose from:

Apples	Nectarines	Prunes
Apricots	Peaches	Raisins
Bananas	Pears	Other fruit
Cherries	Pineapples	Fruit juices
Grapes	Plums	

MILK, YOGURT, AND CHEESE

Milk products are rich in protein, calcium, riboflavin, vitamin B_{12}, magnesium, vitamin A, thiamine, and, if fortified, vitamin D. Milk products need not be high in fat to contain high amounts of calcium. In fact, skim milk contains slightly more calcium than its high-fat counterparts. Do not skimp on low- or nonfat milk products. Even as an adult, you need all the nutrients they supply. Choose from these foods daily:

Buttermilk	Low- or nonfat yogurt
Nonfat or low-fat (1%)	Skim milk
cottage cheese	

Calcium is also found in dark green vegetables.

Women, especially prepubescent girls, need more calcium than men in order to avoid developing the bone-thinning disease osteoporosis.

MEAT, POULTRY, FISH, DRIED BEANS, EGGS, AND NUTS

Meats, poultry, fish, and eggs are good sources of protein, phosphorus, niacin, iron, zinc, and vitamins B_6 and B_{12}. However, Americans eat more meat than is necessary for good health. Limit your meat consumption to no more than 4 to 6 ounces a day.

Choose often from the following:

White meat chicken with no skin	Fish
White meat turkey with no skin	Shellfish

Choose less often (or not at all) from the following:

Beef	Lamb	Veal
Ham	Pork	Eggs

Eat organ meats such as liver, pancreas, and brain rarely, if at all. They are loaded with cholesterol. Pancreas and brain are also high in fat.

Cooked dried beans or peas, as well as nuts and seeds, may be substituted for meat, poultry, fish, and eggs. However, as these plant foods lack vitamin B_{12}, this vitamin must be supplied by other foods. Nuts and seeds are high in fat and should be eaten in moderation, if at all.

WARNING: Before you count a food as meeting your grain requirement, be sure it is mostly complex carbohydrate. For example, don't count a croissant as a grain. A croissant is made of flour (complex carbohydrate) and lots of butter (fat — about 110 calories of fat). Croissants are not exactly in the complex carbohydrates category. Don't include cookies, cake, or crackers, either. Don't include foods that have all the nutrients processed out of them, such as pretzels. (There is nothing wrong with eating a pretzel or two, but it isn't really adding to your health.)

Don't count ice cream or frozen yogurt as dairy. They are often more sugar than dairy. Remember, you want to meet the Food Guide Pyramid requirements to benefit your health, not to impress anyone. You want to eat an abundance of foods that are rich in fiber, vitamins, and minerals — foods that will enhance your long-term health.

Remember:

1. To ensure a well-balanced and healthy diet, you should consume daily at least:
   a. 6–11 servings of grains

Table 5. Minimum Basic Nutritional Requirements

FOOD GROUP	RECOMMENDED	DAILY SERVINGS	SERVING SIZE
Fruits and			½ to 1 cup
Vegetables	All fruits* and vegetables**	2–4	1 fruit
		3–5	½ to 1 cup
Dairy		2–3 (adults)	
		3–4 (children)	
	1% low-fat cottage cheese		½ cup
	Dry-curd cottage cheese		½ cup
	Skim milk		1 cup
	1% low-fat milk		1 cup
	Nonfat yogurt		1 cup
Grain		6–11	
	Whole-grain bread		1 slice
	Bagels		1
	Rice		½ cup
	Bulgur		½ cup
	Whole-grain cereals		1 oz
	Pasta		½ cup
Meat		2	
Poultry	Chicken breast w/o skin**		(2–3 oz)
	Turkey breast w/o skin		
Fish	All fin fish**		(3–4 oz)
	Shellfish**		
	Tuna, water-packed		
	Sardines (in fish oil)		
Meat			
alternatives	Dried beans, peas, lentils		½ cup

*Fresh preferred over canned.
**Not fried.

    b. 3–5 servings of vegetables

    c. 2–4 servings of fruits

    d. 2–3 servings of nonfat or low-fat dairy.

2. You should consume 25–30 grams of fiber daily.

3. Repeat to yourself: **I MUST EAT TO LOSE. I MUST EAT TO LOSE. I MUST EAT TO LOSE. OF COURSE, I MUST EAT NUTRITIOUS, LOW-FAT FOODS TO LOSE.**

13. *Choose to Lose* for Children

"I can't believe how easy good nutrition and good eating habits are to obtain. My children are now interested in what they eat. I am a true advocate of *Choose to Lose*. So is my husband."

Mary Rose Robbins, Derry, New Hampshire

IF YOU are overweight, there is an excellent chance that your children and your spouse are too. You probably share the same taste in foods. Start your children on the thin road early; good eating habits begin in childhood. Don't let your plump toddlers become your chubby children and your obese adolescents. It's not fun to be a fat kid. Fat children are often ostracized. Fat children often suffer discrimination. Fat children almost always become fat adults. If you live *Choose to Lose* and bring your family into your new lifestyle, your children will grow up lean and healthy. It sounds easy and it is. But it will take an effort on your part. There's a big, fat world out there, waiting to corrupt your children, and you will have to give them the tools to keep it at bay.

Fitting into a Fat Culture

Your children are not unique in being overweight. The United States is filled with fat kids. More than one-fourth of all children are obese.

Why not? Your children became fat because they were born into a fat, sedentary culture. They entered a world where fast foods, snack foods, convenience foods, and carry-out are the basic fare. Kids no longer run up to the rec center every afternoon for a pickup game of softball, football, or basketball. They are driven to organized soccer games once a week. Walking or riding a bike is unheard of. Children are chauffeured from activity to activity. Television programs and video games offer hours of fascinating inactivity. No wonder so many children are overweight and physically unfit.

176

Facts about Obesity in Children and Teenagers Today

- Between 25 and 30 percent of children are obese, about a 54 percent increase in the last 15 years.
- Between 20 and 25 percent of teenagers are obese, about a 40 percent increase in the last 15 years.
- Between 50 and 95 percent of obese adolescents become obese adults. The chances of an obese teen attaining normal weight in adulthood is 1 in 28.
- Obese children and teenagers have an increased prevalence of irregular periods, hypertension, respiratory problems, and hyperinsulinemia. They often suffer from peer and adult discrimination, social isolation, low self-esteem, depression, and a negative body image.

Lifestyle Puts Your Children at Risk

The two main reasons they became fat and flabby — eating a high-fat diet and lack of exercise — are lifestyle behaviors that, if carried through adulthood, will increase their risks for all sorts of horrendous adult diseases. Even normal-weight adults are more likely to suffer heart disease if they were fat children. Does the future look bleak? Before you gather up your children and jump off the nearest cliff, rest assured that turning the situation around is not difficult, and will even be fun and delicious. What's more, it will benefit not only your overweight children but you and the rest of your family as well.

Bring in the New

The most effective way to change your overweight children's eating habits is to ease the whole family into a new low-fat regime. Do this subtly and gradually. Don't single out and focus attention on the child with the problem. Make low-fat eating a family affair. Prepare the *Choose to Lose* and *Eater's Choice* recipes, but make no grand announcement that you are cooking healthfully. Just present the finished product and, within a few minutes, you'll hear requests for seconds.

Real Men Eat Low-Fat. If you have a recalcitrant spouse — "Diet food is for the birds!" — don't tell him that you are cooking low-fat. Just do it. Serve him *Bar-B-Que Chicken* (page 231). He'll lick the plate clean. Make him *Potato Skins* (page 241). He'll ask for seconds and thirds. When he realizes that the large watermelon he called his belly has become flat as a board, that his cholesterol has dropped 50 points, and that he has never eaten so well, he won't complain.

Involve the Troops. If you happen to have a family that will look on a new healthy lifestyle as an adventure, disregard the last paragraphs. Involve them. Have them choose low-fat recipes. Better yet, have them prepare the recipes, too.

Reward the Whole Family. Don't worry about resistance. The food will sell itself. You'll love *Tomato-Rice Soup* (page 222) because it's so quick and easy to make. They'll love it because it tastes so good. They'll think *Keema Matar* on *Indian Rice* (*Eater's Choice*) sounds strange, but watch them vie for the last biteful.

Add new vegetables to your repertoire. Steam them until they are crisp, but still tender. Don't even think butter and cheese. Reduce the added fat until you are using almost none. Try low-fat soups. They're filling and satisfying and will keep your kids from leaving the table hungry for high-fat snacks.

For your daughters in particular, be sure to include lots of low- or nonfat dairy and green, leafy vegetables. The years of childhood and adolescence are the time females need to consume a lot of calcium to build strong bones to reduce their risk of osteoporosis later in life. When you're old, eating calcium has less effect on preventing osteoporosis.

If the most advanced cooking you have ever attempted is opening a frozen-food carton, get ready for a pleasurable experience. Cooking is fun. Have a positive attitude and you will enjoy it. It's one job where you always get a reward — your culinary creation.

Rewards of Eating Together. A major reason people eat so poorly is that they eat on the run. They grab a burger and fries at a fast-food restaurant. They gobble up Chinese food out of paper cartons. Their porcelain is Styrofoam. Their silver is plastic. They never really enjoy a meal because they don't focus on the food. They drive and eat, watch TV and eat, read and eat. Sad. Life doesn't have to be that way. One of the joys of eating real food is that you sit down as a family and eat together. You actually talk to one another. Sitting together at the same time may seem impossible as everyone has a different meeting, sporting event, club date, to attend. Again, all you have to do is plan. Instead of scheduling yourself (and your children) to the hilt so you have no time to breathe, make dinner with the family a priority.

The Snack Law

VERY IMPORTANT!! Make sure that your kids don't take snacks — even healthy snacks — too close to dinner. A full child will reject all but junk food. A hungry child will be willing to try your luscious, low-fat meals. If you have a fussy eater, snacking may be the reason.

You're the Boss. Even though you have introduced a divine cuisine and your children are hungry, you may meet resistance. BE FIRM. If they balk at a new type of soup or chicken dish, ask them to try just a bite. They'll change their tune after a taste. If they refuse to eat, don't force them, but don't make them another dish or feed them later. You will only be rewarding their defiant behavior and spoil their chance to discover how wonderful low-fat food can be. Don't get into a power struggle over food. Look at it this way. Not eating dinner one night won't kill them, but eating a diet of high-fat snacks may.

Keep Out the Old

Don't sabotage your efforts to introduce healthy eating by allowing high-fat competition to interfere. Don't bring high-fat chips, crackers, cookies, ice cream, cake, cold cuts, into the house. Don't let your kids bring them in either. They don't need it. Tell them your house is a junk food–free zone. If you hear complaints, remember — you're the boss. Do keep plenty of fruit, nonfat flavored yogurt, carrot sticks, nonfat pretzels, and air-popped popcorn for them to snack on (but not too close to dinner).

TV: A High-Fat Habit

Television is a convenience just like fast-food and frozen dinners. You plop your children in front of the TV and can forget about them for hours. But watching TV is a fattening habit. Scientific studies have shown that the prevalence of obesity in twelve- to seventeen-year-olds increases by 2 percent for each hour of TV watched daily. This is no surprise. Children who watch TV are getting no exercise except for the constant movement of their hand from the bowl of chips to their mouth. Limit the amount of time your children sit in front of the television if you want them to be lean and healthy.

Just Say No. The ads on Saturday morning cartoons are not for carrots or whole-wheat bread. Limiting your children's TV-watching time will probably also limit their high-fat demands. Remember, your goals for your children are not the same as the goals of the advertising industry. Just because your kid has been brainwashed to ask for a certain candy bar, why should you buy it? When your children whine that they want that cute Lunchables Fun Pack (170–260 fat calories) or the fried chicken frozen dinner with cartoons on the front (320 fat calories), just say no. Would you buy them bars of strychnine? You don't have to give them everything they want. Think of their health first. They'll still love you even if you don't buy them everything they ask for.

But Not for Me

You may be reading this section and instead of fantasizing about all the wonderful food you will be eating, you are thinking, "I can't do this. I don't have time." If you are truly interested in helping your overweight children become thin and in ensuring your family's long-term good health, you have to make time. You can do it. It just takes planning. Plan ahead so that you have lots of good, healthy food to make satisfying meals. They don't have to be elaborate. Enlist your family's help in preparing meals and cleaning up. You will love your new life.

A MORE DIRECT APPROACH

In addition to quietly changing your family's meals and snacks into nutritious treats, you may want to confront your children's weight problem more directly. This may be tricky. Never make children feel that they are bad or inferior because they are overweight. Be matter-of-fact. Remember at all times that this is *their* problem. Eating is one area over which they have complete control. You cannot force them to eat right, but you can help them develop skills to make better choices. If, at any time, you feel a resistance to your help, stop. Weight loss is an area where pressuring and pushing has disastrous consequences.

For some of you, a nonintervention policy will take a strong resolve. Either you have been fat all your life and you don't want your children to suffer the emotional pain you have or you are thin and don't want your children to be unhappy. In either case, it doesn't matter what you want. The child has to want to lose weight. Let go and your child will be much more successful.

Teens

If you have overweight teenagers, encourage them to read this book. (Even thin teenagers can learn a lot from reading *Choose to Lose.*) Knowing that fat makes fat and how much fat lurks in the food they eat will have a profound effect on their food choices. By giving your teens control over their diet, *Choose to Lose* will free you from being a food cop and improve your relationship. You may even find your roles reversed with your teens keeping you true to *your* Fat Budget.

If your teens have stopped growing, they can use the adult tables in this book to determine their own Fat Budget. Otherwise, they can read the following instructions on determining a Fat Budget.

Children over Nine

If your children are capable and interested, try to explain why fat makes them fat and carbohydrates don't. Use the instructions on page 182 and work with them to determine their Fat Budgets. Then introduce them to the fast-food and snack sections of the Food Tables for a real eye-opener. Go over other relevant sections of the Food Tables to give them a better understanding of why their food choices are so important. Use pages 121–34 to teach them how to read food labels.

Children under Nine

You may want to determine a Fat Budget and keep food records of your young child's intake so you know how much fat he or she is really consuming. This could be helpful in identifying foods or food patterns to change. However, if keeping track means counting the peas on his spoon as they enter his mouth, a more casual approach will probably be more effective.

DETERMINING A FAT BUDGET

Because there are no ideal height-weight tables for children as there are for adults, you will have to figure out your child's Fat Budget or, if she is old enough she can figure out her own. You will start by discovering approximately how many total calories she eats a day. Then you will take 20 percent of that number to determine her Fat Budget.

1. Keep a record (or have your child keep a record) of your child's food intake for 3 days (2 weekdays and 1 weekend day). Read "The Nitty-Gritty of How to Keep a Food Record" (page 448) to find out exactly how to do it. (You may want to order an inexpensive Choose to Lose Passbook for keeping the food record. See the order form at the back of the book.) Be exact. Make sure your child's diet is typical of her normal daily food intake. She should not try to look "good."

2. Next figure out her average daily total caloric intake by taking an average of her final total calorie subtotal* entries for the 3 days. If your child wants to do this, have her add her 3 final subtotals together and divide by 3 to determine her average daily total caloric intake. Have her look at Kate's worksheet for an example.

Your child's **average daily total caloric intake** is _____.

3. To determine her Fat Budget, have her take 20 percent of her average daily total caloric intake (Step 2 above).

20% × _____ = _____ fat calories = Fat Budget.
          average daily
      total caloric intake

Your child's **Fat Budget** is _____ fat calories a day.

Here is an example to help clarify the procedure. Meet Kate.

Kate's Fat Budget Worksheet

a. Kate looked at her final total calorie subtotal entry for Thursday and saw that she had consumed 1800 total calories for that day. She found she had consumed 2200 total calories on Friday and 2000 total calories on Saturday.

b. She added these 3 final total calorie subtotals: 1800 + 2200 + 2000 = 6000 total calories.

---

*If you have not kept a total calorie subtotal, you may add up the total calories that she ate each day to get a total caloric intake for the whole day. You will then add these 3 total caloric intakes and divide by 3 to get an average daily total caloric intake.

c. To find an average total caloric intake for the 3 days, she divided the 6000 total calories by 3. 6000 ÷ 3 = 2000 total calories a day.

Kate's **average daily total caloric intake** is **2000** total calories. She knows she must eat at least 2000 total calories each day.

d. To find her Fat Budget, she multiplies 20 percent times her average daily total caloric intake of 2000.

20% × 2000 (average total caloric intake) = **400** fat calories = Kate's Fat Budget.

e. Kate must reduce her fat intake to no more than 400 fat calories a day (less would be fine), but she must eat at least 2000 total calories a day. She must replace the fat she is eliminating with calories of nutritious complex carbohydrates.

Note to Zealous Parents

When you reduce the fat in your child's diet, be sure to replace the fat removed with complex carbohydrates (not empty calories) so that your child gets enough calories to grow and develop normally and so she is *never* hungry. Because complex carbohydrates have twice as much bulk as fat for a given number of calories, your child will be eating much more food. Don't be alarmed. Low-fat food is not fattening.

Fat Budget Applied

When your child knows her Fat Budget, she may get a kick out of leafing through the Food Tables. Her Fat Budget will make her judge foods more critically and make better choices. She may also enjoy learning how to read a food label (see pages 121–34) so she can compare the fat contents of different products to her own Fat Budget. She probably will stop at this level of expertise, but you may be surprised by how ably she applies what she learned to new situations.

Keeping Track. If you have a child (more likely a teenager) who wants to keep track of her fat intake, she should be encouraged to do so. She will probably like the idea of having a passbook (it looks like an adult's checkbook) for her own. Have her read the Appendix on keeping a food record (page 448) or read it yourself and help her get started. She should follow the preceding instructions to determine her Fat Budget.

Let your child be in control of adhering to her Fat Budget. To be blunt, don't nose into her food records. What she writes down is her business alone. She must own the problem and accept responsibility. Only if she is in control will she be successful.

You do not want to make eating into a BIG THING. You want eating healthfully to be a natural part of your children's lives. You can do your part by being supportive and by providing a profuse variety of delicious, nutritious low-fat foods to keep your children full and happy.

Note to Overzealous Parents

In your zeal to keep your children thin, don't eliminate all fat from their diets. For proper growth and development, young children require a diet that is about 20 percent total fat and filled with vitamins, minerals, and fiber found in fruits, vegetables, and whole-grains. (Frankly, drastically reducing children's fat intake is a rare problem. The more widespread and serious problem is allowing children to eat 40 to 50 percent of their calories as fat.)

Remember:
1. Feed the entire family nutritious foods.
2. Don't single out overweight children for special attention or foods.
3. Don't make food an issue.
4. Don't feed children even healthy snacks too close to mealtimes.
5. Use tables to determine Fat Budgets for children who have stopped growing.
6. For children who are still growing, base their Fat Budget on total caloric intake as determined from 3-day food records; be sure to replace fat with complex carbohydrates and not let total calories drop.
7. Repeat to yourself: **WE MUST EAT TO LOSE. WE MUST EAT TO LOSE. WE MUST EAT TO LOSE. OF COURSE, WE MUST EAT NUTRITIOUS, LOW-FAT FOODS TO LOSE.**

14. Answers to Questions You Might Ask

Reaching a Plateau

Q. I have been following *Choose to Lose* for several weeks and seem to have reached a standstill in my weight loss. Should I give up?

A. Never! In the first few weeks of following *Choose to Lose* you will be replacing the fat you are losing with the new muscle you are building from exercising. In the long run, added muscle will help you burn fat. In the short run, because the muscle you are building may weigh as much or more than the fat you are losing, you may not see the loss registered on the scale. Throw away your scale. Your fat loss will be evident in the way your clothes fit.

Do not give up now. First of all, no matter what your weight loss, *Choose to Lose* is the healthiest way to eat. You are reducing your risks for all sorts of diseases. Second, you *will* lose weight. This is only a temporary plateau. Hang on. See the next answer, too.

Not Losing

Q. I have been doing *everything* you recommended. Why am I not losing weight?

A. The explanation for your weight loss standstill may be found in your answers to these questions.

   1. **Are you keeping track of everything you eat?**
      If you don't write down everything you eat honestly and accurately, you may *think* you are eating a perfect diet, but you may be consuming more fat than you realize. Perhaps you go to a fast-food restaurant and order a grilled chicken sandwich. You may assume it has only 31 fat calories because that is the cost of a chicken breast plus a bun. When you look it up in the Food

Tables, you will see that a grilled chicken fillet sandwich really contains 153 fat calories. What a difference! Fat is pervasive (and hidden) throughout our food supply. It accumulates fast and furiously.

2. **Are you eating above your minimum total caloric intake?**

You must eat to lose weight. This is the hardest concept for chronic dieters to accept. They are so afraid that eating a lot of food will make them fat, they still (no matter how many times we beg and plead and jump up and down and yell) limit the amount of calories they eat. As a result, they slow down their metabolism and are hungry and dissatisfied. Thus they lose much more slowly and usually give up before they see any results. Take a chance. Eat! What have you got to lose but fat?

3. **Are you meeting your minimum total caloric intake with nutrient-dense foods or with a lot of nonfat ersatz food?**

If you fulfill the minimum nutritional requirements as suggested by the Food Guide Pyramid, you will be a success at losing fat. Besides being chock full of vitamins, minerals, and fiber, these foods will keep you full. If you fulfill your minimum total caloric intake with essentially empty calories (nonfat cakes, cookies, frozen yogurt, etc.), you may find you lose very slowly or not at all.

Some nonfat food may not be as nonfat as we are led to assume. One of our readers called because although she was following *Choose to Lose* to the letter and maintaining her weight, she wasn't losing. The mystery was solved when she told us she ate 3 large nonfat frozen yogurts every day. Eating 3 large frozen yogurts is pushing the system. She really had no way of knowing how much fat was in the nonfat frozen yogurt. We found out recently that Colombo's peanut butter nonfat frozen yogurt (our very favorite in all the world) was not *really* nonfat. Colombo had been allowed to call it nonfat* because the basic frozen yogurt was nonfat. However, the peanut oil flavoring they add contains 23 fat calories for a 4-fluid-ounce (half cup) serving or 41 fat calories for a 7-fluid-ounce serving. The fat adds up quickly.

---

*Colombo now calls its peanut butter frozen yogurt low-fat.

Another problem with eating too many fat-free cookies, cakes, crackers, and ice cream is that they take the place of more nutritious foods. You are denying yourself the vitamins, minerals, and fiber that you need for good health. Fiber is almost totally missing in these products. Fiber fills you up and keeps you regular. We have found that people who overload on fat-free food are often not successful at losing fat.

4. **Are you eating out often?**
   Even though we can advise you what questions to ask and what requests to make to optimize low-fat eating when you dine out, it is still a dangerous activity. You never *really* know whether your vegetables were steamed with no fat as you asked. You can't be sure the rice is not riddled with butter. For the scary truth about eating out, see pages 67–71 in Chapter 4, "Where's the Fat?" and Restaurant Foods and Fast Foods in the Food Tables. If you are eating out once a week or more (eating out isn't limited to going to a special restaurant: carry-out, breakfast in the office cafeteria, lunch at a sub shop, pizza deliveries, etc., all count as eating out), you may find your weight loss progress going nowhere.

5. **Are you exercising aerobically for at least 20 to 30 minutes every day?**
   Exercise is an essential part of fat loss. The more muscle you build by exercising aerobically, the more fat you will burn. You can lose without exercising, but it is much slower and much less permanent.

Weighing In

Q. How often should I weigh in?

A. We recommend weighing yourself once every six months. Better yet, once a year. Best yet, not at all. The point is that weighing yourself doesn't show you anything about your fat loss. Short-term changes in your weight don't discriminate among loss of water, muscle, or fat. In fact, because the muscle you are building by exercising may weigh as much or more than the fat you are losing, you may reach a plateau and not lose weight for a while. If you just looked at the scale, you might become discouraged and go back to your old high-fat ways when, in fact, you should feel encouraged because you have succeeded in building fat-burning muscle. The best advice is to throw away your scale.

But if throwing away your scale would be like tearing a rib from your chest, at least try to overcome the urge to weigh yourself daily (or more likely, hourly). Weigh yourself no more than once a week, or once every other week, for a more realistic reflection of your fat loss. Try to weigh yourself on the same day of the week, at the same time of the day, wearing the same amount of clothing, and using the same scale.

Your best bet is to take Choose to Lose Leader Jan Bishop's advice: Measure your fat loss progress by trying on a pair of slacks that are too tight to wear in public. In a few weeks, try them on again. When this pair fits perfectly, find another pair that is snug and watch it become looser and looser. This way you will see your real progress, not a number on a scale.

Who Can Eat That Much?

Q. I know you say I must eat more than my minimum daily total caloric intake, but at the end of the day I find I hardly ever top 1200 total calories. Do I have to force myself to eat enough food?

A. Surprisingly, eating enough food is *the* most difficult part of following *Choose to Lose*. Start slowly. After all, you probably have been eating almost no food in terms of bulk (but not in terms of fat!) for many years. Set the minimum nutritional requirements of the Food Guide Pyramid as your goal. Add a fruit, a grain, a vegetable, one at a time, until you are fulfilling the recommendation. Nancy Ochsner of Woodland Park, Colorado, thought of this great idea: Each morning, place your fruit, vegetables, grain, and dairy requirements for the day on a plastic tray in the refrigerator and make sure you have emptied it by the end of the day.

Are you eating real dinners? We have soup, a chicken, turkey, or seafood entree on rice, a steamed vegetable or two, sometimes a sweet potato and/or a white potato. Are you eating only a piece of broiled chicken and a salad for dinner? Do you see why we have no trouble accumulating enough calories? Are you including healthy snacks? We enjoy 12 cups of air-popped popcorn every day. Sometimes Ron has 24! Try harder and you will reach and surpass your minimum daily total caloric intake in no time.

Too Little Fat?

Q. I have cut down my fat intake to almost nothing. Is it dangerous to eat too little fat?

A. From a health standpoint it is almost impossible to eat too little fat. Mainland Chinese eat a 10 percent fat diet and they are much healthier than we. If you are eating according to the recommendations of the Food Guide Pyramid, you are probably getting adequate fat. The problem with eating almost no fat is that such martyrlike behavior cannot be endured for long and soon you're off *Choose to Lose* and back to Choose to Gain.

Cholesterol

Q. I have high blood cholesterol. Will it hurt me to follow *Choose to Lose?*
A. Following *Choose to Lose* is a great way to lower your blood cholesterol level. By reducing total fat, you will automatically be reducing saturated fat, which is the main culprit in raising blood cholesterol. We recommend reading our book *Eater's Choice: A Food Lover's Guide to Lower Cholesterol* to learn everything you need to know about heart disease, diet, and cholesterol, but following *Choose to Lose.*

Fading Away to Nothing

Q. If I keep following *Choose to Lose,* will I eventually become emaciated?
A. You only wish! The Fat Budget you determined is the maximum amount of fat you should consume to reach your goal weight and to stay there.

Men — It Just Ain't Fair!

Q. How come my husband loses 10 pounds for every 5 pounds I lose?
A. It really isn't fair. Men naturally have more muscle mass than women so they burn fat more readily. Men's fat often congregates around their middles (apple shape) which may make it easier for them to lose than women, whose fat more often accumulates around the hips and thighs (pear shape). In addition, many men don't have the hang-ups many women have about eating and losing weight. They just do it.

Diet Drinks Versus Regular

Q. Fat — not sugar — makes fat. So can I *really* drink regular cola without gaining weight?
A. Absolutely. Neither regular nor diet drinks are fattening, but neither

are good drink choices, either. Diet drinks have the added disadvantage of containing unhealthy additives. Try the best drink choices instead — skim milk, water, and real fruit juices.

Are Fat Calories Part of My Total Caloric Intake?

Q. When I eat a food, I write down the number of total calories and the number of fat calories it contains. Are those fat calories a *part* of my total caloric intake, or an addition to it?

A. The number of fat calories you eat is a part of your total caloric intake. Say you eat 2000 total calories today. These total calories are the sum of calories from fat, protein, and carbohydrates. You are concerned about reducing your fat calorie intake, so you are keeping track of your fat calories separately, but those fat calories are still a part of your total caloric intake. If, for example, you ate 300 fat calories today, those 300 fat calories would be part of the 2000 total caloric intake. The rest of your total caloric intake for today (2000 total calories − 300 fat calories = 1700 total calories) would be divided between carbohydrate and protein calories.

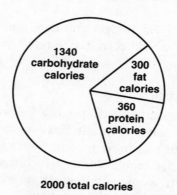

2000 total calories

Individual foods are also made up of calories from carbohydrate, protein, and fat. For example, 200 total calories in a food might break down as follows: 55 fat calories + 45 protein calories + 100 carbohydrate calories = 200 total calories.

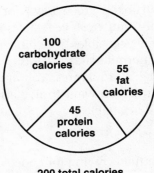

200 total calories

Keeping Records

Q. I hate keeping any type of records. Do I *really* have to keep track of the foods I eat forever?

A. It is a pain in the neck to write down everything you eat. However, only if you record what you eat and determine the cost in fat calories will you know what foods are making you fat and if you are making enough changes to lose weight. You will *not* have to keep records forever. Pretty soon you will know the combinations of foods you like to eat that fit into your Fat Budget. You can stop keeping records when you are consistently eating comfortably within your budget and your records no longer teach you anything.

Boiled Chicken

Q. I love to eat. How can I stay on this diet if I have to eat boiled chicken and Jell-O?

A. We hate to be rude, BUT DIDN'T YOU READ THIS BOOK?!!! We never eat boiled chicken and Jell-O. We eat *Indonesian Chicken with Green Beans* and *Turkey with Capers* and *Calzone* and *Chili Non Carne.* Low-fat cooking does not have to be bland and dull. With herbs and spices, and garlic and onions and ginger and vegetables and fruits and vinegars, you can make sublime low-fat food.

Fruit and/or Vegetables

Q. I don't like fruits or vegetables. What can I eat?

A. When is the last time you tried fruits or vegetables? Are you remembering the overcooked green beans or peas that your mom used to make? Try steaming fresh vegetables until they are crisp but tender. Try fruits and vegetables you haven't eaten before. Bake sweet potatoes or butternut squash. Try Bosc pears and tangerines. Be open to new tastes and textures. You are no longer a little kid showing your power. If you want to live a long, healthy life, you need to eat fruits and vegetables.

Chocolate

Q. Once a month I get a mad craving for chocolate. How can I handle it?

A. The beauty of *Choose to Lose* is that you never have to feel deprived or guilty. Unless you are a chocoholic who loses control after one whiff, limit yourself to a small piece or two during that time of the month. You can balance the cost with lower-fat choices the rest of the day. See "Splurging" (page 144).

High-Fat Cravings

Q. Will I ever get over the need for high-fat foods?

A. You won't believe it now, but if you are like many, many Choosers to Lose, you will lose your high-fat taste. The french fries you thought were divine will seem greasy; the creamy New England chowder you adored will turn your stomach. It takes about 12 weeks to change your tastes. If, however, you are constantly subjecting yourself to high-fat foods, you may never give up the high-fat taste.

Bingeing

Q. On every diet I've tried (and there is not one I haven't) I always end up bingeing and giving up the diet. Will this happen to me on *Choose to Lose*?

A. Although we can't guarantee you won't turn into a wild woman and eat an entire bag of potato chips, we strongly believe that this will never happen when you follow *Choose to Lose*. Following *Choose to Lose* discourages this type of behavior for two reasons.

1. You are encouraged to eat a tremendous amount of food so you are not hungry. On the other diets you followed, you limited calories and thus were starving. You were justified in going crazy and eating everything in sight because you were ravenous.

2. You are allowed to fit in high-fat splurges. You can fit in a few chocolate chip cookies, so you don't need to fantasize about the chocolate chip cookies you aren't eating and then madly devour the whole jar of peanuts to compensate. You know you can have that piece of chocolate candy tomorrow so you don't have to eat the whole box today.

Water

Q. Every other diet I've been on required drinking at least 8 glasses of water a day. Why don't you stress drinking water?

A. Drinking water is an essential part of many diets for two reasons. The first is that when you eat a low-calorie, high-protein diet, you need to flush out the excess nitrogen waste from your kidneys to prevent kidney disease and kidney failure.

    The second reason is to fill you up because on low-calorie diets you are always famished. Although we see nothing wrong with drinking water, *Choose to Lose* does not require drinking any special amount or any at all. When you are hungry, we want you to eat real food, which provides you with vitamins, minerals, and fiber, not take a few unsatisfying sips from your water jug.

Portion Control

Q. I was taught that limiting portion size is the key to weight loss. Why do you stress eating large amounts of food?

A. The only nutrient you need to limit is fat. If you are eating nutritious, fiber-rich nonfat and low-fat foods and staying within your Fat Budget, you can — and should — eat large portions. Eating small portions that limit total calories will defeat your fat-loss goals. It will slow your metabolism, reduce your intake of vitamins, minerals, and fiber, and make you hungry.

Slowing Down to Eat Less

Q. Many other diet programs teach behavioral modification techniques to help you eat slower. Why don't you discuss these?

A. Putting your fork down between mouthfuls, chewing your food 50 times between bites — these devices are tedious, boring, quickly abandoned, and, most important, unnecessary. They have been developed to make people eat less food. We believe in eating a lot of food (see the answer to the previous question) as fast as you wish.

Young Children

Q. If I follow *Choose to Lose* and feed my young children a low-fat diet, will it stunt their growth?

A. The American Heart Association recommends that all children above the age of two eat a low-fat diet. This is because the conditions that precipitate diseases such as heart disease begin in childhood. The plaque that clogs your arteries and gives you a heart attack at age 55 started accumulating when you were a young child. Children develop food tastes and food habits at a young age. Teach them to eat healthfully at a young age and you are giving them the greatest gift.

Epilogue:
Choose to Lose for Life

"I have followed this diet for the last 8 months and have lost 75 lbs and feel great. I have tried so many diets but yours made so much sense and seemed to be so healthy. It was something I could follow and, better yet, it is a way of eating that I could continue for the rest of my life so I can keep the weight off. Thanks again. I feel terrific. I have more energy and, best of all, I look better than I ever looked before."

Barbara La Sante, Bronx, New York

Choose to Lose is more than a diet. It is an education. It is a way of life. Not only will you learn how to make the right food choices to keep you lean forever, but a whole new world of eating will open up to you as you replace fat with complex carbohydrates. Your life will become richer and your palate will expand as you explore new foods and recipes that fit into your Fat Budget. Eating lots of food and little fat as well as exercising will increase your energy and make you feel great.

You will be amazed at how you will change, not only in size and shape, but in attitude. In the beginning, you may find yourself hungrily eyeing a croissant. But instead of gobbling it down, you will see a number pop out at you: *croissant = 110 fat calories*, and then you'll ask yourself, "Is that soggy croissant worth more than a third of my Fat Budget? Wouldn't French bread taste just as good and leave not a trace of fat in my fat stores?" You'll begin to prefer low-fat choices. You may find it hard to believe, but you may eventually lose your craving for high-fat food.

At first, you may find it almost impossible to eat enough food. At the end of the day you will be happy to reach your minimum daily caloric intake. Very soon you will wolf down loads of nutritious, low-fat foods naturally, without effort — only delight.

195

KEEP THOSE MUSCLES MOVING

As part of your new start on life you have made aerobic exercise a regular part of your day. Be sure to keep exercising even after you achieve your goal size. Not only will exercising help you maintain the new you, it is beneficial for the many reasons discussed in Chapter 11.

What Next?

After you achieve your desired weight, you should continue eating the *Choose to Lose* way for the rest of your life. Following the three *Choose to Lose* strategies — reducing fat in your diet by eating below your Fat Budget (the Fat Budget you use to reach your desirable and healthy weight is also your lifetime maintenance budget); eating large amounts of nutritious, low-fat foods such as fruits, vegetables, low- or nonfat dairy, and lean meats; and exercising aerobically every day for at least 20 to 30 minutes — you will be able to maintain your new weight forever.

If, however, you find that you are beginning to gain back the weight you lost, have no fear. If you have not been paying close attention, it is easy for fat to sneak back into your diet. Even though you *know* you have de-fatted your food choices, you really must start keeping track again (see "Answers to Questions You Might Ask," Chapter 14, pages 185–94). Reread *Choose to Lose* and write down all the foods you eat for a few days or weeks. Look for the sources of fat so you can make the right choices and changes. Be sure you are eating below your Fat Budget and exercising aerobically every day. Be sure you are eating enough nutritious, high-fiber foods. Soon you will be lean once again.

PREDICTORS OF SUCCESS

Make the behaviors in the following list a part of your life and you will greatly increase your success in achieving your weight loss goals. Keep them in mind as you change your life to create the "new you."

✔ Focus on health, not weight loss.
✔ Focus on body-size changes, not scale changes.

✔ Replace high-fat foods with low-fat foods.
✔ Eat enough total calories by eating more fruits, vegetables, whole-grains, and low- or nonfat dairy.
✔ Eat real, full meals.
✔ Eat within your Fat Budget.
✔ Budget in an occasional high-fat splurge.
✔ Eat out rarely.
✔ Cook! Prepare *Choose to Lose, Eater's Choice,* or other low-fat recipes.
✔ Exercise aerobically at least 20 to 30 minutes every day.
✔ Have patience!

IT'S UP TO YOU

Soon you will be seeing the New You in the mirror. Not only will the New You be lean, the New You will be full of energy, vim, and vigor. The New You will be full of confidence and high self-esteem because taking control of your diet is the first step to taking control of your life.

You've got the tools. It's your move. Remember, this is for life. Go to it and have fun!

POSTSCRIPT:
HOW *CHOOSE TO LOSE* DIFFERS FROM *EATER'S CHOICE*

In 1987, the first edition of *Eater's Choice: A Food Lover's Guide to Lower Cholesterol* was published. It was one of the first books to deal with the problem of high cholesterol. It was (and still is) the only book of its kind. It focuses on food. It is specific and quantitative so that you know you have made enough changes in your diet to lower your blood cholesterol.

The approach is simple and effective. You first determine your personal Sat-Fat Budget because the main culprit in the diet that raises blood cholesterol level is saturated fat. Thus, by limiting saturated-fat intake, you lower your blood cholesterol. Knowing your Sat-Fat Budget and the sat-fat calories of the foods you want to eat, you can eat any combination of foods as long as you stay within your budget and still lower your blood cholesterol level.

Since *Eater's Choice* was published, thousands of people have lowered their cholesterol levels and thus their risk for heart disease. Many have lost weight as a side effect. Limiting saturated fat will cause you to lose weight because foods that are high in saturated fat are even higher in total fat. When you limit total fat, you lose weight.

As we mentioned in the Introduction, we wrote *Choose to Lose* because so many people following *Eater's Choice* lost weight. However, we realized that just lowering saturated fat does not cause weight loss in every individual. Some foods, such as margarine, most vegetable oils (olive, corn, sunflower, and safflower), and peanut butter are low in saturated fat and would fit easily into a cholesterol-lowering diet. But because they are so high in total fat, consuming them without keeping track could make you gain weight.

Choose to Lose uses the same simple approach as *Eater's Choice*, but instead of a Sat-Fat Budget, you determine a Fat Budget. Knowing your Fat Budget and the fat calories of the foods you choose to eat, you can eat any combination of foods as long as you stay within your budget and still lose weight. With either plan you need never feel deprived, because you can always eat your favorite foods, you learn to appreciate new, healthy foods, you feel better than you ever did, and you look great. As a side effect of *Choose to Lose* you will probably lower your cholesterol because when you reduce total fat, in many instances you also reduce your intake of saturated fat.

Two Weeks of Meal Plans

WE CREATED the following meal plans to show you how easy it is to fit delicious food into your Fat Budget and how to save fat calories for a splurge. These are only *sample* meal plans, not menus designed to be repeated twenty six times each year until you are ninety-nine years old. It is your body and your taste buds, and you will have to devise meal plans that suit you and your Fat Budget. Don't worry. It will be fun.

The first week of meal plans are for three different Fat Budgets: 246, 315, and 398 fat calories a day. Remember, the minimum total caloric intake on which the budgets are based (1228, 1579, 1989) is a floor. They are the number of calories needed to satisfy the basal metabolic rate. An additional 400 or more calories are needed to fuel physical activity. Therefore, the total calories for each menu are at least 400 calories greater than the number used to determine the Fat Budget. The second week of meal plans illustrates how to save up calories for a splurge following a sample budget of 304 fat calories (a 20 percent Fat Budget based on a minimum daily caloric intake of 1521).

At the bottom of each meal plan you can see how it meets the minimum nutritional requirements of 2 to 4 servings of fruits, 3 to 5 servings of vegetables, 6 to 11 servings of grain, and 2 to 3 servings of dairy.

The recipes for dishes printed in italics can be found in *Choose to Lose* or *Eater's Choice*.

Key to Abbreviations

Amt:	amount	lg:	large	sm:	small
br:	breast(s)	med:	medium	sv:	serving(s)
c:	cup(s)	min:	minimum	T:	tablespoon(s)
Cal:	caloric	oz:	ounce(s)	t:	teaspoon(s)
D:	dairy	pc:	piece(s)	Tot:	Total
F:	fruit	pkg:	package(s)	V:	vegetable
G:	grain	sl:	slice(s)		

Meal Plans — Week 1

Sunday — Week 1	FAT BUDGET: 246 MIN TOT CAL INTAKE: 1228			FAT BUDGET: 315 MIN TOT CAL INTAKE: 1579			FAT BUDGET: 398 MIN TOT CAL INTAKE: 1989		
		CALORIES			CALORIES			CALORIES	
	AMT	TOT	FAT	AMT	TOT	FAT	AMT	TOT	FAT
Breakfast									
Buttermilk Waffle	2	276	26	3	414	39	3	414	39
Maple syrup	1 T	33	0	1 T	50	0	1 T	50	0
Honeydew melon	¹⁄₁₀	46	0	¹⁄₁₀	46	0	⅕	92	0
Skim milk	1 c	86	4	1 c	86	4	1 c	86	4
Coffee or tea	1 c	0	0	1 c	0	0	1 c	0	0
Lunch									
Tomato-Rice Soup	1 c	93	0	1 c	93	0	1½ c	140	0
Blackened Chicken	1 br	130	13	1 br	130	13	2 br	260	26
Whole-wheat bread	1 sl	70	18	1 sl	70	18	2 sl	140	18
Baked potato	1 sm	75	0	1 med	112	0	1 med	112	0
Nonfat yogurt	2 T	14	0	2 T	14	0	2 T	14	0
Steamed broccoli	½ c	20	0	½ c	20	0	1 c	40	0
Margarine	½ t	17	17	½ t	17	17	½ t	17	17
Sliced fresh peaches	1 c	74	0	1 c	74	0	1 c	74	0
Skim milk	1 c	86	4	1 c	86	4	1 c	86	4
Coffee or tea	1 c	0	0	1 c	0	0	1 c	0	0
Dinner									
Grapefruit	½	38	0	½	38	0	½	38	0
Chili Non Carne	1 c	117	5	1½ c	176	8	2 c	234	10
Tossed salad	1 c	10	0	1 c	10	0	1 c	10	0
Italian dressing	1 T	69	64	1 T	69	64	1½ T	104	96
Steamed Zucchini Matchsticks	1 c	34	0	1 c	34	0	1 c	34	0
Margarine	½ t	17	17	½ t	17	17	½ t	17	17
Onion Flat Bread	2 sl	166	14	2 sl	166	14	3 sl	249	21
Coffee or tea	1 c	0	0	1 c	0	0	1 c	0	0
Mandelbrot	2 pc	92	36	2 pc	92	36	3 pc	138	54
Snack									
Skim milk	1 c	86	4	1 c	86	4	1 c	86	4
Bran Chex	⅔ c	90	0	⅔ c	90	0	⅔ c	90	0
Banana	1	105	5	1	105	5	1	105	5
TOTALS		1844	210		2095	243		2630	315

F: 4 V: 5 G: 6 D: 3	F: 4 V: 5.5 G: 7 D: 3	F: 5 V: 6 G: 10 D: 3

Meal Plans — Week 1

Monday — Week 1	FAT BUDGET: 246 MIN TOT CAL INTAKE: 1228			FAT BUDGET: 315 MIN TOT CAL INTAKE: 1579			FAT BUDGET: 398 MIN TOT CAL INTAKE: 1989		
		CALORIES			CALORIES			CALORIES	
	AMT	TOT	FAT	AMT	TOT	FAT	AMT	TOT	FAT
Breakfast									
Apricot Oat Muffin	1	135	32	2	270	64	2	270	64
Strawberries, fresh	1 c	45	0	1 c	45	0	1 c	45	0
1% cottage cheese	½ c	90	10	½ c	90	10	¾ c	135	15
Skim milk	1 c	86	4	1 c	86	4	1 c	86	4
Coffee or tea	1 c	0	0	1 c	0	0	1 c	0	0
Lunch									
Chickpea Sandwich on pita bread	1	195	39	1	195	39	2	390	78
Tangerine	1	35	0	1	35	0	1	35	0
Nonfat fruit yogurt	—			—			1 c	190	0
Oatmeal Cookies	1	65	25	2	130	50	2	130	50
Skim milk	—			1 c	86	4	1 c	86	4
Coffee or tea	1 c	0	0	1 c	0	0	1 c	0	0
Dinner									
Tortilla Soup	1 c	144	10	1½ c	216	15	1½ c	216	15
Indonesian Chicken with Green Beans	1 sv	135	14	1 sv	135	14	1½ sv	202	21
White rice	1 c	224	0	1 c	224	0	1 c	224	0
Acorn squash	½ sm	70	0	½ sm	70	0	½ sm	70	0
Steamed broccoli	1 c	92	0	1 c	92	0	1 c	92	0
Margarine	½ t	17	17	½ t	17	17	½ t	17	17
Whole-wheat bread	1 sl	70	9	1 sl	70	9	1 sl	70	9
Nonfat yogurt	1 c	110	0	1 c	110	0	1 c	110	0
Blueberries, fresh	1 c	80	0	1 c	80	0	1 c	80	0
Coffee or tea	1 c	0	0	1 c	0	0	1 c	0	0
Snack									
Skim milk	1 c	86	4	1 c	86	4	1 c	86	4
Popcorn, air-popped	6 c	180	0	8 c	240	0	10 c	300	0
TOTALS		**1859**	**164**		**2277**	**230**		**2834**	**281**
	F: 3	V: 3	G: 8	D: 4	F: 3	V: 3	G: 10	D: 4	F: 3 V: 4 G: 13 D: 4

Meal Plans — Week 1

Tuesday — Week 1	FAT BUDGET: 246 MIN TOT CAL INTAKE: 1228			FAT BUDGET: 315 MIN TOT CAL INTAKE: 1579			FAT BUDGET: 398 MIN TOT CAL INTAKE: 1989		
		CALORIES			CALORIES			CALORIES	
	AMT	TOT	FAT	AMT	TOT	FAT	AMT	TOT	FAT
Breakfast									
Whole-wheat toast	2 sl	140	18	2 sl	140	18	3 sl	210	27
Jelly	1 t	17	0	2 t	34	0	3 t	51	0
Cantaloupe	½	94	0	½	94	0	½	94	0
1% cottage cheese	½ c	90	10	½ c	90	10	½ c	90	10
Skim milk	1 c	86	4	1 c	86	4	1 c	86	4
Coffee or tea	1 c	0	0	1 c	0	0	1 c	0	0
Lunch									
Tuna sandwich:									
Tuna, water-packed	3 oz	90	14	3 oz	90	14	6 oz	180	28
Low-fat mayonnaise	2 t	30	30	2 t	30	30	1 T	45	45
Rye bread	2 sl	130	18	2 sl	130	18	4 sl	260	36
Carrot	1	31	0	1	31	0	1	31	0
Orange	1	60	0	1	60	0	1	60	0
Coffee or tea	1 c	0	0	1 c	0	0	1 c	0	0
Dinner									
Tarragon Squash Soup	1 c	122	3	1½ c	183	5	1½ c	183	5
Turkey Mexique	1 sv	153	23	1 sv	153	23	1 sv	153	23
White rice	1 c	224	0	1 c	224	0	1 c	224	0
Tossed salad	1 c	10	0	1 c	10	0	1 c	10	0
Thousand Island dressing	1 T	59	50	1½ T	89	75	1½ T	89	75
Sweet potato	1	118	0	1	118	0	1	118	0
Spinach, cooked	1 c	41	0	1 c	41	0	1 c	41	0
Margarine	½ t	17	17	½ t	17	17	½ t	17	17
Pear	1	98	0	1	98	0	1	98	0
Skim milk	1 c	86	4	1 c	86	4	1 c	86	4
Coffee or tea	1 c	0	0	1 c	0	0	1 c	0	0
Snack									
Popcorn, air-popped	6 c	180	0	8 c	240	0	10 c	300	0
Skim milk	1 c	86	4	1 c	86	4	1 c	86	4
TOTALS		1962	195		2130	222		2512	278

F: 3   V: 4   G: 8   D: 4 | F: 3   V: 4   G: 9   D: 4 | F: 3   V: 4   G: 13   D: 4

Meal Plans — Week 1

Wednesday — Week 1	FAT BUDGET: 246 MIN TOT CAL INTAKE: 1228			FAT BUDGET: 315 MIN TOT CAL INTAKE: 1579			FAT BUDGET: 398 MIN TOT CAL INTAKE: 1989		
		CALORIES			CALORIES			CALORIES	
	AMT	TOT	FAT	AMT	TOT	FAT	AMT	TOT	FAT
Breakfast									
Whole-wheat toast	1 sl	70	9	1 sl	70	9	1 sl	70	9
Jelly	1 t	17	0	1 t	17	0	1 t	17	0
Raisin bran cereal	¾ c	120	9	¾ c	120	9	1½ c	240	18
Skim milk	1 c	86	4	1 c	86	4	1½ c	129	6
Banana	1	105	5	1	105	5	1	105	5
Orange juice	—			1 c	111	0	1 c	111	0
Coffee or tea	1 c	0	0	1 c	0	0	1 c	0	0
Lunch									
Turkey sandwich:									
Turkey breast	3 oz	114	6	3 oz	114	6	6 oz	228	12
Lettuce, tomato		10	0		10	0		10	0
Low-fat mayonnaise	2 t	30	30	2 t	30	30	4 t	60	60
Whole-wheat bread	2 sl	140	18	2 sl	140	18	4 sl	280	36
Apple	1	81	0	1	81	0	1	81	0
Honey Graham Cracker	—			2	116	24	2	116	24
Skim milk	1 c	86	4	1 c	86	4	1 c	86	4
Coffee or tea	1 c	0	0	1 c	0	0	1 c	0	0
Snack									
Popcorn, air-popped	6 c	180	0	6 c	180	0	8 c	240	0
Dinner									
Carrot Soup	1 c	85	17	1½ c	128	26	1½ c	128	26
Scallop Curry	1 sv	197	46	1 sv	197	46	1 sv	197	46
White rice	1 c	224	0	1 c	224	0	1 c	224	0
Tossed salad	1 c	10	0	1 c	10	0	1 c	10	0
Russian dressing, reduced-calorie	1 T	23	6	1½ T	34	9	1½ T	23	9
Zucchini, steamed	½ c	18	0	½ c	18	0	½ c	18	0
Vinegar	1 t	17	0	1 t	17	0	1 t	17	0
Baked potato	1	145	0	1	145	0	1	145	0
Nonfat yogurt	2 T	14	0	2 T	14	0	4 T	28	0
Fresh sliced peaches	½ c	37	0	1 c	74	0	1 c	74	0
Coffee or tea	1 c	0	0	1 c	0	0	1 c	0	0
Snack									
Nonfat vanilla yogurt	½ c	80	5	1 c	160	9	1 c	160	9
Fresh strawberries	½ c	22	0	1 c	44	0	1 c	44	0
TOTALS		1911	159		2331	199		2841	264

F: 4 V: 4 G: 8 D: 2.5 | F: 6 V: 4.5 G: 8 D: 3 | F: 3 V: 4 G: 13 D: 3.5

Meal Plans — Week 1

Thursday — Week 1	FAT BUDGET: 246 MIN TOT CAL INTAKE: 1228			FAT BUDGET: 315 MIN TOT CAL INTAKE: 1579			FAT BUDGET: 398 MIN TOT CAL INTAKE: 1989		
		CALORIES			CALORIES			CALORIES	
	AMT	TOT	FAT	AMT	TOT	FAT	AMT	TOT	FAT
Breakfast									
Apple Oat Muffin	—			1	125	32	2	250	64
Grapefruit	½	38	0	½	38	0	½	38	0
Wheatena	1 sv	100	9	1 sv	100	9	1 sv	100	9
Margarine	½ t	17	17	½ t	17	17	½ t	17	17
Skim milk	1 c	86	4	1 c	86	4	1 c	86	4
Coffee or tea	1 c	0	0	1 c	0	0	1 c	0	0
Lunch									
Ted Mummery's Turkey Barbecue	1 sv	131	5	1 sv	131	5	2 sv	262	10
Whole-wheat pita	1	165	9	1	165	9	2	330	18
Carrot	1	31	0	1	31	0	1	31	0
Peach	1	37	0	1	37	0	1	37	0
Coffee or tea	1 c	0	0	1 c	0	0	1 c	0	0
Snack									
Popcorn, air-popped	6 c	180	0	8 c	240	0	10 c	300	0
Dinner									
Cucumber Soup	1 c	78	2	1 c	78	2	1 c	78	2
Spaghetti à la Sicilia	1 sv	275	10	1 sv	275	10	1½ sv	412	15
Parmesan cheese	1 T	23	14	1 T	23	14	1 T	23	14
Sesame Chicken	1 sv	160	20	1 sv	160	20	1 sv	160	20
Tossed salad	1 c	10	0	1 c	10	0	1 c	10	0
Italian dressing	1 T	69	64	1 T	69	64	1 T	69	64
Italian bread	2 sl	170	0	2 sl	170	0	2 sl	170	0
Margarine with garlic	¾ t	25	25	1 t	33	33	1 t	33	33
Butternut squash	½	86	0	½	86	0	½	86	0
Cheesecake	1 sl	120	16	1 sl	120	16	1 sl	120	16
Coffee or tea	1 c	0	0	1 c	0	0	1 c	0	0
Snack									
Raisin bran cereal	¾ c	120	9	¾ c	120	9	¾ c	120	9
Skim milk	1 c	86	4	1 c	86	4	1 c	86	4
Banana	—			1	105	5	1	105	5
TOTALS		2007	208		2305	253		2923	304

F: 2 V: 3.5 G: 10 D: 3 | F: 3 V: 3.5 G: 11 D: 3 | F: 3 V: 3.5 G: 13 D: 3

Meal Plans — Week 1

Friday — Week 1	FAT BUDGET: 246 MIN TOT CAL INTAKE: 1228			FAT BUDGET: 315 MIN TOT CAL INTAKE: 1579			FAT BUDGET: 398 MIN TOT CAL INTAKE: 1989		
		CALORIES			CALORIES			CALORIES	
	AMT	TOT	FAT	AMT	TOT	FAT	AMT	TOT	FAT
Breakfast									
Nonfat yogurt with	½ c	62	0	1 c	124	0	1 c	124	0
cut-up fresh fruit	¾ c	60	0	¾ c	60	0	¾ c	60	0
Apricot Oat Muffin	—			1	135	32	1	135	32
Whole-wheat toast	2 sl	140	18	1 sl	70	9	1 sl	70	9
Jelly	2 t	34	0	1 t	17	0	1 t	17	0
Skim milk	1 c	86	4	1 c	86	4	1 c	86	4
Coffee or tea	1 c	0	0	1 c	0	0	1 c	0	0
Lunch									
Asparagus Pasta	1 sv	253	26	1 sv	253	26	1 sv	253	26
Carrot	1	31	0	1	31	0	1	31	0
Cardamom Bread	1 sl	98	15	2 sl	196	30	2 sl	196	30
Blueberries	½ c	41	0	½ c	41	0	1 c	82	0
Coffee or tea	1 c	0	0	1 c	0	0	1 c	0	0
Snack									
Apple	1	81	0	1	81	0	1	81	0
Dinner									
Cantaloupe Soup	1 c	80	0	1½ c	120	0	1½ c	120	0
Fish Baked in Olive, etc.	1 sv	150	19	1 sv	150	19	1½ sv	225	28
Potato Skins	1 sv	66	9	1 sv	66	9	2 sv	132	18
Steamed carrots	½ c	35	0	½ c	35	0	1 c	70	0
Margarine	½ t	17	17	½ t	17	17	1 t	33	33
Whole-wheat bread	1 sl	70	9	1 sl	70	9	2 sl	140	18
Cucumber Salad	½ c	20	0	1 c	40	0	1 c	40	0
Oatmeal Cookies	—			1	65	25	2	130	50
Frozen nonfat vanilla yogurt	1 c	160	0	1 c	160	0	1 c	160	0
Fresh strawberries	½ c	22	0	1 c	44	0	1 c	44	0
Coffee or tea	1 c	0	0	1 c	0	0	1 c	0	0
Snack									
Skim milk	1 c	86	4	1 c	86	4	1 c	86	4
Wheat Chex	⅔ c	100	9	⅔ c	100	9	⅔ c	100	9
Banana	1	105	5	1	105	5	1	105	5
TOTALS		**1797**	**135**		**2152**	**198**		**2520**	**266**

| F: 5 V: 4 G: 7 D: 2.5 | F: 6 V: 4.5 G: 7 D: 3 | F: 8 V: 6 G: 8 D: 3 |

Meal Plans — Week 1

Saturday — Week 1	FAT BUDGET: 246 MIN TOT CAL INTAKE: 1228			FAT BUDGET: 315 MIN TOT CAL INTAKE: 1579			FAT BUDGET: 398 MIN TOT CAL INTAKE: 1989		
		CALORIES			CALORIES			CALORIES	
	AMT	TOT	FAT	AMT	TOT	FAT	AMT	TOT	FAT
Breakfast									
Cinnamon French Toast	3 sl	318	27	3 sl	318	27	4 sl	424	36
Maple syrup	2 T	105	0	2 T	105	0	2 T	105	0
Skim milk	1 c	86	4	1 c	86	4	1 c	86	4
Pineapple slice, ¾" thick	1	42	0	2	84	0	2	84	0
Coffee or tea	1 c	0	0	1 c	0	0	1 c	0	0
Lunch									
Cajun Chicken in a	1 sv	196	28	1 sv	196	28	2 sv	392	56
whole-wheat pita	1	165	9	1	165	9	2	330	18
Fresh strawberries	½ c	22	0	½ c	22	0	½ c	22	0
Nonfat vanilla yogurt	1 c	160	9	1 c	160	9	1 c	160	9
Carrot	1	31	0	1	31	0	1	31	0
Coffee or tea	1 c	0	0	1 c	0	0	1 c	0	0
Snack									
Fresh sliced peaches	1 c	74	0	1 c	74	0	1 c	74	0
Dinner									
Tarragon Squash Soup	1 sv	122	3	1 sv	122	3	1½ sv	183	5
Lemon Chicken	1 sv	176	13	1	176	13	1½ sv	264	20
White rice	1 c	224	0	1.c	224	0	1 c	224	0
Sweet potato	1 med	59	0	1 med	59	0	1 med	59	0
Tossed salad	1 c	10	0	1 c	10	0	1 c	10	0
Low-calorie Russian dressing	1 T	23	6	1 T	23	6	1 T	23	6
Cinnamon Sweet Cake	—			1	148	61	1	148	61
Coffee or tea	1 c	0	0	1 c	0	0	1 c	0	0
Snack									
Popcorn, air-popped	6 c	180	0	8 c	240	0	10 c	300	0
Skim milk	1 c	86	4	1 c	86	4	1 c	86	4
TOTALS		2079	103		2329	164		3005	219

F: 3 V: 4 G: 9 D: 3	F: 4 V: 4.5 G: 10 D: 3	F: 4 V: 6 G: 12 D: 3

Meal Plans — Week 2
Fat Budget: 304 with Splurge
Minimum total calories: 1521 Total Calories

Sunday — Week 2	AMOUNT	CALORIES TOTAL	FAT
Breakfast			
Buttermilk Waffles	3	414	39
Maple syrup	1 T	50	0
Apricots	3	50	0
Skim milk	1 c	86	4
Coffee or tea	1 c	0	0
Lunch			
Apricot Chicken Divine	1 sv	215	23
White rice	1 c	224	0
Steamed broccoli	1 c	40	0
Vinegar	1 t	0	0
Baked potato	1	112	0
Coffee or tea	1 c	0	0
Banana	1	105	5
Snack			
Popcorn, air-popped	6 c	180	0
Dinner			
Barley-Vegetable Soup	1 c	100	0
Focaccia	2 sl	232	26
Spaghetti Squash with Tomato Sauce	1 sv	117	10
Italian bread	1 sl	85	0
Tossed salad	1 c	10	0
Low-calorie Italian dressing	1 T	16	14
Skim milk	1 c	86	4
Coffee or tea	1 c	0	0
Snack			
Nonfat vanilla yogurt	1 c	160	0
Fresh sliced peaches	½ c	37	0
	TOTALS	2319	125
	Fat Budget:		304
	Saved:		179

Meal Plans — Week 2
Fat Budget: 304 with Splurge
Minimum total calories: 1521 Total Calories

Monday — Week 2		CALORIES	
	AMOUNT	TOTAL	FAT
Breakfast			
1% cottage cheese	1 c	164	20
Fresh sliced strawberries	1 c	90	0
Whole-wheat toast	2 sl	140	18
Jelly	2 t	34	0
Grapefruit	½	38	0
Skim milk	1 c	86	4
Coffee or tea	1 c	0	0
Lunch			
Turkey sandwich:			
Turkey breast	3 oz	114	6
Lettuce, tomato		10	0
Mustard	1 t	5	0
Whole-wheat bread	2 sl	140	18
Carrot	1	31	0
Apple	1	81	0
Skim milk	1 c	86	4
Coffee or tea	1 c	0	0
Snack			
Popcorn, air-popped	6 c	180	0
Dinner			
Vegetable Soup with Spinach, Potatoes, Rice, and Corn	1 c	129	12
Scallop Creole	1 sv	177	18
White rice	1 c	224	0
Steamed Zucchini Matchsticks	1 c	34	0
Steamed cauliflower	1 c	24	0
Coffee or tea	1 c	0	0
Snack			
Nonfat vanilla yogurt	1 c	160	0
Blueberries	1 c	80	0
	TOTALS	2027	100
	Fat Budget:		304
	Saved:		204
	Carry-over:		179
	New carry-over:		383

Meal Plans — Week 2
Fat Budget: 304 with Splurge
Minimum total calories: 1521 Total Calories

Tuesday — Week 2	AMOUNT	CALORIES TOTAL	FAT
Breakfast			
Bagel	1	200	18
Preserves	1 T	50	0
Nonfat strawberry yogurt	1 c	125	0
Melon chunks	1 c	57	0
Coffee or tea	1 c	0	0
Lunch			
Curried Tuna Salad with Pears	1 sv	175	23
Whole-wheat pita bread	1	165	9
Carrot	1	31	0
Orange	1	60	0
Skim milk	1 c	86	4
Coffee or tea	1 c	0	0
Dinner			
Oriental Noodle Soup	1 c	64	8
Bar-B-Que Chicken	1 br	173	13
White rice	1 c	224	0
Mashed potatoes (skim milk)	1 c	160	0
Indian Vegetables	1 sv	72	7
Tossed salad	1 c	10	0
Low-calorie French dressing	1 T	22	8
Whole-wheat bread	1 sl	70	9
Coffee or tea	1 c	0	0
Snack			
Skim milk	1 c	86	4
Honey Graham Crackers	3	174	36

TOTALS		2004	139
Fat Budget:			<u>304</u>
Saved:			165
Carry-over:			<u>383</u>
New carry-over:			548

Meal Plans — Week 2
Fat Budget: 304 with Splurge
Minimum total calories: 1521 Total Calories

Wednesday — Week 2		CALORIES	
	AMOUNT	TOTAL	FAT
Breakfast			
Oatmeal	1 c	300	50
Raisins	1 T	31	0
Margarine	½ t	17	17
Skim milk	1 c	86	4
Whole-wheat toast	2 sl	140	18
Banana	1	105	5
Coffee or tea	1 c	0	0
Lunch			
Baked chicken breast sandwich:			
Chicken breast (no skin)	3 oz	142	28
Lettuce, tomato, mustard		10	0
Rye bread	2 sl	130	18
Carrot	1	31	0
Peach	1	37	0
Popcorn, air-popped	6 c	180	0
Coffee or tea	1 c	0	0
Dinner			
Zucchini Soup	1 c	80	0
Cajun Chicken	1 sv	196	28
White rice	1 c	224	0
Baked potato	1 lg	145	0
Steamed broccoli	1 c	46	0
Margarine	½ t	17	17
Skim milk	1 c	86	4
Coffee or tea	1 c	0	0
Snack			
Nonfat yogurt with fruit	1 c	190	5

TOTALS	2193	194
Fat Budget:		304
Saved:		110
Carry-over:		548
New carry-over:		658

Meal Plans — Week 2
Fat Budget: 304 with Splurge
Minimum total calories: 1521 Total Calories

Thursday — Week 2	AMOUNT	CALORIES TOTAL	FAT

Breakfast

	AMOUNT	TOTAL	FAT
English muffin	2	280	18
Jelly	1⅓ T	75	0
Grapefruit	½	38	0
Cocoa:			
cocoa powder	1 t	5	0
sugar	2 t	30	0
skim milk	1 c	86	4

Lunch

Chili Non Carne	1 c	117	5
Chopped lettuce, tomatoes, onions	¼ c	10	0
French bread	2 sl	200	0
Skim milk	1 c	86	4
Orange	1	60	0
Coffee or tea	1 c	0	0
Frozen nonfat yogurt	1 c	160	0
Strawberries	½ c	22	0

Dinner

Sour Cherry Soup	1 c	165	0
Broiled Ginger Fish	1 sv	194	35
White rice	1 c	224	0
Hot and Garlicky Eggplant	1 sv	25	5
Baked potato	1 med	112	0
Nonfat yogurt	2 T	14	0
Tossed salad	1 c	10	0
Low-calorie French dressing	1 T	22	8
Grapefruit sections	½ c	37	0
Coffee or tea	1 c	0	0
Mandelbrot	1	46	18

Snack

Raisin bran cereal	¾ c	120	9
Skim milk	1 c	86	4

		TOTAL	FAT
TOTALS		2224	110
Fat Budget:			304
Saved:			194
Carry-over:			658
New carry-over:			852

Meal Plans — Week 2
Fat Budget: 304 with Splurge
Minimum total calories: 1521 Total Calories

Friday — Week 2		CALORIES	
	AMOUNT	TOTAL	FAT
Breakfast			
Wheatena	1 c	200	18
Margarine	½ t	17	17
Skim milk	1 c	86	4
Orange	1	60	0
Whole-wheat toast	2 sl	140	18
Coffee or tea	1 c	0	0
Lunch			
Fruit Salad with Cottage Cheese		280	10
1% cottage cheese	½ c		
Blueberries	½ c		
Peach	1		
Cantaloupe	¼		
Honeydew melon	⅙		
Bran Muffin	2	232	46
Coffee or tea	1 c	0	0
Snack			
Popcorn, air-popped	6 c	180	0
Dinner			
Ginger-Carrot Soup	1 c	80	6
Chicken Marrakesh	1 sv	132	13
Indian Rice	1 c	188	13
Sweet Potatoes with Oranges, Apples, and Sweet Wine	1 sv	125	0
Whole-wheat bread	1 sl	70	9
Coffee or tea	1 c	0	0
Fig Newton cookie (Nabisco)	2	100	18
Snack			
Bran Chex	⅔ c	90	9
Skim milk	1 c	86	4
Banana	1	105	5
	TOTALS	2171	190
	Fat Budget:		304
	Saved:		114
	Carry-over:		852
	New carry-over:		966

Meal Plans — Week 2
Fat Budget: 304 with Splurge
Minimum total calories: 1521 Total Calories

Saturday — Week 2 Splurge Day	AMOUNT	CALORIES TOTAL	FAT
Breakfast			
Oatmeal	1 c	300	50
Pumpernickel toast	2 sl	160	18
Jelly	1 T	50	0
Orange	1	60	0
Nonfat flavored yogurt	1 c	160	0
Skim milk	1 c	86	4
Coffee or tea	1 c	0	0
Lunch			
Chicken with Rice, Tomatoes, and Artichokes	1 sv	274	12
Pear	1	98	0
Carrot sticks	½ cup	15	0
Skim milk	1 c	86	4
Coffee or tea	1 c	0	0
Dinner			
Sirloin steak	6 oz	354	132
Baked potato	1	145	0
Sour cream	2 T	52	46
French bread rolls	2	200	0
Tossed salad	1½ c	15	0
Blue cheese dressing	2 T	154	144
Cheesecake	1 sl	280	162
Coffee or tea	1 c	0	0
Snack			
Pepto-Bismol	2 T	0	0

TOTALS	2489	572
Fat Budget:		304
Saved:		−268
Carry-over:		966
New carry-over:		698

RECIPES

Recipes

WE LOVE to eat, our sons love to eat, our families love to eat, our guests love to eat — that is why we developed the delicious, low-fat recipes in *Eater's Choice* and *Choose to Lose*. You don't have to eat Jell-O, boiled chicken, or broth to lose weight. You can eat *Cajun Chicken* and *Ginger-Carrot Soup* and *Potato Skins* and *Turkey with Capers*. The following recipes are generally quick and easy to make. Try them. They will make reaching and maintaining your desirable and healthy weight a pleasure. Be sure to check out the recipes in *Eater's Choice*, too. You will find an additional 216 quick and easy, tasty, low-fat treats.

Be advised: Because the Goor oven is not necessarily calibrated to your oven, and your chicken breasts or swordfish steaks may be thicker or thinner than ours, etc., consider the baking time in the recipes an estimate. If the recipes tell you to bake a dish for 45 minutes, check your oven at 30. Your food may be ready.

A Note to Sodium and Sugar Watchers

If you are monitoring your sodium or sugar intake, you may want to cut down on the amount of salt or sugar in some of these recipes.

NOTE: Q indicates recipes that are quick and easy to prepare. But beware: Some Q recipes require marinating for several hours or overnight. Always read recipes before beginning!

Tips

- Read Chapter 9 for hints on cooking low-fat.
- Use freshly ground black pepper. There really is a difference between the stale, tasteless pepper that comes in a can and the bright taste of freshly ground pepper. It is definitely worth buying a pepper mill (not necessarily expensive) and whole peppercorns (available in the spice section of your grocery store).
- Fresh garlic is available at grocery stores and is far superior to garlic powder or garlic salt. It will stay fresh for weeks in the refrigerator.
- Fresh ginger root is available at many grocery stores and is easily kept for months in the refrigerator in a jar filled with sherry. When you are ready to cook, cut off the amount you need and peel and discard the outer covering. Use ginger root with superior results in recipes (except cakes and breads) that call for ginger.
- Grate a whole nutmeg (available in the spice section of your grocery store) with a hand grater for a fresher, nuttier taste.
- In any recipe that calls for canned chicken broth, either strain the broth by skimming off the surface with a fine tea strainer or use a gravy skimmer. If the fat is hardened (keep it in the refrigerator and the fat will congeal), just lift it off with a spoon.
- When using white flour, use unbleached white flour. When flour is bleached, it loses many of its important nutritional qualities.

Soups

CAULIFLOWER SOUP [Q]

Cauliflower Soup is a treasure. It is simple and quick to make and has a wonderful, delicate taste.

1 large head cauliflower
1 can chicken broth (10¾ oz), strained
2 stalks celery, diced
2 green onions, sliced
1 teaspoon olive oil
2 tablespoons unbleached white flour
1–2 cups water

Remove and discard cauliflower stem. Steam flowerets until tender. Reserve about ½ to 1½ cups and set aside. (You need about 4–5 cups cauliflower for the soup itself. Make sure you don't reserve too much!)

Purée cauliflower and chicken broth in blender. Set aside.

Sauté celery and green onions in oil until tender.

Reduce heat to medium and stir in flour.

Stir in cauliflower purée. Slowly mix in 1 cup of water, stirring constantly until soup thickens. If soup is too thick, stir in remaining water, ¼ cup at a time. Continue cooking until warmed through.

Cut reserved flowerets into bite-size pieces, add to soup, and serve.

Makes 6 one-cup servings (approximately)
Per serving: 47 Total calories; 7 Fat calories

BARLEY-VEGETABLE SOUP

A hearty soup that improves as it ages. Make it in the morning or the night before so it will have time to thicken.

½ cup pearl barley
2 quarts homemade chicken stock, or 3 cans (10¾ oz each) chicken broth, strained, + 3 cans water
1 small onion, cut into fourths
1 carrot, cut into thirds
1 stalk celery, cut into 1-inch slices

1 teaspoon thyme
1 bay leaf
Freshly ground pepper to taste
3–5 carrots, sliced
2 stalks celery, sliced
½ zucchini, sliced
½ cup onion, chopped
2 cups fresh spinach, chopped

Place barley, chicken stock, onion quarters, carrot thirds, celery slices, thyme, and bay leaf in a large soup pot and bring to a boil. Reduce heat, cover, and simmer for about 1 hour or until barley is tender.

Add sliced carrots, celery, zucchini, and chopped onion and cook until tender.

Add spinach a few minutes before serving.

Makes 9 one-cup servings
Per serving: 100 Total calories; 0 Fat calories

CANTALOUPE SOUP Q

Cantaloupe is an excellent source of vitamins A and C and fiber as well as being just plain delicious. Combined with ginger, orange juice, and buttermilk, cantaloupe makes a refreshing and unusual summer soup.

2 cantaloupes, chilled if possible
¼ cup orange juice
1 teaspoon chopped ginger root

3 tablespoons sweet vermouth
½ cup buttermilk

Halve melons, discard seeds, scoop out meat, and place it in blender. Add orange juice, ginger, vermouth, and buttermilk, and blend. If cold, serve immediately. Otherwise, chill.

Makes 6 one-cup servings
Per serving: 80 Total calories; 0 Fat calories

CARROT SOUP [Q]

Carrot soup is a great spur-of-the-moment soup because it is simple to make and you probably have the ingredients on hand. It is thick and tasty — wonderful to warm the soul and body on a nippy winter day.

1 medium onion, chopped
3 small cloves garlic, minced
1 teaspoon thyme
12 carrots, sliced (about 6 cups)
2 potatoes, peeled and sliced
    (about 2 cups)

1 bay leaf
Freshly ground pepper to taste
2 cans (10¾ oz each) chicken
    broth, strained

In a soup pot or large casserole, combine onion, garlic, and thyme.
Mix in carrots, potatoes, bay leaf, and pepper.
Add chicken broth and enough water to cover vegetables.
Bring soup to a boil. Reduce heat, cover, and simmer for 30 minutes.
Remove bay leaf and purée soup in blender.

Makes 11 one-cup servings
Per serving: 69 Total calories; 0 Fat calories

CUCUMBER SOUP [Q]

Cucumber soup gets a gold star for excellence. It is as refreshing as a dip in a cool lake on a hot day. It is simple, quick, and impressive.

2 cucumbers
2 cups nonfat yogurt
1 can (10¾ oz) chicken broth,
    strained

1 clove garlic, crushed
Walnuts, for garnish

Peel cucumbers and cut into bite-size cubes. Salt heavily and set aside.
Spoon yogurt into a medium casserole and stir until smooth.
Stir in chicken broth. Mix in garlic.
Rinse salt off cucumbers, add them to yogurt mixture, and add salt to taste.
Chill in refrigerator for several hours. Garnish with chopped walnuts.

Makes 5 one-cup servings
Per serving: 78 Total calories; 0 Fat calories
Per walnut half: 12 Total calories; 10 Fat calories

GINGER-CARROT SOUP Ⓠ

This soup can be eaten either cold or warm. The lime and ginger give it an interesting flavor.

1 tablespoon minced ginger root
2 cloves garlic, minced
½ cup chopped onion
1 teaspoon olive oil
5 cups sliced carrots

2 cans (10¾ oz each) chicken broth, strained, + 1 can water
¼ cup fresh lime juice (approximately)
Nonfat yogurt, for garnish

In a soup pot or large casserole, sauté ginger root, garlic, and onion in olive oil. Add a splash of water and cook vegetables until tender. Stir in carrots.

Add chicken broth and water and simmer until carrots are tender (about 20 minutes).

Add lime juice and purée soup in blender until smooth.

Chill or serve warm. Top each bowl with a large dollop of yogurt.

Makes 7 one-cup servings
Per serving: 80 Total calories; 6 Fat calories

TOMATO-RICE SOUP Ⓠ

If you hate wasting the juice that remains in the can after you have used only the tomatoes, this recipe will appeal to you. Each time you use canned tomatoes, accumulate their juice in a storage container in the freezer for future soups.

6 cups juice from canned tomatoes
1 tablespoon grated onion
1 pinch ground cloves

½ cup long-grain rice
1 cup frozen peas
1 cup frozen corn

Combine tomato juice, onion, cloves, and rice and bring to a boil. Reduce heat and simmer for about 20 minutes, until rice is tender.

Add peas and corn and cook about 5 minutes more.

Makes 8 one-cup servings
Per serving: 93 Total calories; 0 Fat calories

GINGER SQUASH SOUP Q

½ cup chopped onion
2 tablespoons minced ginger root
6 cups butternut squash, peeled, seeded, and cut into thin slices
2 cans chicken broth (10¾ oz each), strained

1 cup water
½ teaspoon salt (optional)
4 cloves garlic
2–3 tablespoons fresh lime juice
Salt and freshly ground black pepper to taste

In a large soup pot, combine onion, ginger root, and squash.
Add broth, water, salt, and garlic, and bring to a boil.
Reduce heat and simmer, covered, until squash is tender, about 15 minutes.
Purée in blender or food processor.
Return to pot and stir in lime juice, salt, and pepper.
Add more water, a tablespoon at a time, if soup is too thick.

Makes 7 one-cup servings
Per serving: 52 Total calories; 0 Fat calories

ORIENTAL NOODLE SOUP Q

This is a great last-minute soup. The dried Chinese noodles can be stored forever. The tofu and snow peas should be fresh.

2 cans chicken broth (10¾ oz each), strained, + 2 cans water
2 ounces cellophane noodles*
1 tablespoon soy sauce

¼ teaspoon white pepper
1 cake tofu,* cubed
1 green onion, sliced
10–15 snow peas

Bring broth and water to a boil in a soup pot. Add cellophane noodles.
Simmer about 10 minutes, until noodles are soft.
Add soy sauce and white pepper. Simmer a minute or two.
Add tofu, green onion, and snow peas and serve.

Makes 6 one-cup servings
Per serving: 64 Total calories; 8 Fat calories

---

*Available at Oriental food stores and some supermarkets.

SOUR CHERRY SOUP ☐Q

Sour Cherry Soup is a sweet soup. It is ideal for a luncheon or dinner party and *very* simple to make. It has no fat but does have a lot of sugar.

2 cans (1 lb each) undrained sour cherries packed in water
¾ cup sugar
1 stick cinnamon

2 tablespoons unbleached white flour
6 tablespoons cold water
2 cups water

Remove about 12 cherries from one can and put aside for garnish. (Or buy another whole can of cherries.)

In a medium saucepan, cook cherries with their juice, sugar, and cinnamon stick for 10 to 15 minutes.

In a small bowl, mix flour and 3 tablespoons of the cold water until smooth. Blend in remaining 3 tablespoons cold water.

Remove cinnamon stick from cooked cherries and set aside.

Pour cherry mixture into blender. Add flour mixture and blend until soup is smooth.

Return soup to saucepan, add 2 cups water, and heat just to boiling.

Return cinnamon stick to soup and chill.

Garnish each bowl of soup with a few cherries before serving.

Makes 6 one-cup servings
Per serving: 165 Total calories; 0 Fat calories

TORTILLA SOUP ☐Q

This is an instantaneous soup that always gets rave reviews.

6 corn tortillas*
1 medium onion, diced
3 cloves garlic, minced
1 teaspoon olive oil
2 tablespoons chili powder
1 teaspoon oregano
1 large can (28 oz) heavy concentrated crushed tomatoes

1 can (10¾ oz) chicken broth, strained, + 1 can water
1 green pepper, diced
1 cup frozen corn
Salt and pepper to taste

---

*Corn tortillas can be found in the refrigerator section of most supermarkets. Be sure they contain no lard or other saturated fat.

About 15 minutes before you serve soup, heat tortillas in a slow oven (325°F), until crisp.

In a soup pot, sauté onion and garlic in oil. Add a splash of water and cook vegetables until soft.

Stir in chili powder and oregano.

Stir in tomatoes, chicken broth, and water.

Bring to a boil and simmer for a few minutes.

Add green pepper and corn.

Add salt and pepper to taste.

For each serving, break a tortilla into small pieces and place at the bottom of a soup bowl. Ladle soup over the tortilla and serve.

Makes 7 one-cup servings
Per serving: 144 Total calories; 10 Fat calories

VEGETABLE SOUP WITH SPINACH, POTATOES, RICE, AND CORN Q

This soup is great! So quick, so easy, and so tasty.

2 cloves garlic, minced
1 teaspoon olive oil
5 ounces fresh spinach, torn into bite-size pieces
1 can chicken broth (10¾ oz), strained, + 2 cans water
½ teaspoon salt, optional
2 small potatoes, peeled and cubed
¼ cup long-grain rice
1 cup frozen corn

In soup pot, sauté garlic in oil until soft.

Stir in spinach and cook for about 1 minute.

Add broth, water, salt, potatoes, and rice, and bring to a boil.

Reduce to a simmer and cook for about 15 minutes or until potatoes are tender and rice is cooked.

Add corn and cook for about 1 minute.

Makes 5 one-cup servings
Per serving: 129 Total calories; 12 Fat calories

ZUCCHINI SOUP Q

One of the greatest recipes known to mankind. Hot or cold, summer or winter, for family or company, zucchini soup is delicious — and easy. You can even prepare it 20 minutes before you eat. If you want to make more and freeze it, just add a few more zucchini and more broth. This recipe is very flexible. Add more or less of any ingredient, and it will still taste superb.

3 large or 4 medium zucchini
   (or more or less), sliced
½ cup chopped onion
¼ cup long-grain rice
Chicken stock to cover zucchini,
   or 2 cans (10¾ oz each)
   chicken broth, strained, +
   water to cover zucchini

1 teaspoon salt
1 teaspoon curry powder
   (approximately)
1 teaspoon Dijon mustard
   (approximately)
½–1 cup nonfat yogurt

In a large soup pot, combine zucchini, onion, rice, chicken stock, water, and salt (add more water, if necessary, to cover zucchini).

Simmer for 15 minutes or until zucchini are tender.

Purée in blender, adding curry powder, mustard, and yogurt to taste. Eat warm or cool.

This soup freezes well. Reheat frozen soup for best results. Eat immediately or cool for later.

Makes 8 (approximately) one-cup servings
Per serving: 80 Total calories; 0 Fat calories

Poultry

APRICOT CHICKEN DIVINE Q

One-quarter cup of nonfat yogurt (0 fat calories) replaces ¼ cup of sour cream (108 fat calories) to create this divine chicken.

4 skinned chicken breasts	½ tablespoon Dijon mustard
¼ cup unbleached white flour	¼ cup nonfat yogurt
½ teaspoon salt (optional)	1 tablespoon slivered almonds
¼ cup apricot preserves	

Preheat oven to 375°F.

Shake chicken in a plastic bag filled with flour and salt until chicken is coated.

Place chicken in a single layer in a shallow baking pan and bake for 25 minutes.

Combine apricot preserves, mustard, and yogurt.

Spread apricot mixture on chicken and bake for 10–15 minutes more or until done.

Just before serving, brown almonds lightly in toaster oven.

Sprinkle almonds over chicken and serve over rice.

Serves 4
Per serving: 215 Total calories; 23 Fat calories

CAJUN CHICKEN

8 boned and skinned chicken breasts

½ cup unbleached white flour
½ teaspoon salt, optional

Seasoning Mix (Use more or less of the peppers for a hotter or milder taste.)

¾ teaspoon oregano
½ teaspoon thyme
½ teaspoon basil
½ teaspoon salt
½ teaspoon paprika

¼ teaspoon freshly ground black pepper
½ teaspoon cayenne pepper
¼ teaspoon white pepper

3 cloves garlic, minced
¾ cup chopped onion
2 stalks celery, diced
1 green pepper, chopped
1 tomato, coarsely chopped
1 tablespoon olive oil

1 can (10¾ oz) chicken broth, strained
1 small can (8 oz) tomato sauce
1 potato, peeled and diced
2 bay leaves

Preheat oven to 350°F.

Shake chicken in a plastic bag filled with flour and salt until chicken is coated. Place chicken in a single layer in baking pan and bake for 25 to 30 minutes until cooked through.

Meanwhile, cook potatoes in a small amount of water until tender. Set aside.

While chicken is baking, combine oregano, thyme, basil, salt, paprika, and peppers, and set aside.

In a large frying pan, sauté garlic, onion, celery, green pepper, and tomato in oil. Add a splash of water and cook vegetables until soft.

Mix in seasoning mixture and let simmer for about a minute.

Mix in broth and tomato sauce. Bring to a boil, then simmer for 5 minutes.

Lower heat and add chicken breasts, potato, and bay leaves. Cook until potatoes are soft.

NOTE: If you find the finished dish too "hot" for your taste, dilute with an additional can of tomato sauce.

Serves 8
Per serving: 196 Total calories; 28 Fat calories

INDONESIAN CHICKEN WITH GREEN BEANS Q

A beautiful dish — green beans set against ochre-colored sauce — and very tasty. This is one of our all-time favorites.

6 boned and skinned chicken breasts
½ cup unbleached white flour
¼ teaspoon freshly ground black pepper
½ teaspoon salt (optional)
1 pound green beans, washed and cut into bite-size pieces
10 cloves garlic, minced
1 tablespoon minced ginger root

1 small onion, chopped
1 teaspoon olive oil
Juice of 1 lime (preferred) or lemon
1 tablespoon double black soy sauce*
2 teaspoons brown sugar
2 teaspoons turmeric
½ teaspoon salt (optional)
½ cup water

Preheat oven to 375°F.

Shake chicken in a plastic bag with flour, pepper, and ½ teaspoon salt until chicken is completely coated.

Place chicken in a single layer in a baking pan and bake until fully cooked, about 20–30 minutes. Set aside. You may bake the chicken the night before and refrigerate it until ready to add to sauce.

Cook green beans in a pot of boiling water for 5–10 minutes until tender but still crisp. Set aside.

Cut chicken into bite-size pieces. Set aside.

Sauté garlic, ginger root, and onion in olive oil until soft.

Add lime juice, soy sauce, brown sugar, turmeric, ½ teaspoon salt, and ¼ cup of the water.

Slowly add remaining water, if necessary. Sauce should not be watery.

Add chicken and green beans and stir until completely covered with sauce.

Serve over rice.

8 servings
Per serving: 135 Total calories; 14 Fat calories

---

*Double black soy sauce is available at Oriental food stores and some supermarkets. You can make your own by mixing 2 teaspoons soy sauce with 1 teaspoon dark molasses.

LEMON CHICKEN [Q]

A delicate blending of tart and sweet, Lemon Chicken can't help but become one of your most popular family or company dishes.

4 boned and skinned chicken breasts
Juice of 2 lemons
½ cup unbleached white flour
½ teaspoon salt (optional)
¼ teaspoon freshly ground pepper

¼ teaspoon paprika
1 tablespoon grated lemon peel
2 tablespoons brown sugar
1 tablespoon fresh lemon juice
1 tablespoon water
1 lemon, sliced thin

Place chicken in a bowl or casserole. Cover with lemon juice and marinate in refrigerator for several hours or overnight, turning chicken periodically.

Preheat oven to 350°F.

Combine flour, salt, pepper, and paprika in plastic bag.

Remove chicken breasts from marinade and coat each with flour by shaking it in the plastic bag.

Place chicken in the baking pan in a single layer.

Either peel the yellow (zest) from a lemon and chop it fine in your food processor (a mini food chopper makes a perfect grater), or grate the zest with a hand grater. Mix grated peel with the brown sugar.

Sprinkle the lemon zest–sugar mixture evenly over the chicken breasts. Combine lemon juice and water and sprinkle evenly over chicken.

Put 1 lemon slice on each chicken breast and bake chicken for 35 to 40 minutes or until it is cooked through.

Serves 4
Per serving: 176 Total calories; 13 Fat calories

EAST INDIAN CHICKEN [Q]

4–5 skinned chicken breasts
¼ cup orange marmalade
1½ tablespoons cider vinegar
1 tablespoon granulated sugar
½ tablespoon brown sugar

¼ teaspoon salt (optional)
¼ teaspoon cumin
¼ teaspoon ginger
1½ teaspoons Worcestershire sauce

Preheat oven to 350°F.

Place chicken in a shallow baking pan in one layer.

In a medium-small bowl, combine the remaining ingredients and pour them evenly over the chicken breasts.

Bake 20 to 30 minutes or until breasts are cooked through.

Serves 4 or 5
Per serving: 71 Total calories; 13 Fat calories

BAR-B-QUE CHICKEN Q

Bar-B-Que chicken is a popular main dish with food lovers of all ages. It also makes a great sandwich. Place the barbecued chicken on a slice of bread, top with sauce, a slice of tomato, a few slices of onion, and another slice of bread.

2 tablespoons Dijon mustard
¼ cup vinegar
¼ cup molasses
½ cup ketchup
½ teaspoon Worcestershire
  sauce

2 cloves garlic, minced
Dash of Tabasco sauce
8 skinned chicken breasts or
  thighs*

In a large bowl, mix together Dijon mustard, vinegar, molasses, ketchup, Worcestershire sauce, garlic, and Tabasco for marinade. Pour about half the marinade over the chicken and refrigerate the rest to use later.

Marinate chicken for an hour (or less, if you haven't planned ahead).

Remove chicken and reserve remaining marinade.

Barbecue or broil chicken for 10 minutes.

Turn and coat chicken with marinade and cook until done.

Heat reserved marinade. Spoon over chicken before serving.

Serves 8

	Total calories	Fat calories
1 breast	173	13
1 thigh	126	24

---

*For a barbecue, you may want greater quantities of chicken. Just double, triple, quadruple, etc., the recipe.

CHICKEN MARRAKESH Q

4 boned and skinned chicken
  breasts
3 tablespoons fresh lemon juice
1 tablespoon grated lemon peel
1 clove garlic, minced

2–3 teaspoons thyme
½ teaspoon salt (optional)
½ teaspoon freshly ground
  pepper
1 lemon, thinly sliced

Place chicken in a bowl or casserole.

Mix together lemon juice, lemon peel, garlic, thyme, salt, and pepper and pour over chicken. Marinate chicken in refrigerator for at least 3 hours.

Preheat oven to 350°F.

Remove chicken from marinade and place in shallow baking dish.

Pour marinade over chicken and bake chicken for 20 to 30 minutes or until cooked through.

Garnish with lemon slices.

Serves 4
Per serving: 132 Total calories; 13 Fat calories

BLACKENED CHICKEN Q

Ron is in seventh heaven when he bites into a chunk of chicken and the chicken bites back. The spicier it is, the better he likes it. He likes Blackened Chicken a lot.

Spice Mix

1 teaspoon thyme
1 teaspoon basil
½ teaspoon onion powder
¼ teaspoon salt (optional)
½ teaspoon cayenne pepper

½ teaspoon paprika
½ teaspoon white pepper
¼ teaspoon freshly ground
  black pepper

5 skinned chicken breasts

Combine seasonings on a small plate. Roll each breast in seasonings, coating it on both sides, and set it aside on a large plate. For a milder chicken, use less seasoning on each breast.

Either grill on a cast-iron pancake griddle or barbecue grill, broil, or bake chicken until cooked through. Don't overcook.

NOTE: If you are using a cast-iron griddle, don't let it get too hot or it will char the chicken. You may need to turn on your exhaust fan to clear the hot spices from the air.

5 servings
Per serving: 130 Total calories; 13 Fat calories

CHICKEN WITH RICE, TOMATOES, AND ARTICHOKES Q

4 boned and skinned chicken
   breasts
2 cloves garlic, minced
½ cup chopped onion
1 teaspoon olive oil
1 large can (28 oz) tomatoes,
   chopped
2 cups water
½ teaspoon thyme

½ teaspoon oregano
½ teaspoon salt (optional)
¼ teaspoon freshly ground
   pepper
1 bay leaf
2 cups uncooked long-grain rice
1 jar (11½ oz) artichoke hearts,
   packed in water

Cut chicken into bite-size pieces and set aside.

In a large casserole, sauté garlic and onion in olive oil. Add a splash of water and cook vegetables until soft.

Stir in tomatoes and their liquid, water, thyme, oregano, salt, pepper, and bay leaf and bring to a boil.

Add chicken and rice, cover casserole, and reduce heat to low.

Cook for 25 minutes or until rice is tender, most liquid is absorbed, and chicken is cooked through.

Stir in artichokes and serve.

Serves 8
Per serving: 274 Total calories; 12 Fat calories

SESAME CHICKEN BROCHETTES Q

6 boned and skinned chicken
   breasts
¼ cup soy sauce
½ cup dry white wine or
   vermouth

1 clove garlic, minced
1 tablespoon sesame seeds,
   lightly toasted

Cut chicken breasts into 1-inch cubes and place in a bowl or casserole.

Combine soy sauce, wine, and garlic and pour over chicken. Marinate in refrigerator for at least 30 minutes.

Preheat oven to broil or prepare grill.

Remove chicken from marinade and reserve marinade.

Skewer chicken and broil or grill until cooked through, basting occasionally with marinade.

Sprinkle sesame seeds over chicken and serve over rice.

Heat marinade and spoon over chicken and rice.

6 servings
Per serving: 160 Total calories; 20 Fat calories

TURKEY MEXIQUE Q

A great dish with a chili taste.

1 cup chopped onion	1½ cups chicken broth, strained
2 teaspoons minced garlic	3 tablespoons tomato paste
2 teaspoons olive oil	3 cups diced turkey breast, raw
1–2 tablespoons chili powder	or cooked
1 tablespoon cumin seed	1 green pepper, diced
½ teaspoon salt	¼ cup stuffed green olives,
1 tablespoon unbleached white	sliced
flour	½ cup water

In a large skillet, sauté onion and garlic in olive oil. Add a splash of water and cook vegetables until soft.

Stir in chili powder, cumin seed, salt, and flour.

Add chicken broth and tomato paste and blend well.

Cook for 5 minutes over low heat.

Stir in turkey, green pepper, and olives and heat through. (If turkey is raw, cook until it turns white and is fully cooked.)

If sauce is too thick, add water 2 tablespoons at a time until desired consistency is reached.

Serve over rice.

Serves 6
Per serving: 146 Total calories; 16 Fat calories

TURKEY WITH CAPERS [Q]

You may sauté turkey cutlets, but this takes a lot of fat. Flouring turkey cutlets, then grilling them on a cast-iron pancake griddle with no added fat produces cutlets that are also tender but have almost no fat calories.

1 pound turkey breast cutlets	3 tablespoons red wine vinegar
½ cup unbleached white flour	2 tablespoons Dijon mustard
1 clove garlic, minced	1 cup chicken broth, strained
¼ cup chopped onion	2 tablespoons tomato paste
1 teaspoon olive oil	⅓ cup chopped parsley
3 tablespoons capers, drained	

Place cutlets between two pieces of wax paper and pound with meat mallet or rolling pin until thin.

Place flour on a plate. Dip each cutlet in flour, coating it on both sides, and set it on a large plate.

Heat cast-iron griddle. Cover it with cutlets. Turn cutlets when their edges start turning white. Remove cutlets as soon as they are no longer pink. Don't let them overcook! Turkey can become tough if cooked too long. Set them aside.

In a large skillet, sauté garlic and onion in olive oil until soft.

Stir in capers, vinegar, Dijon mustard, chicken broth, and tomato paste. Add parsley.

Add turkey cutlets and mix until they are covered with sauce.

4 servings
Per serving: 174 Total calories; 18 Fat calories

Fish and Shellfish

BROILED GINGER FISH Q

1 cup flour
1 teaspoon salt (optional)
½ teaspoon freshly ground
  pepper
4 six-ounce fish fillets
  (monkfish, haddock, etc.)

2 teaspoons margarine
4 teaspoons diced ginger root
Lemon slices to cover fillets

Set oven to broil and grease broiler pan with oil.
Combine flour, salt, and pepper on a large plate.
Dredge fillets in flour, covering both sides.
Dot fillets with margarine, sprinkle them with ginger, and cover with lemon slices.
Broil for 5 to 15 minutes or until fish flakes easily.

Serves 4
Per serving: 194 Total calories; 35 Fat calories

FISH BAKED IN OLIVE, CHILI PEPPER, AND TOMATO SAUCE Q

¾ cup chopped onion
2 cloves garlic, minced
1 teaspoon olive oil
1 tablespoon cornstarch
1 can (16 oz) tomatoes,
  chopped, juice reserved
⅓ cup sliced stuffed green olives

1 teaspoon chopped red or
  green chili pepper
1½ pounds flounder fillets (or
  other mild fish)
Salt to taste (optional)
1 tablespoon fresh lemon juice

Preheat oven to 375°F.

In a medium skillet, sauté onion and garlic in olive oil. Add a splash of water and cook vegetables until soft.

Mix in cornstarch.

Add tomatoes and their juice and mix until well blended.

Cook over medium-high heat until sauce thickens.

Stir in olives and chili pepper.

Spoon half the sauce into a baking pan large enough to hold the fillets in one layer. Place fillets over sauce.

Salt fillets and sprinkle them with lemon juice.

Cover fillets with remaining sauce and bake for 10 minutes or until they flake easily.

Serves 6
Per serving: 150 Total calories; 19 Fat calories

SCALLOP OR SHRIMP CURRY Q

Delight your guests or family with this unusual curry. The apples and lime create a unique combination of sweet and sour tastes.

1 cup chopped onion
1 apple, peeled, cored, and
  chopped
2 cloves garlic, minced
1–3 teaspoons curry powder
1 tablespoon olive oil
¼ cup unbleached white flour
½ teaspoon salt (optional)
¼ teaspoon cardamom
¼ teaspoon freshly ground
  pepper

1 can (10¾ oz) chicken broth,
  strained
1 tablespoon fresh lime juice
1¼ pounds bay scallops or
  shrimp, shelled and deveined
1 cup sliced mushrooms
10–15 snow peas (optional)
½–1 cup water

In a large skillet, sauté onion, apple, garlic, and curry powder in olive oil until tender.

Remove skillet from heat and blend in flour, salt, cardamom, and pepper.

Stir in chicken broth and lime juice until curry sauce is well blended.

Bring curry sauce to a boil, reduce heat, and simmer, uncovered, for about 5 minutes. Stir occasionally.

Meanwhile, place scallops or shrimp in a pot of boiling water and cook until just tender (5–10 minutes). Drain and set aside.

When curry sauce is finished cooking, add shellfish, mushrooms, and snow peas. If sauce is too thick add water, ¼ cup at a time, until desired consistency is achieved. Serve over rice.

Serves 6
Per serving: 187 Total calories
                          Fat calories
    with shrimp   35
    with scallops   25

SCALLOP OR SHRIMP CREOLE Q

2 green peppers, chopped
1 cup chopped onion
2 cloves garlic, minced
2 teaspoons olive oil
1 teaspoon brown sugar
¼ teaspoon freshly ground
   pepper
½ teaspoon thyme
¼ teaspoon cayenne pepper
1 bay leaf

½ teaspoon salt (optional)
2 large cans (28 oz each)
   tomatoes, drained, juiced, and
   chopped
½ cup sliced celery
1½ cups sliced mushrooms
3 tablespoons chopped parsley
1 pound bay scallops or shrimp,
   shelled and deveined

Sauté green peppers, onion, and garlic in olive oil. Add a splash of water and cook vegetables until soft.

Add brown sugar, pepper, thyme, cayenne pepper, bay leaf, and salt and stir well.

Stir in tomatoes and cook over low heat for 30 minutes or until sauce is thick.

Add celery and mushrooms and cook for a few minutes more.

Mix in parsley and scallops or shrimp and cook for 5 to 10 minutes or until shellfish is cooked through.

Serve immediately so shellfish will not overcook.

Serve over rice.

Serves 6
Per serving: 177 Total calories
                          Fat calories
    with shrimp   28
    with scallops   18

Vegetables

INDIAN VEGETABLES

This recipe makes a large pot of colorful, tasty vegetables, which may be eaten warm or cold. Try it as a main dish served over rice.

2 teaspoons olive oil
1 teaspoon black mustard
    seeds*
3 cloves garlic, chopped
1 medium onion, chopped
1 green pepper, chopped
2–3 potatoes, peeled and cubed
1 small eggplant, peeled and
    cubed
1½ teaspoons turmeric
1 teaspoon salt (optional)
¼ cup water
1 teaspoon cumin

1 teaspoon coriander
1 teaspoon garam masala*
Any vegetables, for example:
    1 head broccoli, cut into
        flowerets (about 3 cups)
    1 cup or more cauliflower
        flowerets
    6 carrots, sliced
    1 cup or more green beans,
        cut in half
    1 cup sliced celery
    1 zucchini, sliced
1 cup water

In a large pot, heat olive oil and add black mustard seeds.

When the mustard seeds begin to pop, add garlic, onion, and green pepper and cook until soft.

Stir in potatoes and eggplant.

Add turmeric and salt and mix until vegetables are covered with turmeric sauce.

---

*Available at Indian or Oriental food stores.

Add ¼ cup water, reduce heat to low, cover the pot, and cook for 10 minutes.

Stir in cumin, coriander, garam masala, and vegetables.

Add 1 cup water and increase heat to medium.

After 10 minutes, lower heat and cook until vegetables are tender.

Serves 12
Per serving: 72 Total calories; 7 Fat calories

HOT AND GARLICKY EGGPLANT Q

1 medium eggplant (about 1 pound)

5 small, dried black Chinese mushrooms*

1 tablespoon chili paste with garlic*

1 tablespoon vinegar

½ tablespoon soy sauce

½ tablespoon double black soy sauce*

2 tablespoons dry sherry

½ teaspoon sugar

1 large green pepper, chopped

1 teaspoon olive oil

½ cup water

Slice eggplant into bite-size pieces. Salt generously and set aside for about 20 minutes.

Meanwhile, place mushrooms in a small bowl and cover them with boiling water.

After about 15 minutes, remove mushrooms. Squeeze out the excess water and discard stems. Slice mushrooms and set aside.

Wash off the salt and bitter juices of the eggplant. In a vegetable steamer, cook eggplant until soft. Set aside.

Combine chili paste with garlic, vinegar, soy sauces, sherry, and sugar and set aside.

In a large skillet, sauté green pepper and mushrooms in oil. Add a splash of water and cook until tender.

Stir in eggplant.

Mix in soy sauce mixture until vegetables are covered and then stir in water.

Simmer for about 5 minutes.

Makes 8 half-cup servings
Per serving: 25 Total calories; 5 Fat calories

---

*Available at Oriental food stores.

CURRIED WHIPPED POTATOES ⃞Q

You need not add butter or margarine to make delectable whipped potatoes. In this recipe, sautéed onions, mustard seed, and cumin make them special and exotic. Leave the sautéed onions out of this recipe and you have plain but scrumptious whipped potatoes at 0 fat calories per serving.

4 potatoes (about 2 pounds)
¾ cup chopped onions
1 teaspoon olive oil
½ teaspoon mustard seed
½ teaspoon cumin
1–4 tablespoons skim milk
Salt and freshly ground black pepper to taste

Peel potatoes, slice thinly, and place in a medium saucepan with water to cover. Bring to a boil and boil until tender.

Meanwhile, sauté onions in olive oil. Lower heat to medium and stir in mustard seed and cumin. Cook a few moments until onions are soft.

Drain potatoes. Beat potatoes with an electric mixer. Add milk, one tablespoon at a time, until potatoes are whipped.

Mix in onions and salt and pepper to taste.

4 servings
Per serving: 168 Total calories; 10 Fat calories

POTATO SKINS ⃞Q

Leslie Goodman-Malamuth of the Center for Science in the Public Interest devised this recipe as a substitute for the high-fat potato skins you often find in restaurants. Not only is this recipe quick and easy, the resulting potatoes are scrumptious.

4 large potatoes
1 teaspoon olive oil (optional)
Paprika to taste

Preheat oven to 450°F.

Scrub potatoes well, cut them lengthwise into six wedges the size and shape of dill pickle spears, and dry them on a paper towel.

In a large bowl, toss potato spears with olive oil until they are well covered.

Spread potatoes on a baking sheet, dust them with paprika, and bake for 20 to 30 minutes or until fork-tender.

Serves 6 (So good, 2 people can easily finish them off!)
Per serving: 66 Total calories; 7 Fat calories

SWEET POTATOES WITH ORANGES, APPLES, AND SWEET WINE Q

4 cups sweet potatoes cut into
½-inch slices
1 cup diced apple
1 orange, peeled and cut into
bite-size pieces

2–3 tablespoons brown sugar
¼ cup plum wine or other
sweet wine
3 whole cloves

Preheat oven to 375°F.

Place sweet potato slices in a saucepan with water to cover. Bring to a boil. Reduce heat, cover, and simmer until just tender.

Drain sweet potatoes and place in a casserole.

Mix apple, orange, brown sugar, wine, and cloves.

Pour mixture over sweet potatoes.

Bake, covered, for 30 minutes or until apples are tender.

Serves 6
Per serving: 125 Total calories; 0 Fat calories

ACORN SQUASH Q

3 medium acorn squash*
1 cup boiling water
3 teaspoons margarine
(optional)

Freshly ground black pepper to
taste

Preheat oven to 400°F.

Cut each squash in half and scoop out seeds and fibers.

Slice a small piece off the bottom of each half so that they will not roll over.

Place squash halves, cut-side down, in a shallow casserole.

Pour boiling water into the casserole and cover it tightly with aluminum foil.

Bake for 45 minutes or until squash is soft when pierced with a fork.

Turn squash cut-side up and fill each half with ½ teaspoon margarine.

---

*Butternut squash may also be cooked this way and is delicious. Its dull cream exterior conceals a beautiful, deep orange interior.

Bake for 5 minutes more.
Grind pepper over squash and serve.

6 servings

	Total calories	Fat calories
Per serving	40	0
with margarine	55	15

STEAMED ZUCCHINI MATCHSTICKS Q

So light, so tasty — you don't even need to add salt, spices, or fat. But you may want to crush garlic into one teaspoon of melted margarine and combine it with the vegetables.

2 small zucchini (or ½ small zucchini per person)
1 thick carrot, peeled

1 teaspoon margarine (optional)
1 clove garlic (optional)

Cut zucchini and carrot into 2-inch lengths.
Place a zucchini section on a cutting surface, skin-side down.
Holding the sides of the section, slice lengthwise at ⅛-inch intervals. Hold the slices together.
Roll the section one-quarter turn, making sure the slices stay together.
Again, make parallel slices, ⅛ inch apart lengthwise.
Result: zucchini matchsticks.
Repeat for remaining sections of zucchini and carrot.
Place zucchini sticks on top of carrot sticks in a vegetable steamer and steam until just tender (about 1 or 2 minutes).

Serves 4

	Total calories	Fat calories
Per serving	17	0
with margarine	24	7

Pizza, Chili, Pasta, and Rice

FOCACCIA Q

The whole-wheat flour in this pizza makes it healthier and gives it a crunchy texture. Try it! It's easy.

Dough
1½ teaspoons dry active yeast	2½ cups whole-wheat flour
½ teaspoon honey	¾ teaspoon salt (optional)
1 cup warm water	1 tablespoon olive oil

Tomato Sauce
1 large can (28 oz) tomatoes, or 3 large tomatoes	½ teaspoon oregano
2 cloves garlic, minced	¼ teaspoon basil
1 small onion, chopped	Ground hot cherry peppers (optional)
1 teaspoon olive oil	

The Dough

Place yeast, honey, and warm water in food processor or large bowl. Let proof (get bubbly).

Add flour, salt, and olive oil and process or knead until smooth and elastic, adding flour if needed.

Place dough in an oiled bowl, cover with a towel, and let rise in a warm place for about 1 hour.

Punch down dough and let it rest on floured counter for 10 minutes.

Grease a 10 × 15-inch cookie sheet with oil. Roll dough out (or press with your hands) onto the cookie sheet.

Pinch a rim around the edge. Cover with a towel and let rise for 30 minutes.

Meanwhile, make the tomato sauce.

The Tomato Sauce

If using canned tomatoes, drain liquid and chop tomatoes. If using whole tomatoes, chop fine.

In a medium skillet, sauté garlic and onion in olive oil until tender. Stir in tomatoes, oregano, and basil and let simmer until thick (about 10–15 minutes).

Preheat oven to 400°F.
Spread the sauce over the dough.
Add hot cherry peppers, if desired.
Bake for 20 to 25 minutes.

Makes 12 pieces
Per piece: 113 Total calories; 18 Fat calories

CHILI NON CARNE [Q]

This is a great chili recipe. It is filled with nutritious vegetables that provide texture but do not interfere with the delicious chili taste. Eat it hot in a bowl mixed with chopped onion, tomatoes, and lettuce, or spoon it into pita bread with chopped onion, lettuce, and tomatoes.

¾ cup chopped onion
2 cloves garlic, minced
1 teaspoon olive oil
2 tablespoons chili powder
¼ teaspoon basil
¼ teaspoon oregano
¼ teaspoon cumin
2 cups finely chopped zucchini
1 cup finely chopped carrot
1 large can (28 oz) tomatoes
    + 1 small can (14½ oz)
    tomatoes, drained and
    chopped

1 can (15 oz) kidney beans,
    undrained
2 cans (15 oz each) kidney
    beans, *drained* and
    thoroughly rinsed
Chopped onions, tomatoes,
    lettuce, or green peppers, for
    garnish

In a large pot, sauté onion and garlic in olive oil. Add a splash of water and cook until soft.

Mix in chili powder, basil, oregano, and cumin.

Stir in zucchini and carrots until well blended. Cook for about 1 minute over low heat, stirring occasionally.

Stir in chopped tomatoes, undrained kidney beans, and drained kidney beans.

Bring to a boil. Reduce heat and simmer for 30 to 45 minutes or until thick.

Top with chopped onions, tomatoes, and lettuce or green peppers.

Makes 8 one-cup servings
Per serving: 117 Total calories; 5 Fat calories

SPAGHETTI SAUCE À LA SICILIA [Q]

Make a basic tomato sauce and add steamed eggplant and mushrooms for an appetizing spaghetti sauce that needs no ground meat.

1 small eggplant, peeled and cubed
6 cups Basic Tomato Sauce (see below)
2 cups sliced mushrooms
12 ounces spaghetti

Salt eggplant and cover with a heavy plate. After 15 minutes, wash off salt and steam eggplant until tender. Set aside.

In a medium saucepan, heat 6 cups of tomato sauce.

Stir in eggplant and mushrooms, cook 5 minutes more.

While spaghetti sauce is cooking, prepare spaghetti according to package directions.

Pour tomato sauce over spaghetti and serve.

Serves 6
Per serving: 275 Total calories; 10 Fat calories

Basic Tomato Sauce

1 cup chopped onion
2 teaspoons olive oil
4 large cans (28 oz each) tomatoes, drained
1 can (6 oz) tomato paste
2 teaspoons basil
1 teaspoon salt (optional)

In a large saucepan, cook onion in olive oil until soft.

Chop tomatoes and stir in tomato paste. (Tomatoes can easily be chopped and tomato paste blended in a food processor.)

Add to onions.

Stir in basil and salt.

Simmer until thick (at least 1 hour).

This tomato sauce freezes well.

Makes 16 half-cup servings
Per serving: 32 Total calories; 5 Fat calories

ASPARAGUS PASTA ⬚Q

Asparagus-pasta makes a delightful luncheon dish, first course for an elegant meal, or light dinner. No one consuming this dish will believe how incredibly simple it is to make.

1 pound asparagus, sliced into 1-inch pieces	¼ teaspoon thyme
3 tablespoons Dijon mustard	2 tablespoons chopped parsley
1 tablespoon olive oil	¾ pound very thin spaghetti or pasta of your choice
¼ cup thinly sliced shallots	Salt and pepper to taste
1 clove garlic, minced	1 cup sliced mushrooms
2 anchovy fillets, chopped	

In a large pot of boiling water, cook asparagus until tender and still bright green (about 3 minutes).

Combine mustard, olive oil, shallots, garlic, anchovies, thyme, and parsley. Set aside.

Cook pasta. Drain, but reserve 1 cup of the cooking water.

Combine pasta with dressing. Add asparagus and mushrooms and mix well. Add some of the cooking water if too dry. Add salt and pepper to taste.

Serves 6
Per serving: 253 Total calories; 26 Fat calories

Variation: Follow the above recipe but add two boned and skinned chicken breasts that have been steamed and cut into bite-size pieces.

Serves 6
Per serving: 296 Total calories; 30 Fat calories

INDIAN RICE [Q]

1 teaspoon olive oil	1 teaspoon coriander
2 cloves garlic, minced	¼ teaspoon cinnamon
1 tablespoon minced ginger root	¼ teaspoon ground cloves
¾ cup chopped onion	¼ teaspoon salt (optional)
¼ teaspoon cardamom	1½ cups long-grain rice
¼ teaspoon caraway seeds	3¾ cups water

In a medium saucepan, heat olive oil.

Add garlic, ginger, onion, and a splash of water and cook until soft.

Mix in cardamom, caraway seeds, coriander, cinnamon, cloves, salt, and rice and blend well.

Add water, cover, and bring to a boil. Reduce heat and cook until all water is absorbed (about 25 minutes).

Makes 12 half-cup servings
Per serving: 91 Total calories; 5 Fat calories

Salads

DIJON CHICKEN-RICE SALAD Q

3¾ cups water
1½ cups long-grain rice
½ teaspoon salt (optional)
3 tablespoons Dijon mustard
3 tablespoons white vinegar
1 tablespoon olive oil

1½–2 cups diced green and/or
  red pepper
¼ cup pitted black olives, sliced
¼ cup sliced green onion
3 cooked chicken breasts, diced

In a medium saucepan, bring water to a boil.

Add rice and salt, reduce heat, cover, and simmer for 20 to 25 minutes or until water is absorbed.

Place rice in a bowl.

Combine mustard, vinegar, and olive oil and mix into rice.

Add green pepper, olives, green onion, and chicken and mix well.

Tastes best when tepid. If the salad is too dry, mix in a little water, 1 tablespoon at a time.

Makes 6 one-and-a-half-cup servings
Per serving: 267 Total calories; 34 Fat calories

CUCUMBER SALAD Q

2 cucumbers, peeled and sliced
  thin
1 medium onion, sliced thin
1 teaspoon salt (optional)

1 teaspoon sugar
1 teaspoon dill weed
1 cup white vinegar

Mix cucumbers and onion together in a ceramic or glass bowl.

Add salt, sugar, and dill weed to vinegar and pour over cucumbers and onion.

Chill 1 hour.

Serves 6
Per serving: 20 Total calories; 0 Fat calories

POTATO SALAD [Q]

4–5 Russet (red) potatoes
½ cup nonfat yogurt
3 tablespoons reduced-calorie
  mayonnaise

1 teaspoon tarragon
1 tablespoon white vinegar
1 teaspoon Dijon mustard
½ teaspoon salt (optional)

Scrub potatoes thoroughly. Steam until tender.
Meanwhile, combine remaining ingredients. Set aside.
Cut potatoes into chunks (do not remove skin).
Pour sauce over potatoes so they are thoroughly coated.
Serve warm or cold.

Serves 6
Per serving: 105 Total calories; 14 Fat calories

CURRIED TUNA SALAD WITH PEARS [Q]

1½ tablespoons reduced-calorie
  mayonnaise
2 tablespoons nonfat yogurt
¼–½ teaspoon curry powder

2 cans (6½ oz each) water-
  packed tuna, drained
¼ cup diced pear
Lettuce

Combine mayonnaise, yogurt, and curry powder.
Mix into tuna fish.
Stir in pear.
Serve over lettuce.

Serves 3
Per serving: 175 Total calories; 23 Fat calories

FRUIT SALAD WITH COTTAGE CHEESE OR YOGURT [Q]

This high-protein, low-fat dish makes a filling lunch. Round it off with a piece of homemade bread and, for dessert, home-popped popcorn.

Spring or Summer Fruits

¼ cantaloupe   1 peach
½ cup blueberries   ⅙ honeydew melon

Fall or Winter Fruits

½ Golden Delicious apple   ½ Bosc pear
1 kiwi   ½ orange

½ cup 1% cottage cheese or
  nonfat yogurt

Cut fruit into bite-size pieces and place in bowl.
Mix in cottage cheese or yogurt.

Serves 1

	Total calories	Fat calories
Spring or summer salad:		
with cottage cheese	280	10
with nonfat yogurt	250	0
Fall or winter salad:		
with cottage cheese	270	10
with nonfat yogurt	245	0

Sandwiches and Dips

FAUX GUACAMOLE Q

Your guests will never imagine that the dip they are eagerly devouring was made with asparagus. What a buy. A great-tasting treat at a cost of 0 total fat calories.

2 tablespoons yogurt cheese*
1 pound asparagus
1 clove garlic, crushed
¼ teaspoon cayenne pepper
¼ teaspoon chili powder
1 tablespoon fresh lemon juice

2 ounces diced green chili peppers**
1 cup chopped tomatoes
1 tablespoon chopped onion
Whole-wheat pita bread

Prepare yogurt cheese a day in advance (see box on page 253).

Snap off the bottom ends of the asparagus and discard. Find a frying pan that will hold the asparagus in one layer and fill it with an inch of water. Bring the water to a boil and add the asparagus. Cook until soft. Drain asparagus and purée with garlic in blender or food processor.

Mix in cayenne pepper, chili powder, lemon juice, yogurt cheese, chili peppers, tomatoes, and onion. Chill for several hours.

Serve with toasted whole-wheat pita pockets divided into quarters or Bagel Chips (recipe follows).

---

*See box on page 253.
**Available in small cans in most supermarkets.

Makes 1½ cups (approximately)

	Total calories	Fat calories
Per tablespoon	7	0
with pita bread quarter	33	0

YOGURT CHEESE Q

Yogurt cheese made with nonfat yogurt may be substituted for sour cream and cream cheese in some recipes, greatly reducing the fat calories. It is easy to make. Place nonfat yogurt (without gelatin) in a coffee filter (or cheesecloth) in a coffeepot or in a strainer over a bowl. Cover and refrigerate overnight. As the yogurt drains, it condenses. About half the yogurt will become cheese. Pour off whey and keep cheese in a covered container in the refrigerator. Add herbs, green onions, or Dijon mustard to make a flavored cheese.

Calories per tablespoon: 7 Total calories; 0 Fat calories

BAGEL CHIPS Q

A great crunchy snack — eat them alone or with dips.
Bagels (plain, onion, garlic, etc.)

Flavor Options
1 clove garlic
Chili powder

Cajun Seasoning Mix (page 228)
Cinnamon and sugar

Preheat oven to 200°F.

Cut bagel into ¼–⅜-inch-thick slices. They will look like very thin bagels. (Halve or quarter slices if you want smaller bagel chips.) Place pieces on cookie sheet on one layer.

Either press garlic and spread over bagel slices, sprinkle chili powder or spice mix over them, leave them plain, or for a sweet treat, sprinkle on a mix of cinnamon and sugar.

Bake for 1–2 hours.

Per bagel chip: 38 Total calories; 2 Fat calories

CHICKPEA SANDWICH OR DIP Q

1 can chickpeas
2 cloves garlic
⅓ cup parsley
1 tablespoon tahini (sesame
  seed paste)*
Juice of 1 lemon (about ¼ cup)

4 six-inch whole-wheat pita
  bread pockets
Chopped tomatoes, green
  onions, and lettuce, for
  garnish

Drain chickpeas. Reserve liquid. In blender or food processor, chop garlic and parsley.

Add chickpeas, tahini, and lemon juice.

Blend until smooth, adding more chickpea liquid if spread is too stiff. Make sandwiches by spooning chickpea spread into pita bread pockets.

Garnish with chopped tomatoes, green onions, and lettuce.

Makes 4 sandwiches

Use as a dip for vegetables, crackers, squares of pita, etc.

Makes about 1½ cups

	Total calories	Fat calories
Per sandwich	195	35
Per tablespoon	20	4

BABA GHANOUSH Q

1 medium eggplant
¼ cup or more fresh lemon
  juice
3 tablespoons tahini (sesame
  seed paste)*

1–2 cloves garlic
¼ cup chopped parsley
Salt to taste

Peel eggplant, cut into bite-size pieces, and salt heavily. Set aside for 15 minutes. Rinse and squeeze eggplant and steam in vegetable steamer until soft.

Purée eggplant in food processor or blender.

---

*Available at Mideast food shops and many supermarkets.

Blend in lemon juice and tahini.

Just before you serve, crush garlic into purée and mix in parsley and salt.

Taste. Add more lemon juice if you wish.

Serve with whole-wheat or plain pita bread cut into pieces.

Makes about 2 cups
Per tablespoon: 12 Total calories; 7 Fat calories

TED MUMMERY'S TURKEY BARBECUE

We discovered a most wonderful turkey barbecue while at a health conference in Steven's Point, Wisconsin. Ted Mummery, the owner of La Claire's Frozen Yogurt, Inc., has kindly allowed us to share his recipe with you. It's delicious in a whole-wheat pita pocket or on an onion bagel or a roll.

5–6 lbs turkey breast
4 cans (14½ oz each) stewed
  tomatoes
2 large cans (12 oz each)
  tomato paste
1 cup water
½ cup brown sugar
⅓ cup dark molasses
½ cup apple cider vinegar
1 teaspoon hickory salt*
  (optional) or 1 teaspoon salt

1 heaping teaspoon garlic
  powder
1½ heaping teaspoons onion
  powder
1 heaping teaspoon basil
1½ heaping teaspoons oregano
1 heaping teaspoon cayenne
1 teaspoon all-purpose
  seasoning
½ teaspoon white pepper

Preheat oven to 350°F.

Remove skin and fat from turkey breast.

Bake turkey with breast down until fully cooked, about 1½–2½ hours. (You may do this the night before.) Refrigerate.

Mix tomatoes, tomato paste, and water in blender or food processor for a few moments. You want to chop the tomatoes, not purée them.

---

*Ted recommends 3 teaspoons of hickory salt. If you are eating this barbecue often, we suggest eliminating the hickory salt as it contains an unhealthy ingredient — smoke (charcoal).

Place in 5-quart Crockpot. (You may also cook barbecue in a large pot on the stove.) Stir in remaining ingredients. Set Crockpot on automatic or cook in pot at low heat for about 2 hours.

Pull turkey from bones and cut into bite-size pieces. Add turkey to sauce and cook for about another hour.

Makes 30 half-cup servings
Per serving: 131 Total calories; 5 Fat calories

Breads, Muffins, and Waffles

CARDAMOM BREAD

1 tablespoon active dry yeast
2 tablespoons brown sugar
¼ cup warm water
2–4 cups unbleached white
   flour

1 teaspoon salt
¼–½ teaspoon cardamom*
2 tablespoons olive oil
1 cup skim milk

Combine yeast, brown sugar, and water in a large bowl or a food processor. Let proof (get bubbly).

Add 2 cups flour, salt, and cardamom and mix.

Add skim milk and olive oil and mix.

Knead dough 10 minutes or process 15 seconds or until dough is smooth and elastic, adding more flour if necessary.

Place dough in a large oiled bowl, cover with a towel, and let rise in warm place for 1 hour or until doubled in bulk.

Roll into loaf and place in loaf pan greased with margarine.

Cover with a towel and let rise for 1 hour or until doubled in bulk.

Preheat oven to 425°F.

Bake loaves for 10 minutes.

Reduce heat to 350°F and bake for 30 minutes more or until loaves are golden brown and sound hollow when tapped.

Makes 1 loaf

	Total calories	Fat calories
Per ½-inch slice	98	15
Per loaf	1663	255

---

*For a totally different taste, substitute 1 teaspoon cinnamon.

ANADAMA BREAD

This version of the New England bread has whole-wheat flour added to it to make it healthier while retaining its wonderful taste and texture.

1 tablespoon active dry yeast	1–1½ teaspoons salt
Pinch of sugar	2 tablespoons olive oil
¼ cup warm water	1 cup water
¾ cup corn meal	3 tablespoons molasses
1½ cups whole-wheat flour	
1½ cups unbleached white flour (approximately)	

Dissolve yeast with pinch of sugar in ¼ cup warm water in a large bowl or a food processor. Let proof.

Mix in corn meal, whole-wheat flour, 1 cup of the white flour, and salt.

Stir in olive oil, 1 cup warm water, and molasses.

Knead dough 10 minutes or process 15 seconds or until dough is smooth and elastic, adding more white flour if necessary.

Place dough in a large oiled bowl, cover with a towel, and let rise in a warm place for 1 hour or until doubled in bulk.

Form into a loaf and place in a loaf pan greased with margarine. Cover and let rise for 1 hour or until doubled in bulk.

Preheat oven to 400°F.

Bake loaf for 15 minutes.

Reduce heat to 350°F and bake about 30 minutes more or until loaf is golden brown and sounds hollow when tapped.

Makes 1 loaf

	Total calories	Fat calories
Per ½-inch slice	113	15
Per loaf	1919	257

CUMIN WHEAT BREAD

Although this is a totally whole-wheat bread, it is not the least bit heavy. It is a favorite with young children as well as adults.

1 tablespoon dry yeast	1 teaspoon salt
¼ cup warm water	½ teaspoon whole cumin seeds
2 tablespoons honey	1½ tablespoons olive oil
3½ cups whole-wheat flour	1 cup skim milk

In a large mixing bowl or the bowl of a food processor, combine yeast, water, and honey. Let proof.

Mix in 2 cups of the flour, the salt, and cumin seeds.

Add oil and milk and mix or process well, adding more flour until dough is fairly stiff.

Knead dough 10 minutes or process for 15 seconds or until dough is smooth and elastic, adding more flour if necessary.

Form dough into a ball. Place in an oiled bowl. Cover and let rise for about 1 hour.

Roll dough into a loaf and place in loaf pan greased with margarine. Cover with towel and let rise for 1 hour.

Preheat oven to 375°F and bake for 50–60 minutes or until bread is golden and sounds hollow when tapped.

Makes 1 loaf

	Total calories	Fat calories
Per ½-inch slice	107	15
Per loaf	1814	252

ONION FLAT BREAD

1 tablespoon active dry yeast	1 teaspoon + a few shakes salt
1 pinch sugar	1 teaspoon margarine (optional)
1 cup warm water	1 cup chopped onions
2½–3 cups unbleached white flour*	1 teaspoon paprika

Place yeast, sugar, and water in a large bowl or a food processor. Let proof.

---

*For a slightly different taste, use 1 cup of whole-wheat flour, along with 1½–2 cups unbleached white flour.

Mix in 2 cups flour and salt. Knead for 10 minutes or process for 15 seconds, until smooth and elastic, adding flour if necessary.

Place dough in an oiled bowl, cover with a towel, and let rise in a warm place for an hour or until doubled in bulk.

Punch dough down and split in half. Let rest for 5 minutes.

Meanwhile, grease two 9-inch cake pans with margarine.

Melt the teaspoon of margarine.

Press dough into cake pans.

Spread margarine over the tops and press onion into the surface.

Let rise about 45 minutes or until doubled in bulk.

Preheat oven to 450°F.

Sprinkle tops with paprika and a few shakes of salt.

Bake 20–25 minutes, until lightly browned.

Makes 2 loaves, 8 slices per loaf
Per loaf: 667 Total calories; 56 Fat calories
Per slice: 83 Total calories; 7 Fat calories

Per loaf without margarine: 622 Total calories; 11 Fat calories
Per slice without margarine: 78 Total calories; 1 Fat calorie

SESAME BREADSTICKS

Beware! These breadsticks are habit-forming.

1 teaspoon active dry yeast
¼ cup warm water
⅔ cup whole-wheat flour
2 or more cups unbleached white flour
1 teaspoon salt, optional

⅔ cup nonfat skim milk
1 tablespoon olive oil
1 egg white
2 teaspoons water
1 tablespoon sesame seeds

Place yeast and warm water in a large bowl or a food processor. Let proof.

Mix in flours and salt.

Add milk and olive oil, and knead for 10 minutes or process until dough is smooth and elastic, adding more flour if necessary.

Place dough in a bowl, cover with a towel, and let rise 1 hour.

Preheat oven to 400°F.

On a lightly floured surface, roll the dough into a quarter-inch-thick rectangle.

Cut the dough into half-inch strips. (If you prefer thicker breadsticks, cut the dough into one-inch strips.)

Roll each strip in your palms to make a breadstick and lay it on an ungreased baking sheet. Place the sticks about a half inch apart.

Beat the egg white and water together and brush onto breadsticks.

Sprinkle sesame seeds evenly over breadsticks.

Count the breadsticks so you can calculate their fat calories.

Bake for 20 to 30 minutes or until golden brown. Cool on a rack.

Makes about 35 six-inch sticks
To determine the total calories and fat calories for each breadstick, divide the number of breadsticks into the following numbers:
Total calories: 1423; Fat calories: 196
For example, 196 fat calories divided by 35 breadsticks = 6 fat calories each.

BRAN MUFFINS

Wheat bran, made from the outer coverings of wheat kernels, is rich in vitamins, minerals, and insoluble dietary fiber. Insoluble dietary fiber promotes regularity and is believed to protect against colon cancer.

1 cup whole-wheat flour	1 cup buttermilk
1 cup wheat bran	1 egg, beaten
3 tablespoons brown sugar	3 tablespoons molasses
1/4 teaspoon salt	2 tablespoons olive oil
1 teaspoon baking soda	1/3 cup raisins
1/2 teaspoon baking powder	

Preheat oven to 400°F. Grease a 12-cup muffin tin with margarine.

Combine whole-wheat flour, wheat bran, brown sugar, salt, baking soda, and baking powder. Set aside.

In a mixing bowl, mix buttermilk, egg, molasses, and oil.

Add dry ingredients and mix until just moistened.

Fold in raisins.

Fill muffin tin and bake for about 15 minutes or until golden brown and a cake tester comes out clean.

Makes 12 muffins
Per muffin: 116 Total calories; 23 Fat calories

APRICOT OAT MUFFINS Q

½ cup orange juice
1 cup dried apricots, chopped
(easily done in food
processor)
¼ cup brown sugar
1 cup oat bran

¼ cup wheat germ
¾ cup whole-wheat flour
2 teaspoons baking powder
2 tablespoons olive oil
½ cup skim milk
1 egg

Preheat oven to 400°F. Grease a 12-cup muffin tin with margarine.

In a small saucepan, heat orange juice until boiling. Mix in apricots and brown sugar.

Remove saucepan from heat and cool apricot mixture slightly.

In a medium bowl, combine oat bran, wheat germ, whole-wheat flour, and baking powder. Set aside.

In a mixing bowl, beat together oil, skim milk, and egg.

Add dry ingredients and apricot-orange juice mixture to milk mixture and mix until just moistened.

Fill muffin tin and bake for 15 minutes or until golden brown and a cake tester comes out clean.

Makes 12 muffins
Per muffin: 135 Total calories; 32 Fat calories

CINNAMON FRENCH TOAST

2 egg whites
3 tablespoons skim milk
½ teaspoon vanilla
½ teaspoon ground cinnamon

Pinch of grated nutmeg
3 slices whole-wheat bread or
French bread
2 teaspoons margarine
(optional)

In a shallow dish, mix egg whites, skim milk, vanilla, cinnamon, and nutmeg.

Soak both sides of bread in mixture.

Heat a large frying pan or a cast-iron griddle.* Spread margarine over it if necessary.

---

*Use a cast-iron griddle, which requires little or no margarine to keep the French toast from sticking, to reduce the fat even more.

Add bread. Reduce heat to medium.
Turn bread after 2 minutes. Cook until golden brown and crispy.

Serves 3
Per serving: 106 Total calories; 29 Fat calories
Per serving without margarine: 86 Total calories; 9 Fat calories

BUTTERMILK WAFFLES

1 egg white at room
   temperature
1 cup whole-wheat flour
1 cup unbleached white flour
2 teaspoons baking powder

½ teaspoon salt
1 cup buttermilk
1 cup skim milk
2 teaspoons olive oil

Preheat waffle iron.
Beat egg white until stiff but not dry. Set aside.
In a medium bowl, combine whole-wheat flour, white flour, baking
powder, and salt.
Add buttermilk and skim milk. *Do not overmix.*
Fold in egg white. Fold in oil.
Place batter on waffle iron in amounts specified by your waffle iron
instructions. Cook accordingly.

Makes 8 Belgian waffles

	Total calories	*Fat calories*
Total batter	1102	107
Per square*	138	13

---

*Because waffle irons come in many sizes, this recipe may make more or fewer than 8 waffle squares. Divide 1102 by the number of waffle squares you make to figure out the total calories per square (for example, 1102 ÷ 8 = 138). Divide 107 by the number of waffle squares to figure out the fat calories per square (for example, 107 ÷ 8 = 13.4).

Desserts

The desserts in *Choose to Lose* are a mixture of very, very low-fat recipes like *Cheesecake!* (16 fat calories per slice), *Cocoa Angel Food Cake* (0 fat calories per slice), *Cocoa Oatmeal Cookies* (5 fat calories per cookie), *Glazed Cinnamon Buns* (18 fat calories per bun), and *Key Lime Pie* (27 fat calories per slice), and some lower-than-their-high-fat-counterparts desserts but not really low-fat, such as *Pineapple Pound Cake* (47 fat calories per slice), *Cinnamon Sweet Cakes* (61 fat calories per square), and *Tante Nancy's Apple Crumb Cake* (60 fat calories per slice). Enjoy them, but go easy on either type.

COCOA ANGEL FOOD CAKE

¾ cup cake flour
¼ cup unsweetened cocoa
1¼ cups sugar
1¼–1½ cups egg whites (about 10–12)

1 teaspoon cream of tartar
1 teaspoon vanilla
½ teaspoon almond extract

Preheat oven to 350°F.

Sift together three times: cake flour, cocoa, and ¼ cup of the sugar. Set aside.

Sift remaining 1 cup sugar and set aside.

Whip egg whites until foamy. Add cream of tartar. Continue beating until whites are stiff but not dry.

Fold in sugar a little at a time.

Fold in vanilla and almond extract.

Sift flour-cocoa mixture over batter (¼ at a time) and fold into batter.

Pour batter into an ungreased 10-inch tube pan and bake for 45 minutes or until a cake tester comes out clean.

Invert the tube pan and let cake cool.

Makes 12 slices
Per slice: 119 Total calories; 0 Fat calories

CHEESECAKE!

I never believed you could make a cheesecake low in fat. With this recipe I have become a believer. While not *exactly* the same as real cheesecake, this low-fat version is delicious.

NOTE: Start this cake more than a day in advance because it takes 24 hours to make the yogurt cheese and then you need to chill the cake for a few hours after you bake it.

Yogurt Cheese (page 253), made from two 32-oz containers vanilla nonfat yogurt

Graham Cracker Crust (page 267), made with 1 tablespoon or no margarine

Filling

Yogurt cheese	2 tablespoons cornstarch
½ cup sugar	5 egg whites

The day before you plan to serve the cheesecake, prepare the yogurt cheese. But instead of draining the yogurt overnight, drain it for 24 hours to create a cheesecake consistency.

When the yogurt cheese is ready, prepare the Graham Cracker Crust in a 9-inch pie plate.

Preheat oven to 325°F.

Place yogurt cheese in a large bowl. In a small bowl, mix sugar and cornstarch together and then add to yogurt cheese. Blend. Mix in egg whites. Blend well, but do not beat air into the batter.

Pour batter into crust and bake about 60–70 minutes, until center is set. Cool slightly and then refrigerate until chilled. You may top with fruit topping.

Makes 12 slices
Per slice:

	Total calories	Fat calories
Crust made with 1 tablespoon margarine	120	16
Crust made with no fat	112	8

If you use a commercial crust, divide total and fat calories of crust by 12 and add to filling (70 total calories/slice and 0 fat calories) to determine amounts per slice.

TANTE NANCY'S APPLE CRUMB CAKE

Apple Crumb Cake is luscious. The crust is thick, crunchy, and sweet. The slightly tart apples melt in your mouth.

2–2½ pounds tart apples*
 (about 6–7 large), peeled,
 cored, and sliced
⅓ cup water
¼ cup sugar

2 cups unbleached white flour
¾ cup sugar
1½ teaspoons baking powder
½ cup margarine
1 egg yolk

Preheat oven to 350°F. Grease an 8-inch springform pan with margarine.

In a large pot, cook apple slices with water and ¼ cup sugar until apples are tender but not mushy. Drain and reserve.

In a small bowl, mix flour, ¾ cup sugar, and baking powder.

With a pastry blender, cut in ½ cup margarine.

Cut in egg yolk.

Reserve 1 cup of flour mixture for the topping. Press remainder into bottom and sides of pan.

Spoon drained apples into pan.

Cover with reserved topping.

Bake for about 1 hour or until crust is golden brown.

Makes 12 slices
Per slice: 220 Total calories; 60 Fat calories

---

*You can use as few as 5 large apples, but more is better. Or substitute 2–2½ pounds peaches or 4 cups blueberries.

GRAHAM CRACKER CRUST [Q]

Not only do Honey Graham Crackers make a delicious cookie, Honey Graham Cracker crumbs make a delicious pie crust, particularly for lemon meringue or Key lime pie. Make your own graham cracker crumbs and graham cracker crust using the Honey Graham Crackers recipe on page 272. To reduce fat, use no margarine.

8 homemade graham cracker crumbs (1¼ cups)	1 teaspoon sugar
	1 tablespoon margarine

Preheat oven to 375°F.

In food processor or blender, crush 8 graham crackers into fine crumbs.

Combine crumbs and sugar and pour into pie plate.

Melt margarine and mix into crumbs.

Press crumbs into pie plate to make a crust.

Bake 8 minutes, or until lightly browned.

Makes one pie crust
Per crust: 600 Total calories; 186 Fat calories
  with no added margarine: 510 Total calories; 96 Fat calories

KEY LIME PIE [Q]

This pie is as pretty to look at as it is delightful to eat. It never fails to wow guests and please the most discriminating palate. Many Key lime pies call for 3 egg yolks, but you will use only 1 to create this divine dessert. You can use lemon juice instead of lime juice and call this Lemon Meringue Pie.

Graham Cracker Crust (see above)

Filling
¾ cup sugar
¼ cup unbleached white flour
3 tablespoons cornstarch
¼ teaspoon salt

½–⅔ cup fresh lime juice + water to equal 2¼ cups
1 egg yolk
1 teaspoon margarine

Meringue
5 egg whites, at room temperature

¼ teaspoon cream of tartar
½ cup + 2 tablespoons sugar

The Filling

In a medium saucepan, thoroughly mix sugar, flour, cornstarch, and salt.

Add ¼ cup lime water and blend into a smooth paste.

Add remaining lime water and mix until smooth.

Stir filling over medium heat until it begins to boil and thicken. Remove saucepan from heat.

In a small bowl, combine egg yolk with a small amount of filling and blend until smooth. Mix back into filling in saucepan. (This step is important. If you were to add the egg yolk directly into the hot filling, the egg yolk would curdle.) Stir margarine into the filling and pour into crust. Cool until filling gels.

The Meringue

Preheat oven to 375°F.

Whip egg whites with cream of tartar until stiff but not dry.

Add sugar and continue beating until whites form stiff peaks.

Gently cover lime filling with egg whites, making sure whites cover pie completely.

Bake for 8 to 10 minutes or until meringue is golden brown.

Cool at room temperature.

Makes 10 slices

Per slice, with Graham Cracker Crust*: 210 Total calories; 36 Fat calories. With no added fat in crust: 201 Total calories; 27 Fat calories.

PINEAPPLE POUND CAKE Q

2½ cups unbleached white flour
1½ teaspoons baking soda
½ teaspoon salt
1 can (20 ounces) pineapple chunks in heavy syrup
½ cup margarine

¾ cup sugar
3 egg whites
1 teaspoon vanilla
1 cup nonfat yogurt
¼ cup sugar

Preheat oven to 375°F. Grease a 10-inch tube pan with margarine. Mix flour, baking soda, and salt and set aside.

---

*Based on the Graham Cracker Crust, page 267.

Drain syrup from pineapple chunks, reserving ¼ cup.

Cream margarine and ¾ cup sugar.

Add egg whites and vanilla and beat well.

Add flour mixture and yogurt alternately to sugar mixture and mix well.

Pour half the batter into pan. Spread pineapple evenly over batter. Cover with remaining batter.

Bake for 40 minutes or until a cake tester comes out clean.

Let the cake cool for 5 minutes.

Meanwhile, in a small saucepan, combine reserved pineapple syrup and ¼ cup sugar.

Bring to a boil, reduce heat, and simmer for 3 to 5 minutes.

Remove cake from pan. Pierce it with a fork and spoon juice mixture into holes and over the top of the cake.

Makes 16 slices
Per slice: 177 Total calories; 47 Fat calories

GLAZED CINNAMON BUNS

1 tablespoon active dry yeast
3 tablespoons sugar
½ cup warm water
1½ cups whole-wheat flour
1½ + cups unbleached white
  flour
1 teaspoon salt
1 teaspoon cinnamon
1½ tablespoons olive oil

½ cup nonfat skim milk
1 egg white
⅓ cup firmly packed brown
  sugar
2 teaspoons cinnamon
½ cup raisins
1 cup confectioners' sugar
1–3 tablespoons nonfat skim
  milk

Place yeast, sugar, and water in a large bowl or the bowl of a food processor. Let proof until foamy.

Add 1½ cups of whole-wheat flour, 1½ cups of white flour, salt, oil, 1 teaspoon cinnamon, milk, and egg white and mix or process. Keep adding white flour until dough becomes fairly stiff.

Knead dough for 10 minutes or process for 15 seconds or until dough is smooth and elastic, adding more flour if necessary.

Place dough in bowl you have greased with a drop or two of olive oil, cover with a dish towel, and let rise in a warm place for 1 hour or until doubled in bulk.

When the dough has doubled in size, place it on a lightly floured surface.

Grease a 12-cup muffin tin with margarine. Set aside.

While the dough rests, combine brown sugar, 2 teaspoons cinnamon, and raisins and set aside.

Roll dough into a 9 × 12-inch rectangle.

Sprinkle cinnamon mixture evenly over the dough.

Starting with the long side of the rectangle, roll the dough *tightly* into a jelly roll. Cut it crosswise into 12 even pieces.

Place each piece, cut side up, into a muffin cup. Cover with a towel and let rise 45 minutes.

Preheat oven to 400°F. Bake buns for 15–20 minutes or until nicely browned. Transfer them to a cooling rack.

Place confectioners' sugar in bowl of an electric mixer. Add 1 tablespoon of milk and mix on low speed until smooth. Add more milk very slowly if mixture is too thick.

Spoon glaze over tops of buns.

Makes 12 buns
Per bun: 120 Total calories; 18 Fat calories

CINNAMON SWEET CAKES Q

A family favorite that can be made on the spur of the moment.

¼ cup olive oil	¾ cup whole-wheat flour
1 egg	¾ cup unbleached white flour
½ cup skim milk	2 teaspoons baking powder
½ cup sugar	½ teaspoon salt

Topping

½ cup brown sugar	1 tablespoon margarine
½ cup chopped walnuts	1 teaspoon cinnamon
1 tablespoon unbleached white flour	

Preheat oven to 375°F. Grease an 8 × 8-inch baking pan with margarine.

In a large mixing bowl, beat together oil, egg, and skim milk.

Add sugar, whole-wheat flour, white flour, baking powder, and salt and beat until smooth.

Spoon batter into baking pan. (Batter will be thick.)

To make the topping, combine brown sugar, walnuts, flour, and cinnamon in a small bowl.

Melt margarine and stir into mixture.

Sprinkle topping evenly over batter.

Bake for about 25 minutes or until a cake tester comes out clean.

Makes 16 squares
Per square: 148 Total calories; 61 Fat calories

MANDELBROT Q

These cookies are addictive. Thank you, Esther Krashes!

⅔ cup sugar
¼ cup olive oil
3 egg whites
1 egg

1½ cups unbleached white flour
1 teaspoon baking powder
½ cup coarsely ground almonds
1 teaspoon orange extract

Preheat oven to 350°F.

Lightly grease a cookie sheet with margarine or olive oil.

In a large mixing bowl, cream sugar and olive oil.

Mix in egg whites and egg.

Add flour and baking powder and mix until smooth.

Stir in almonds and orange extract.

Pour onto cookie sheet. Spread into rectangle (8″ × 10″), about ½ inch thick.

Bake for 20 minutes or until lightly browned.

Remove cookie sheet from oven.

Cut dough into strips about 3 inches wide and then score (do not cut through) into bars about ¾ inch wide.

Turn strips over and bake 10 more minutes or until crisp.

Break into bars.

Makes 4 dozen bars
Per bar: 46 Total calories; 18 Fat calories

HONEY GRAHAM CRACKERS [Q]

1 cup whole-wheat flour	2 tablespoons margarine
½ cup unbleached white flour	2 tablespoons light brown sugar
½ teaspoon baking powder	2 tablespoons honey
¼ teaspoon baking soda	½ teaspoon vanilla
Pinch of salt	2 tablespoons skim milk

Preheat oven to 350°F and grease a cookie sheet with margarine.
Combine flours, baking powder, baking soda, and salt, and set aside.
Cream margarine, sugar, and honey in an electric mixer.
Mix in vanilla.
Add flour mixture and milk.
Gather dough together (add a drop of milk if too dry) and knead into
a ball.
Roll dough onto cookie sheet into a rectangle, ⅛ inch thick.
If dough is too sticky, sprinkle it with flour.
Without moving dough, cut into 3-inch squares.
Lightly score a line through the center of each square and pierce each
side several times with a fork.
Bake 10 to 15 minutes, until edges brown. Remove crackers and cool
on a wire rack.
Crackers will become crisp as they cool.

Makes 18 crackers
Per cracker: 58 Total calories; 12 Fat calories

COCOA OATMEAL COOKIES [Q]

These low-fat cookies are one of the many wonderful recipes found in
Delightful Dishes by Friends Against Fat, a cookbook compiled by the
participants of the first *Choose to Lose* course given by Wellness Together
of Garrett County Memorial Hospital, Garrett County, Maryland.
Thank you, Kendra Stemple Todd and your participants!

⅔ cup unbleached flour	1 teaspoon baking soda
⅔ cup sugar	½ teaspoon salt
1 cup rolled oats (oatmeal)	2 egg whites
⅓ cup unsweetened cocoa	⅓ cup corn syrup
1 teaspoon baking powder	1 teaspoon vanilla

Preheat oven to 350°F and grease a cookie sheet with margarine or a cooking spray.

In a large mixing bowl combine flour, sugar, oats, cocoa, baking powder, baking soda, and salt.

Add egg whites, corn syrup, and vanilla. Stir just until the dry ingredients are moistened.

Drop batter by teaspoonfuls onto the cookie sheet and bake for 10 minutes or until set.

Cool for 5 minutes on cookie sheet. Remove immediately or cookies will harden and will be difficult to remove.

Makes about 2 dozen cookies
Per Cookie: 69 Total calories; 5 Fat Calories

MERINGUE SHELLS WITH FRESH STRAWBERRIES AND WARM RASPBERRY SAUCE

Here's a delectable dessert that has no fat. It is extremely simple to prepare and, later, to assemble. Make sure to budget in 1 to 2 hours baking time for the meringue.

Meringue Shells
4 egg whites at room
 temperature
⅛ teaspoon salt
⅛ teaspoon cream of tartar
¾ cup sugar
½ teaspoon vanilla
¼ teaspoon almond extract

Filling
1 pint strawberries, washed, hulled, and halved (actually any berry or cut-up fruit will do)

Sauce
1 package (10 oz) frozen
 raspberries
1 teaspoon cornstarch
½ teaspoon lemon juice

The Meringue
Preheat oven to 275°F. Completely cover your baking sheet with a piece of brown paper. Set aside.

In a very clean mixing bowl, whip egg whites until foamy. Continue whipping as you add salt and cream of tartar. When egg whites form soft peaks, slowly add sugar while continuing to beat until whites are glossy and stiff. Mix in vanilla and almond extract.

On the brown paper, use a spoon or spatula to spread the meringue into 6 shells, 4–5 inches across with a raised edge about 1 inch high. You may also use a pastry tube to squeeze out concentric circles to form a base and sides. The shells should be deep enough to hold the fruit.

Bake for 2 hours. Turn off heat and let meringues sit in closed oven for 2 hours or overnight. Gently remove meringues, as they crack easily.

The Filling
Fill the shell cavity with a mound of strawberries.

The Raspberry Sauce
Thaw raspberries or, if you forgot to plan ahead, place pouch containing raspberries into a bowl of warm water for about 2 minutes to thaw. When partially thawed, purée the raspberries in a blender.

Place cornstarch in a small saucepan. Add 1 tablespoon of purée and mix with cornstarch until smooth. Stir in remaining purée and add lemon juice. Bring to a boil and simmer for 1 minute.

Spoon several tablespoons of the warm sauce over the strawberries. You may also refrigerate the sauce and serve it cold.

6 servings
Per serving: 130 Total calories; 0 Fat calories

FOOD TABLES

CONTENTS

INTRODUCTION TO THE FOOD TABLES

The Food Tables in this new edition of *Choose to Lose* contain both saturated fat calories and total fat calories. Total fat is the sum of saturated fat, monounsaturated fat, and polyunsaturated fat. Each has a different effect on heart health, but all are equally fattening. Knowing both the saturated and total fat calories in a food will help you make more informed choices.

People who are keeping track of saturated fat to lower their blood cholesterol should know how much total fat a food contains. For example, if you are only considering saturated fat you might blithely consume a Wendy's baked potato with broccoli and cheese because it has only 18 sat-fat calories. However, if you had looked at the total fat calories for this "healthy" potato you would see that it contains 126 fat calories. This is a heaping amount of fat — almost half the Fat Budget for a woman wanting to weigh 120 pounds, or about one-third the Fat Budget of a man wanting to weigh 150.

Those who are reducing total fat may also be interested in the amount of saturated fat in foods to help them make healthier choices. For instance, both olive oil, the most heart-healthy of all the fats, and butter, a highly heart-risky food, are 100 percent fat and fattening. However, a tablespoon of olive oil, which has 119 total fat calories, has only 16 sat-fat calories. A tablespoon of butter has 100 fat calories, but has 65 sat-fat calories. By using the Food Tables, you can quickly see that butter is a poorer choice because it is very saturated.

Because products are constantly changing, always look at nutrition labels for the most up-to-date nutrition information. If you don't know where to look for a food in the Food Tables, turn to the Food Tables Index, immediately following the Food Tables. (This is different from the general index at the end of the book.)

The abbreviation "NA" means the sat-fat calories are "not available."

Foods are often measured in grams instead of ounces. To put amounts into perspective, remember that 1 ounce = approximately 28 grams.

BEVERAGES

FOOD	AMOUNT	CALORIES		
		TOTAL	FAT	SAT-FAT
Alcoholic				
Beer	12 fl oz	150	0	0
Lite beer	12 fl oz	100	0	0
Gin, rum, vodka, whiskey				
80–90 proof	1.5 fl oz	95–110	0	0
Other				
brandy Alexander	3 fl oz	254	**52**	32
Irish coffee	8 fl oz	210	**99**	60
piña colada	6 fl oz	392	**103**	85
eggnog	8 fl oz	342	**171**	102
Wine				
dessert	3.5 fl oz	140	0	0
table	3.5 fl oz	75	0	0
Carbonated				
Club soda	12 fl oz	0	0	0
Cola	12 fl oz	160	0	0
Ginger ale	12 fl oz	125	0	0
Lemon-lime	12 fl oz	150	0	0
Orange, grape	12 fl oz	180	0	0

BEVERAGES

FOOD	AMOUNT	CALORIES		
		TOTAL	FAT	SAT-FAT
Cocoa				
Hershey's				
made with whole milk	6 fl oz	135	**58**	34
made with 2% milk	6 fl oz	113	**35**	20
made with skim milk	6 fl oz	87	**5**	0
Swiss Miss with water	1 pkt (28 g)	110	**10**	0
Coffee				
Nescafé cappuccino	1 pkt (27 g)	110	**20**	5
International Coffees				
Cafe Amaretto	6 fl oz prep.	50	**27**	NA
Cafe Français	6 fl oz prep.	60	**27**	NA
Cafe Vienna	6 fl oz prep.	60	**18**	NA
Italian cappuccino	6 fl oz prep.	50	**18**	NA

Coffee Bar Coffees

If whipped cream is added to your coffee, add 60 total calories and 45 fat calories.

Coffee Beanery				
Cafe Mocha				
with whole milk	8 fl oz	94	**45**	NA
with 2% milk	8 fl oz	76	**27**	NA
with skim milk	8 fl oz	54	**0**	NA
Cappuccino				
with whole milk	12 fl oz	296	**81**	NA
with 2% milk	12 fl oz	267	**54**	NA
with skim milk	12 fl oz	232	**9**	NA
Espresso	2.4 fl oz	0	**0**	NA
Latte				
with whipped cream and				
grated chocolate	16 fl oz	350	**180**	NA
with whole milk	16 fl oz	263	**126**	NA
with 2% milk	16 fl oz	211	**72**	NA
with skim milk	16 fl oz	151	**9**	NA
Gloria Jean's (made with 2% milk)				
Cafe Mocha	8 fl oz	222	**36**	NA
grande	16 fl oz	312	**63**	NA
iced	12 fl oz	282	**54**	NA
Espresso	2.7 fl oz	0	**0**	NA
Latte	8 fl oz	76	**27**	NA
grande	16 fl oz	166	**54**	NA

BEVERAGES

FOOD	AMOUNT	CALORIES		
		TOTAL	FAT	SAT-FAT
Starbucks				
Cafe Mocha				
short				
with whole milk	8 fl oz	195	**135**	NA
with 2% milk	8 fl oz	175	**117**	NA
with skim milk	8 fl oz	156	**99**	NA
grande				
with whole milk	16 fl oz	409	**279**	NA
with 2% milk	16 fl oz	365	**243**	NA
with skim milk	16 fl oz	324	**189**	NA
iced	12 fl oz	271	**171**	NA
Cappuccino	8 fl oz	99	**45**	NA
grande	16 fl oz	249	**117**	NA
Espresso	2.7 fl oz	0	**0**	NA
Latte				
short				
with whole milk	8 fl oz	114	**54**	NA
with 2% milk	8 fl oz	90	**36**	NA
with skim milk	8 fl oz	68	**9**	NA
grande				
with whole milk	16 fl oz	247	**117**	NA
with 2% milk	16 fl oz	195	**72**	NA
with skim milk	16 fl oz	146	**18**	NA
Fruit Drinks				
Noncarbonated				
canned	6 fl oz	85–100	**0**	0
frozen	6 fl oz	80	**0**	0
Hot Chocolate	8 fl oz	232	**122**	72
with whipped cream	¼ cup	334	**221**	133
Instant Breakfast Shakes				
Carnation				
Creamy Milk Chocolate	1 pkt (37 g)	130	**10**	5
Creamy Milk Chocolate, sugar-free	1 pkt (21 g)	70	**10**	5
Tea	8 fl oz	0	**0**	0

Dairy drinks (milk, milk shakes, etc.): *see* **DAIRY AND EGGS** and **FAST FOODS.**
Fruit juices: *see* **FRUITS AND FRUIT JUICES.**

DAIRY AND EGGS

		CALORIES		
FOOD	AMOUNT	TOTAL	FAT	SAT-FAT
Butter				
Regular	1 pat	36	**36**	23
	1 tbsp	100	**100**	65
	1 stick (½ cup)	813	**813**	515
Whipped	1 tbsp	67	**67**	38
	1 stick (½ cup)	542	**542**	344

Margarine and other butter substitutes: *see* **FATS AND OILS.**

Cheese				
American	1 oz	106	**80**	50
Blue	1 oz	100	**73**	48
Bonbel (Laughing Cow)	1 oz	70	**50**	36
Brie	1 oz	90	**70**	27
Camembert	1 oz	90	**70**	27
Cheddar	1 oz	114	**85**	54
shredded	¼ cup	110	**80**	54
Colby	1 oz	112	**82**	54
Cottage cheese				
4%	½ cup	110	**43**	23
2% fat	½ cup	102	**20**	14
1% fat	½ cup	90	**10**	7
dry curd	½ cup	80	**9**	4
Cream cheese				
regular	1 tbsp	52	**48**	26
with salmon or strawberries	2 tbsp	100	**80**	54
soft	2 tbsp	100	**90**	63
whipped	1 tbsp	37	**34**	19
Edam	1 oz	101	**71**	45
Feta	1 oz	75	**54**	38
with basil and tomato	1 oz	80	**60**	36
Farmer				
Friendship	1 oz	40	**27**	18
May-Bud	1 oz	90	**63**	41
Gouda	1 oz	101	**70**	45
Gruyère	1 oz	117	**83**	48
Limburger	1 oz	93	**69**	43
Monterey	1 oz	106	**77**	45
Mozzarella				
whole milk	1 oz	80	**50**	36
shredded	1 oz	90	**65**	42
part skim	1 oz	72	**45**	27

DAIRY AND EGGS

FOOD	AMOUNT	CALORIES		
		TOTAL	FAT	SAT-FAT
Muenster	1 oz	104	**77**	49
Neufchâtel	1 oz	74	**60**	38
Parmesan	1 tbsp	23	**14**	9
	1 oz	129	**77**	49
Port du Salut	1 oz	100	**72**	43
Provolone	1 oz	100	**68**	44
Ricotta				
whole milk	½ cup	216	**145**	93
part skim	½ cup	171	**88**	55
Romano	1 oz	110	**70**	49
Roquefort	1 oz	105	**78**	49
String	1 oz	80	**50**	36
Swiss	1 oz	107	**70**	45
Tilsit	1 oz	96	**66**	43
Cheese, Fat-free				
All brands	1 slice (21 g)	25–30	**0**	0
Cream cheese	2 tbsp	30	**0**	0
Mozzarella, shredded	¼ cup (28 g)	45	**0**	0
Cheese, Reduced-Calorie or Lite				
Alouette Lite Herbs & Garlic	2 tbsp	60	**35**	27
Bonbel Light Wedge				
(Laughing Cow)	1 piece (28 g)	50	**30**	18
Cheddar, shredded				
⅓ Less Fat Kraft	¼ cup	90	**50**	36
Sargento	¼ cup	70	**40**	18
Cream cheese				
Philadelphia ⅓ Less Fat	2 tbsp	70	**60**	36
Monterey Jack				
Dorman's	1 slice	120	**60**	41
Kraft	28 g	80	**45**	27
Mozzarella	¼ cup	60	**30**	18
Ricotta	¼ cup	75	**35**	18
Rondelé Soft Spreadable Lite	2 tbsp	60	**35**	23
String (Poly-O)	1 piece (28 g)	80	**50**	36
Weight Watchers, all	1 slice (21 g)	50	**20**	0
Cheese Spreads				
Alouette				
Garlic and Spices	2 tbsp	70	**60**	41
Spinach	2 tbsp	60	**50**	32
Boursin	2 tbsp	120	**110**	45

DAIRY AND EGGS

FOOD	AMOUNT	CALORIES		
		TOTAL	FAT	SAT-FAT
Cheez Whiz (Kraft)	2 tbsp	100	**70**	45
Rondelé Soft Spreadable				
Black Pepper & Garden				
Vegetable	2 tbsp	90	**80**	54
Garlic & Herbs	2 tbsp	100	**80**	54
Cream				
Half-and-half	1 tbsp	20	**15**	10
Light, coffee or table	1 tbsp	29	**26**	16
	1 cup	469	**417**	260
Nondairy				
Frozen				
Rich's Coffee Rich	1 tbsp	25	**15**	0
Powdered				
Coffee Mate	1 tbsp	30	**15**	14
flavored	1⅓ tbsp	60	**25**	23
Refrigerated				
Farm Rich				
fat-free	1 tbsp	10	**0**	0
light	1 tbsp	10	**5**	0
original	1 tbsp	20	**15**	0
Sour cream	2 tbsp	60	**50**	36
	1 cup	493	**434**	270
fat-free	2 tbsp	20	**0**	0
light	2 tbsp	35	**25**	14
Whipping cream				
heavy, fluid	1 cup	821	**792**	493
Whipped	½ cup	205	**198**	123
light, fluid	1 cup	699	**665**	416
nondairy (Cool Whip)	2 tbsp	25	**15**	14
	½ cup	200	**120**	108
Pressurized topping				
whipped light	2 tbsp	30	**20**	14
Reddi Wip	2 tbsp	20	**15**	9
Milk				
1% fat	1 cup	104	**23**	14
2% fat	1 cup	121	**42**	27
Buttermilk	1 cup	99	**0–36**	0–12
Chocolate				
2% milk	1 cup	179	**45**	28
whole milk	1 cup	208	**76**	47

DAIRY AND EGGS

FOOD	AMOUNT	TOTAL	FAT	SAT-FAT
		CALORIES		
Condensed, sweetened	1 tbsp	62	**15**	9
Evaporated				
skim	1 cup	200	**5**	2
	1 tbsp	13	**0**	0
whole	1 cup	340	**172**	104
	1 tbsp	21	**11**	7
Nonfat				
dry	¼ cup	109	**2**	1
instant	to make 1 qt	326	**6**	4
Skim	1 cup	86	**4**	0–3
Whole	1 cup	150	**73**	45
dry	¼ cup	159	**77**	48
Yogurt				
Custard-style				
Whitney's Original 100% Natural, all flavors	6 oz	190	**45**	27
Yoplait, all flavors	6 oz	170	**25**	14
French-style				
La Yogurt				
All flavors but Piña Colada	6 oz	180	**25**	14
Piña colada	6 oz	180	**30**	14
Low-fat				
Astro vanilla				
with apple crisp granola topping	6 oz	230	**35**	23
with chocolate fudge crunch	6 oz	230	**45**	23
with oat bran raisin granola topping	6 oz	230	**40**	23
Breyers	8 oz	250	**25**	14
Colombo	8 oz	120	**40**	23
Dannon, all flavors	8 oz	210	**30**	18
Fruit on the Bottom, all flavors	8 oz	240	**25**	14
Premium	8 oz	150	**35**	23
Lucerne, Pre-Stirred, all flavors	8 oz	250	**25**	14
Whitney's Supreme, all flavors	6 oz	200	**20**	9
Yoplait Original, all flavors	6 oz	170	**15**	9
Yoplait Trix	6 oz	180	**25**	14

DAIRY AND EGGS

FOOD	AMOUNT	CALORIES TOTAL	FAT	SAT-FAT
Nonfat				
Colombo				
fruit flavors	8 oz	190	0	0
other flavors	8 oz	160	0	0
Colombo Light 100, all				
flavors	8 oz	100	0	0
Dannon	8 oz	110	0	0
Blended, all flavors	6 oz	150–160	0	0
Lucerne Light, all flavors	6 oz	90	0	0
Lucerne, Pre-Stirred, all				
flavors	8 oz	180	0	0
Weight Watchers Ultimate				
90, all flavors	8 oz	90	0	0
Yoplait Light, all flavors	6 oz	90	0	0
Egg, chicken				
Whole, large	1 egg	79	50	15
White	1 white	16	0	0
Yolk	1 yolk	63	50	15
Egg substitute				
Egg Beaters™ (Fleischmann's)	¼ cup	30	0	0
Healthy Choice Egg Product	¼ cup	25	<5	0
Scramblers (Morningstar				
Farms)	¼ cup	35	0	0
Simply Eggs	½ cup	80	20	9
	3 tbsp	35	10	0

FAST FOODS

FOOD	AMOUNT	CALORIES TOTAL	FAT	SAT-FAT
Arby's				
Bacon platter	1	593	297	83
Baked potato				
Broccoli and Cheddar	1	417	162	63
Deluxe	1	621	328	163
Mushroom and Cheese	1	515	240	52

FAST FOODS

FOOD	AMOUNT	CALORIES		
		TOTAL	FAT	SAT-FAT
Biscuit				
Bacon	1	318	**162**	39
Ham	1	323	**150**	36
Plain	1	280	**135**	30
Sausage	1	460	**288**	85
Blueberry Muffin	1	240	**63**	9
Croissant				
Bacon and Egg	1	430	**270**	139
Butter	1	260	**140**	94
Ham and Swiss	1	345	**186**	109
Mushroom and Swiss	1	495	**340**	137
Sausage and Egg	1	520	**353**	167
Cheesecake	1 serving	305	**205**	65
Chicken Breast Sandwich	1	445	**203**	27
Chicken Club Sandwich	1	505	**243**	63
Chicken Cordon Bleu				
Sandwich	1	520	**243**	48
Chocolate Chip Cookie	1	130	**36**	18
Cinnamon Nut Danish	1	360	**99**	9
Egg Platter	1	460	**216**	65
Fish Fillet Sandwich	1	526	**243**	63
Fries				
Cheddar Fries	1 sm order	399	**197**	81
Curly Fries	1 sm order	337	**169**	67
French Fries	1 sm order	246	**119**	27
Grilled Chicken Barbecue				
Sandwich	1	385	**118**	32
Grilled Chicken Deluxe				
Sandwich	1	430	**180**	32
Ham n' Cheese Sandwich	1	353	**128**	46
Ham Platter	1	518	**234**	72
Horsey Sauce	1 oz	120	**54**	18
Italian Sub	1	671	**349**	115
Light Sandwiches				
Roast Beef Deluxe	1	294	**90**	32
Roast Chicken Deluxe	1	276	**63**	15
Roast Turkey Deluxe	1	260	**54**	14
Polar Swirl				
Butterfinger	1	457	**163**	76
Heath	1	543	**196**	47
Oreo	1	482	**177**	94
Peanut Butter Cup	1	517	**216**	73

FAST FOODS

FOOD	AMOUNT	CALORIES		
		TOTAL	FAT	SAT-FAT
Polar Swirl (*cont.*)				
Snickers	1	510	170	60
Potato Cakes	1 serving	201	108	20
Roast Beef Sandwich				
Arby Q	1	389	137	50
Bac'n Cheddar Deluxe	1	512	284	78
Beef 'n Cheddar	1	508	239	69
French Dip	1	368	139	50
French Dip 'n Swiss	1	429	171	79
Giant	1	544	237	99
Junior	1	233	97	37
Philly Beef 'n Swiss	1	467	228	87
Regular	1	383	164	63
Super	1	552	255	68
Roast Beef Sub	1	623	288	104
Salads (without dressing)				
Chef	1	205	86	35
Chicken	1	204	65	30
Garden	1	117	47	24
Salad dressings				
Blue Cheese	1 packet	295	281	52
Buttermilk Ranch	1 packet	349	347	50
Honey French	1 packet	322	242	36
Italian, light	1 packet	23	10	1
Thousand Island	1 packet	298	263	39
Sausage platter	1	640	370	120
Shakes				
Chocolate	10.6 fl oz	450	105	25
Jamocha	10.8 fl oz	368	95	23
Vanilla	8.8 fl oz	330	100	36
Soup				
Boston Clam Chowder	1 cup	193	90	40
Cream of Broccoli	1 cup	166	65	34
Potato with Bacon	1 cup	184	79	39
Wisconsin Cheese	1 cup	281	162	81
Toastix	1 serving	420	225	41
Tuna Sub	1	663	333	74
Turnover				
Apple	1	310	165	63
Blueberry	1	320	180	57
Cherry	1	280	160	48
Turkey Sub	1	486	171	48

FAST FOODS

FOOD	AMOUNT	CALORIES		
		TOTAL	FAT	SAT-FAT
Arthur Treacher's				
Chicken, fried	1 serving	369	**198**	36
Chicken Sandwich	1	413	**171**	27
Chips (french fries)	1 serving	276	**117**	18
Chowder	1 serving	112	**45**	18
Cole Slaw	1 serving	123	**72**	9
Fish, broiled	5 oz	245	**126**	NA
Fish, fried	2 pieces	355	**180**	27
Krunch Pup (batter-fried hot dog)	1	203	**135**	36
Lemon Luv (fried pie)	1 serving	276	**126**	18
Shrimp, fried	1 serving	381	**216**	27
Burger King				
Apple Pie	1	311	**126**	36
BK Broiler Chicken Sandwich, no mayo	1	267	**72**	18
BK Broiler Sauce	1	37	**36**	9
Blueberry Mini Muffins	1 serving	292	**126**	27
Breakfast Buddy with sausage, egg, and cheese	1	255	**144**	54
Burger Buddies	1 pair	349	**153**	63
Cheeseburger	1	317	**135**	63
Deluxe	1	390	**207**	72
Double	1	483	**243**	117
Bacon	1	510	**279**	126
Bacon Deluxe	1	584	**342**	144
Chef Salad	1	178	**81**	36
Chicken Sandwich	1	685	**360**	81
Chicken Tenders	6 pieces	236	**117**	27
Chunky Chicken Salad	1	142	**36**	9
Croissan'wich				
Bacon, Egg, and Cheese	1	355	**216**	72
Ham, Egg, and Cheese	1	351	**198**	63
Sausage, Egg, and Cheese	1	534	**360**	126
French Fries, regular	1 serving	372	**180**	45
French Toast Sticks	1 serving	538	**288**	72
Garden Salad	1	95	**45**	27
Hamburger	1	275	**99**	36
Deluxe	1	344	**171**	54
Hash Browns	1 serving	215	**108**	27
Ocean Catch Fish Fillet Sandwich	1	479	**297**	72

FAST FOODS

FOOD	AMOUNT	CALORIES		
		TOTAL	FAT	SAT-FAT
Onion Rings, regular	1 serving	339	**171**	45
Pies				
Cherry	1	360	**117**	36
Lemon	1	290	**72**	27
Ranch Dipping Sauce	1	171	**162**	27
Scrambled Egg Platter (eggs, croissant, hash browns)	1 serving	549	**306**	81
with bacon	1 serving	610	**351**	99
with sausage	1 serving	768	**477**	135
Shakes				
Chocolate	10 fl oz	326	**90**	54
Vanilla	10 fl oz	334	**90**	54
Specialty Sandwiches				
Chicken	1	688	**360**	72
Ham and Cheese	1	471	**216**	81
Whaler Sandwich	1	488	**243**	54
with cheese	1	530	**270**	72
Whopper	1	614	**324**	108
with cheese	1	709	**396**	144
Double Whopper	1	844	**477**	171
with cheese	1	935	**549**	216
Whopper Jr.	1	322	**153**	54
with cheese	1	364	**180**	72

Carl's Jr.

FOOD	AMOUNT	CALORIES		
		TOTAL	FAT	SAT-FAT
Breakfast Burrito	1	430	**234**	108
Carl's Catch Fish Sandwich	1	560	**270**	36
Charbroiler Sandwich				
BBQ Chicken	1	310	**54**	18
Chicken Club	1	570	**261**	72
Cheeseburger				
Western Bacon	1	730	**351**	180
Double	1	1030	**567**	288
Cheesecake	1 piece	310	**153**	72
Chicken Strips	6 pieces	260	**171**	45
Chocolate Cake	1 piece	300	**99**	27
Chocolate Chip Cookie	1	330	**153**	63
Cinnamon Rolls	1 serving	460	**162**	9
CrissCut Fries, regular	1 serving	330	**198**	27
Danish	1	520	**144**	36
French Fries, regular	1 serving	420	**180**	45
French Toast Dips	1 serving	490	**234**	54
Fudge Moussecake	1 piece	400	**207**	99

FAST FOODS

FOOD	AMOUNT	CALORIES		
		TOTAL	**FAT**	**SAT-FAT**
"Great Stuff" Potato				
Bacon and Cheese	1	730	**387**	135
Broccoli and Cheese	1	590	**279**	99
Cheese	1	690	**324**	135
Sour Cream and Chive	1	470	**171**	63
Hamburger	1	320	**126**	45
Carl's Original	1	460	**180**	81
Famous Star	1	610	**342**	117
Super Star	1	820	**477**	216
Hash Brown Nuggets	1 serving	270	**153**	36
Hot Cakes with Margarine	1 serving	510	**216**	45
Muffin				
Blueberry	1	340	**81**	9
Bran	1	310	**63**	<9
Onion Rings	1 serving	520	**234**	54
Roast Beef Club Sandwich	1	620	**306**	99
Roast Beef Deluxe Sandwich	1	540	**234**	90
Santa Fe Chicken Sandwich	1	540	**117**	27
Teriyaki Chicken Sandwich	1	330	**54**	18
Turkey Club Sandwich	1	530	**207**	54
Shakes, regular	1	350	**63**	36
Sunrise sandwich	1	300	**117**	54
Zucchini	1 serving	390	**207**	54
Chick-Fil-A				
Chargrilled Chicken				
Garden salad	1	126	**19**	NA
Sandwich	1	258	**43**	NA
Deluxe	1	266	**44**	NA
Chicken Nuggets	8	287	**135**	NA
Chicken Salad Plate	1	291	**168**	NA
Chicken Salad Sandwich	1	449	**238**	NA
Chick-n-Q Sandwich	1	206	**61**	NA
Fudge Brownie with Nuts	1	369	**172**	NA
Grilled 'n Lites	2 skewers	97	**18**	NA
Icedream	1 reg cone	134	**44**	NA
Lemon Pie	1 slice	329	**46**	NA
Original Chicken Sandwich	1	360	**76**	NA
Church's Fried Chicken				
Catfish, fried	3 pieces	201	**108**	NA
Chicken, fried				
breast	1 serving	278	**153**	NA

FAST FOODS

FOOD	AMOUNT	TOTAL	FAT	SAT-FAT
		CALORIES		
Chicken, fried (*cont.*)				
leg	1 serving	147	**81**	NA
thigh	1 serving	305	**198**	NA
wing	1 serving	303	**180**	NA
Chicken Breast Fillet				
Sandwich	1	608	**306**	NA
Chicken Nuggets				
regular	6 pieces	330	**171**	NA
spicy	6 pieces	312	**153**	NA
Coleslaw	1 serving	83	**63**	NA
Corn on the Cob, buttered	9 oz	165	**27**	NA
Dinner Roll	1	83	**18**	NA
Fish Fillet Sandwich	1	430	**162**	NA
French Fries, regular	3 oz	256	**117**	NA
Hush Puppies	2	156	**54**	NA
Pie				
Apple	1 serving	300	**171**	NA
Pecan	1 serving	367	**180**	NA
Dairy Queen				
Banana Split	1	510	**99**	72
BBQ Beef Sandwich	1	225	**36**	9
Buster Bar	1	460	**261**	81
Chicken Fillet Sandwich,				
breaded	1	430	**180**	36
with cheese	1	480	**225**	63
Chicken Fillet Sandwich,				
grilled	1	300	**72**	18
Chocolate cone				
large	1	350	**99**	72
regular	1	230	**63**	45
Chocolate cone, dipped				
large	1	510	**216**	140
regular	1	340	**144**	90
small	1	190	**81**	54
Dilly Bar	1	210	**117**	54
Double Delight	1 serving	490	**180**	NA
DQ Frozen Cake	1 slice	380	**162**	72
DQ Sandwich	1	140	**36**	24
Fish Fillet Sandwich	1	370	**144**	27
with cheese	1	420	**189**	54
Float	1	410	**63**	41

FAST FOODS

FOOD	AMOUNT	CALORIES		
		TOTAL	FAT	SAT-FAT
Freeze	1	500	108	72
French fries	1 regular	300	126	27
	1 large	390	162	36
Garden Salad, no dressing	1	200	117	63
Hamburger	1	310	117	54
with cheese	1	365	162	81
DQ Homestyle Ultimate				
Burger	1	700	423	189
Double	1	460	225	108
with cheese	1	570	306	162
Single	1	360	144	54
with cheese	1	410	180	81
Heath Blizzard	1 regular	820	324	153
Heath Breeze	1 regular	680	189	54
Hot Dog	1	280	144	54
with cheese	1	330	189	81
with chili	1	320	180	63
Super Hot Dog	1	520	243	100
with cheese	1	580	306	142
with chili	1	570	288	112
quarter pound	1	590	342	144
Hot Fudge Brownie Delight	1	710	261	126
Malt				
Chocolate				
large	20 fl oz	1060	225	NA
regular	14 fl oz	760	162	NA
small	10 fl oz	520	117	NA
Vanilla	1 regular	610	126	72
Mr. Misty Float	1	390	63	41
Mr. Misty Freeze	1	500	108	70
Mr. Misty Kiss	1	70	0	0
Mr. Misty				
large	1	340	0	0
regular	1	250	0	0
small	1	190	0	0
Nutty Double Fudge	1	580	198	90
Onion Rings	1 regular	240	108	27
Parfait	1 serving	430	72	47
Peanut Buster	1 serving	710	288	90
QC Chocolate Big Scoop	1	310	126	90

FAST FOODS

FOOD	AMOUNT	CALORIES		
		TOTAL	FAT	SAT-FAT
Shake				
Chocolate				
large	20 fl oz	990	**234**	128
regular	14 fl oz	710	**171**	111
small	10 fl oz	490	**117**	64
Vanilla	1 regular	520	**126**	72
Soft ice cream, without cone	4 oz	180	**54**	36
Soft ice cream cone				
large	1	340	**90**	63
regular	1	240	**63**	45
small	1	140	**36**	27
Strawberry Blizzard	1 regular	570	**144**	99
Strawberry Breeze	1 regular	420	**9**	<9
Strawberry Shortcake	1 serving	540	**99**	NA
Strawberry Waffle Cone				
Sundae	1	350	**108**	45
Sundae				
Chocolate				
large	8.4 fl oz	440	**90**	58
regular	6 fl oz	310	**72**	45
small	3.5 fl oz	190	**36**	23
Vanilla cone	1 regular	230	**65**	45
Yogurt Cup	1 regular	170	**<9**	<9
Yogurt Strawberry Sundae	1 regular	200	**<9**	<9
Denny's				
Baked Potato	1	180	**0**	NA
Biscuit	1	217	**63**	NA
BLT Sandwich	1	492	**306**	NA
Blueberry Muffin	1	309	**126**	NA
Catfish	1 entree	576	**432**	NA
Chicken Strips	4 oz	240	**90**	NA
Chili	8 oz	238	**135**	NA
Cinnamon Roll	1	450	**126**	NA
Club Sandwich	1	590	**180**	NA
Coleslaw	1 cup	119	**86**	NA
Country Gravy	1 oz	140	**72**	NA
Eggs Benedict	1	658	**320**	NA
French Fries	1 order	303	**142**	NA
French Toast	2 slices	729	**504**	NA
Fried Chicken	1 entree	463	**266**	NA
Fried Shrimp	1 entree	230	**135**	NA

FAST FOODS

FOOD	AMOUNT	CALORIES		
		TOTAL	FAT	SAT-FAT
Grilled Cheese Sandwich	1	454	261	NA
Grilled Chicken	1 entree	192	36	NA
Grilled Chicken Sandwich	1	439	108	NA
Guacamole	1 oz	60	55	NA
Hamburger				
Bacon Swiss	1	819	468	NA
Denny	1	629	340	NA
San Fran	1	872	432	NA
Works	1	944	549	NA
Hash Browns	4 oz	164	18	NA
Liver with Bacon and Onions	1 entree	334	130	NA
Mozzarella Sticks	1	88	60	NA
Omelet				
Denver	1	567	243	NA
Ultimate	1	577	369	NA
Onion Rings	3 rings	258	135	NA
Pancakes	2	272	36	NA
Patty Melt	1	761	423	NA
Rice Pilaf	⅓ cup	89	21	NA
Sausage	1 link	113	90	NA
Soup				
Cheese	1 bowl	309	198	NA
Chicken Noodle	1 bowl	105	30	NA
Clam Chowder	1 bowl	235	126	NA
Potato	1 bowl	141	120	NA
Split Pea	1 bowl	231	45	NA
Stir-fry	1 entree	328	99	NA
Stuffing	½ cup	180	81	NA
Super Bird	1	625	216	NA
Salad				
Chef	1	492	180	NA
Chicken, no shell	1	207	36	NA
Taco, no shell	1	514	180	NA
Tuna	1	340	162	NA
Steak				
Fried Chicken, no gravy	1 entree	252	131	NA
Hamburger	1 entree	669	484	NA
New York	1 entree	582	324	NA
Top Sirloin	1 entree	223	57	NA
Tortilla Shell, fried	1	439	270	NA
Turkey, no gravy	1 entree	505	130	NA

FAST FOODS

| FOOD | AMOUNT | CALORIES | | |
		TOTAL	FAT	SAT-FAT
Veggie Cheese	1	350	**180**	NA
Waffle	1	261	**94**	NA
Domino's Pizza				
12" Pizza				
Cheese	2 slices	360	**90**	45
Deluxe	2 slices	540	**207**	95
Extravaganza	2 slices	510	**216**	104
Pepperoni	2 slices	410	**135**	68
with extra cheese	2 slices	460	**176**	86
Pepperoni Feast	2 slices	460	**171**	81
Pepperoni, Sausage,				
Mushroom	2 slices	460	**180**	81
Sausage	2 slices	430	**149**	68
Vegi Feast	2 slices	390	**117**	59
Dunkin' Donuts				
Cookie				
Chocolate Chunk	1	200	**90**	NA
with nuts	1	210	**99**	NA
Oatmeal Pecan Raisin	1	200	**81**	NA
Croissant	1	310	**171**	NA
Almond	1	420	**243**	NA
Chocolate	1	440	**261**	NA
Donut				
Apple-filled with Cinnamon				
Sugar	1	250	**99**	NA
Bavarian with Chocolate				
Frosting	1	240	**99**	NA
Blueberry-filled	1	210	**72**	NA
Glazed French Cruller	1	140	**72**	NA
Jelly-filled	1	220	**81**	NA
Lemon-filled	1	260	**108**	NA
Glazed Coffee Roll	1	280	**108**	NA
Rings				
Cake	1	270	**153**	NA
Chocolate-frosted Yeast	1	200	**90**	NA
Glazed				
Buttermilk	1	290	**126**	NA
Chocolate	1	324	**189**	NA
Whole-Wheat	1	330	**162**	NA
Yeast	1	200	**81**	NA

FAST FOODS

FOOD	AMOUNT	TOTAL	FAT	SAT-FAT
		CALORIES		
Muffin				
Apple 'n Spice	1	300	72	NA
Banana Nut	1	310	90	NA
Blueberry	1	280	72	NA
Bran with Raisins	1	310	81	NA
Corn	1	340	108	NA
Cranberry Nut	1	290	81	NA
Oat Bran	1	330	99	NA
Hardee's				
Apple Turnover	1	270	108	36
Big Cookie Treat	1	250	117	36
Big Country Breakfast				
Bacon	1	660	360	90
Country Ham	1	670	342	81
Ham	1	620	297	63
Sausage	1	849	630	144
Big Twin	1	450	225	99
Bagel				
Bacon	1	280	81	34
Bacon and Egg	1	330	108	41
Bacon, Egg, and Cheese	1	375	144	68
Egg	1	250	54	24
Egg and Cheese	1	295	90	NA
Plain	1	200	27	5
Sausage	1	350	144	59
Sausage and Egg	1	400	171	68
Sausage, Egg, and Cheese	1	445	207	86
Biscuit	1	257	112	29
Bacon	1	360	189	36
Bacon and Egg	1	410	216	45
Bacon, Egg, and Cheese	1	460	252	72
Canadian Rise 'n Shine	1	482	250	72
Cheese	1	304	142	NA
Chicken	1	430	198	36
Cinnamon 'n Raisin	1	320	153	45
Country Ham	1	350	162	27
Country Ham and Egg	1	400	198	36
Ham	1	320	144	18
Ham and Egg	1	370	171	36
Ham, Egg, and Cheese	1	420	207	54
'N Gravy	1	440	216	54

FAST FOODS

FOOD	AMOUNT	CALORIES TOTAL	FAT	SAT-FAT
Biscuit (*cont.*)				
Rise 'n Shine	1	320	**162**	27
Sausage	1	440	**255**	63
Sausage and Egg	1	503	**280**	72
Steak	1	500	**261**	63
Steak and Egg	1	550	**288**	72
Western Omelet	1	400	**243**	72
Breadstick	1	150	**36**	0
Cheeseburger	1	300	**134**	54
Bacon	1	610	**351**	144
Quarter-pound	1	500	**261**	126
Chicken Fillet Sandwich	1	370	**117**	18
Coleslaw	4 oz	240	**180**	27
Combo Sub	1	380	**54**	27
Cool Twist Sundae (hot fudge)	1	320	**90**	45
Crispy Curls	1 order	300	**144**	27
Fisherman's Fillet Sandwich	1	469	**190**	45
French Fries	1 large	360	**153**	27
	1 regular	230	**100**	18
Fried Chicken				
Breast	1	340	**171**	63
Chicken Stix	6 pieces	210	**81**	18
Leg	1	152	**72**	27
Thigh	1	370	**234**	81
Wing	1	205	**117**	45
Frisco Breakfast Sandwich	1	430	**180**	63
Frisco Chicken Sandwich	1	680	**369**	90
Frisco Club Sandwich	1	670	**378**	108
Grilled Chicken Breast				
Sandwich	1	310	**81**	9
Hamburger	1	260	**90**	36
Big Deluxe	1	503	**270**	108
Frisco Burger	1	730	**423**	153
Ham Sub	1	370	**63**	36
Hash Rounds	1 serving	249	**126**	27
Hot Dog	1	290	**144**	36
Hot Ham 'n Cheese Sandwich	1	330	**108**	45
Mushroom 'n Swiss Burger				
Sandwich	1	509	**243**	117
Muffin				
Blueberry	1	400	**153**	36
Oatbran Raisin	1	410	**144**	27

FAST FOODS

FOOD	AMOUNT	CALORIES		
		TOTAL	FAT	SAT-FAT
Pancakes	1 order	280	**18**	9
with 2 strips of bacon	1 order	350	**81**	27
with a sausage patty	1 order	430	**144**	54
Roast Beef Sandwich				
Big	1	380	**162**	72
Regular	1	280	**99**	36
Roast Beef Sub	1	370	**45**	27
Salad				
Chef	1	215	**117**	72
Green	1	184	**108**	63
Grilled Chicken, no dressing	1	120	**36**	9
Potato	1 small	260	**171**	27
Shrimp 'n Pasta	1 serving	362	**261**	NA
Shakes				
Chocolate	1	390	**90**	54
Peach	1	530	**99**	63
Strawberry	1	390	**72**	45
Vanilla	1	370	**81**	54
Turkey Club Sandwich	1	390	**144**	36
Turkey Sub	1	390	**63**	36
Jack in the Box				
Apple Turnover	1	354	**171**	NA
Breakfast Jack	1	307	**117**	46
Cheeseburger	1	315	**126**	51
Bacon	1	705	**405**	135
Double	1	467	**243**	111
Ultimate	1	942	**621**	238
Cheesecake	1 slice	309	**162**	85
Chicken and Mushroom				
Sandwich	1	438	**162**	45
Chicken Fajita Pita	1	292	**72**	27
Chicken Strips	4 pieces	285	**117**	28
Chicken Supreme Sandwich	1	641	**351**	90
Chicken Wings	6 pieces	846	**396**	96
Country-Fried Steak Sandwich	1	450	**225**	63
Crescent				
Sausage	1	584	**387**	140
Supreme	1	547	**360**	119
Curly Fries	1 serving	358	**180**	42
Double Fudge Cake	1 piece	288	**81**	20
Egg Rolls	3	437	**216**	61

FAST FOODS

FOOD	AMOUNT	CALORIES		
		TOTAL	FAT	SAT-FAT
Fish Supreme Sandwich	1	510	**243**	55
French Fries	1 regular	351	**153**	36
Grilled Chicken Fillet				
Sandwich	1	431	**171**	42
Hamburger	1	276	**108**	37
Grilled Sourdough	1	712	**450**	143
Ham and Swiss	1	638	**351**	NA
Mushroom	1	477	**243**	NA
Swiss and Bacon	1	643	**387**	NA
Hash browns	1 order	156	**99**	23
Jumbo Jack	1	584	**306**	99
with cheese	1	677	**360**	126
Mini Chimichangas	4 pieces	571	**252**	77
Moby Jack	1	444	**225**	NA
Old-Fashioned Patty Melt	1	713	**414**	133
Onion Rings	1 serving	382	**207**	50
Pancake Platter	1	612	**198**	77
Salad				
Chef	1	325	**162**	76
Pasta Seafood	1 serving	394	**198**	NA
Taco	1	503	**279**	121
Scrambled Egg				
Platter	1	560	**288**	78
Pocket	1	431	**189**	68
Shakes				
Chocolate	1	330	**63**	39
Strawberry	1	320	**63**	39
Vanilla	1	320	**54**	32
Sirloin Steak Sandwich	1	517	**207**	45
Sourdough Breakfast				
Sandwich	1	381	**180**	64
Supreme Nachos	1 serving	718	**360**	NA
Taco				
regular	1 serving	191	**99**	34
super	1 serving	288	**153**	53
Toasted Raviolis	7 pieces	537	**252**	72
Tortilla Chips	1 serving	139	**54**	NA
KFC (Kentucky Fried Chicken)				
Buttermilk Biscuit	1	235	**108**	29
Chicken Little Sandwich	1	169	**90**	18
Coleslaw	1 serving	114	**54**	9

FAST FOODS

FOOD	AMOUNT	CALORIES		
		TOTAL	FAT	SAT-FAT
Colonel's Chicken Sandwich	1	482	**243**	51
Corn on the Cob	1 serving	176	**27**	9
Kentucky Fried Chicken				
Extra Tasty Crispy Chicken				
breast	1	344	**189**	45
drumstick	1	205	**126**	27
thigh	1	415	**280**	72
wing	1	230	**153**	36
Hot and Spicy Chicken				
breast	1	382	**225**	54
drumstick	1	207	**126**	27
thigh	1	412	**270**	72
wing	1	244	**162**	36
Hot	6	471	**297**	72
Original Recipe Chicken				
breast	1	276	**126**	36
drumstick	1	150	**81**	18
thigh	1	290	**189**	45
wing	1	181	**108**	27
Kentucky Fried Chicken Dinner				
Original Recipe				
wing and breast	1 dinner	604	**289**	NA
drumstick and thigh	1 dinner	643	**317**	NA
wing and thigh	1 dinner	661	**340**	NA
Extra Crispy				
wing and breast	1 dinner	755	**383**	NA
drumstick and thigh	1 dinner	765	**483**	NA
wing and thigh	1 dinner	902	**434**	NA
Kentucky Fries	1 serving	244	**108**	27
Kentucky Nuggets	6 pieces	280	**162**	38
Long John Silver's				
Baked Chicken	1 order	130	**36**	11
Dinner	1 order	550	**135**	29
Baked Fish	1 order	150	**9**	NA
Dinner	1 order	570	**108**	19
Baked Shrimp	1 order	120	**45**	NA
Batter-Dipped Chicken Sandwich	1	280	**72**	19
Batter-Dipped Fish Sandwich	1	340	**117**	29
Batter-Fried Fish	1 piece	180	**100**	18

FAST FOODS

FOOD	AMOUNT	CALORIES		
		TOTAL	FAT	SAT-FAT
Batter-Fried Shrimp	1 piece	47	**27**	6
Dinner	1 serving	711	**405**	NA
Breaded Clams	1 order	526	**279**	46
Breaded Oysters	1 piece	60	**27**	NA
Breaded Shrimp	1 order	388	**207**	21
Platter	1 order	962	**513**	NA
Chicken Nuggets Dinner	6 pieces	699	**405**	NA
Chicken Plank	1 piece	120	**54**	14
Chicken Planks	2 pieces	240	**108**	29
with fries	2 pieces	490	**234**	51
with fries	3 pieces	885	**459**	86
for kids	2 pieces	560	**261**	57
Chocolate Chip Cookie	1	230	**81**	51
Chowder				
Clam	1 serving			
	(6.6 oz)	128	**45**	16
Seafood	1 cup	140	**54**	18
Clam Dinner	1 order	990	**522**	99
Coleslaw	½ cup	140	**54**	9
Combination entrees, with fries, slaw, 2 hush puppies				
1 fish and 2 chicken	1 order	950	**441**	99
2 fish and 8 shrimp	1 order	1140	**585**	127
2 fish, 5 shrimp, and 1 chicken	1 order	1160	**585**	128
2 fish, 4 shrimp, and 3 oz clams	1 order	1240	**630**	137
Corn Cobbette	1 piece	140	**72**	23
Fish and Chicken				
with fries	1 piece each	550	**288**	61
for kids	1 piece each	620	**306**	67
Fish and Fryes				
2 pieces of fish	1 order	651	**324**	72
3 pieces of fish	1 order	853	**432**	91
Fish Dinner, fried, 3 pieces	1 order	1180	**630**	NA
Fish Sandwich, Homestyle	1 order	510	**198**	44
Fryes	1 order	247	**135**	23
Hush Puppies	1	70	**18**	4
Oatmeal Raisin Cookie	1	160	**90**	18
Ocean Chef Salad	1 order	110	**9**	4
Oyster Dinner	1 order	789	**405**	NA

FAST FOODS

FOOD	AMOUNT	CALORIES		
		TOTAL	FAT	SAT-FAT
Pie				
Apple	1 piece	320	**117**	41
Cherry	1 piece	360	**117**	40
Lemon	1 piece	340	**81**	27
Pumpkin	1 piece	251	**99**	NA
Scallop Dinner	1 order	747	**405**	NA
Saltines	2	25	**9**	NA
Seafood Gumbo	1 cup	120	**72**	19
Seafood Platter	1 order	976	**522**	NA
Seafood Salad	1 order	380	**279**	46
Tartar Sauce	1	50	**45**	9
Walnut Brownie	1	440	**198**	49
McDonald's				
Apple Pie	1	260	**135**	43
Big Mac	1	570	**315**	104
Biscuit with Biscuit Spread	1	330	**164**	68
Bacon, Egg, and Cheese	1	483	**284**	83
Sausage	1	467	**278**	105
Sausage and Egg	1	585	**360**	131
Cheeseburger	1	318	**144**	60
Chef Salad	1	170	**81**	36
Chicken McNuggets	6 pieces	323	**182**	46
Cookies				
Chocolaty Chip	1 box	342	**144**	74
McDonaldland	1 box	308	**99**	38
Danish				
Apple	1	390	**162**	31
Cinnamon Raisin	1	440	**189**	38
Iced Cheese	1	390	**198**	54
Raspberry	1	410	**144**	28
Egg McMuffin	1 order	340	**142**	53
English Muffin with Butter	1 order	186	**45**	21
Filet-O-Fish	1 order	435	**231**	50
Fries				
small	1 order	220	**108**	23
medium	1 order	320	**153**	32
large	1 order	400	**198**	45
Hamburger	1	263	**99**	40
Hash Brown Potatoes	1 order	144	**81**	26
Hotcakes with Syrup and Butter	1 order	500	**90**	34

FAST FOODS

FOOD	AMOUNT	CALORIES		
		TOTAL	FAT	SAT-FAT
McChicken	1	490	**257**	49
McD.L.T.	1 order	680	**396**	133
McLean Deluxe	1	320	**90**	36
with cheese	1	370	**126**	45
Quarter Pounder	1	427	**212**	82
with cheese	1	525	**284**	115
Sausage	1	210	**171**	45
Sausage McMuffin	1	427	**237**	91
with egg	1	517	**296**	115
Scrambled Eggs	1 serving	180	**117**	46
Shake				
Chocolate	1	383	**81**	37
Strawberry	10.2 fl oz	362	**81**	37
Soft Serve and Cone	1 serving	189	**45**	20
Sundae				
Caramel	1	361	**90**	31
Hot fudge	1 order	357	**99**	49
Strawberry	1 serving	320	**81**	29
Pizza Hut				
Hand-Tossed Pizza, medium				
Cheese	2 slices	518	**180**	122
Pepperoni	2 slices	500	**207**	116
Super Supreme	2 slices	556	**225**	117
Supreme	2 slices	540	**234**	124
Pan Pizza, medium				
Cheese	2 slices	492	**162**	81
Pepperoni	2 slices	540	**198**	83
Super Supreme	2 slices	563	**234**	108
Supreme	2 slices	589	**270**	124
Personal Pan Pizza				
Pepperoni	1 pizza	675	**261**	113
Supreme	1 pizza	647	**252**	101
Thin 'n Crispy pizza, medium				
Cheese	2 slices	398	**153**	94
Pepperoni	2 slices	413	**180**	95
Super Supreme	2 slices	463	**189**	94
Supreme	2 slices	459	**198**	99
Red Lobster				
Alaskan Snow Crab Legs	1 order	200	**99**	54
Bay Platter	1	680	**243**	81
Bayou-style Seafood Gumbo	6 oz	180	**45**	9

FAST FOODS

FOOD	AMOUNT	CALORIES		
		TOTAL	FAT	SAT-FAT
Broiled Flounder Fillets	1 order	150	**54**	27
Broiled Rock Lobster	1 order	250	**45**	18
Fish Fillet Sandwich	1	230	**85**	<9
Grilled Chicken Breast	1	170	**54**	18
Grilled Chicken and Shrimp	1 order	490	**180**	54
Grilled Chicken Sandwich	1	340	**90**	36
Grilled Shrimp Skewers	1 order	290	**81**	36
Ice Cream	1 order	260	**126**	81
Live Maine Lobster	1 order	200	**45**	18
Seafood Lover's Platter	1	650	**243**	108
Sherbet	1 order	180	**27**	18
Shrimp				
Cocktail	1	90	**18**	4
in the Shell	6 oz	130	**18**	<9
Scampi	1 order	310	**207**	126
Today's Fresh Catch (for lunch portions, halve the calories and fat calories)				
Atlantic Cod	1 dinner	300	**108**	54
Atlantic Salmon	1 dinner	460	**306**	108
Catfish	1 dinner	440	**270**	108
Coho Salmon	1 dinner	480	**252**	90
Grouper	1 dinner	300	**108**	54
Haddock	1 dinner	320	**108**	54
King Salmon	1 dinner	580	**360**	72
Mahi Mahi	1 dinner	320	**108**	54
Ocean Perch	1 dinner	360	**162**	90
Orange Roughy	1 dinner	440	**270**	54
Rainbow Trout	1 dinner	440	**252**	72
Red Rockfish	1 dinner	280	**108**	54
Sea Bass	1 dinner	360	**144**	72
Snapper	1 dinner	320	**108**	54
Sole	1 dinner	320	**108**	54
Swordfish	1 dinner	300	**162**	108
Walleye Pike	1 dinner	340	**108**	54
Yellow Lake Perch	1 dinner	340	**108**	54
Roy Rogers				
Bacon Bits	1 tsp	24	**9**	NA
Baked Potato, Hot-Topped				
Bacon 'n Cheese	1	397	**198**	NA
Broccoli 'n Cheese	1	376	**162**	NA
Plain	1	211	**0**	NA
Sour Cream 'n Chives	1	408	**189**	NA

FAST FOODS

FOOD	AMOUNT	CALORIES		
		TOTAL	FAT	SAT-FAT
Baked Potato (*cont.*)				
Taco Beef 'n Cheese	1	463	198	NA
with margarine	1	274	63	NA
Biscuit	1	231	108	NA
Breakfast Crescent Sandwich	1	401	243	NA
Bacon	1	431	270	NA
Ham	1	557	378	NA
Sausage	1	449	261	NA
Brownie	1	264	99	NA
Cheddar Cheese	¼ cup	112	81	NA
Cheeseburger	1	563	333	NA
Bacon	1	581	351	NA
Chicken				
breast	1	324	171	NA
breast and wing	1	466	261	NA
leg	1	117	63	NA
thigh	1	282	180	NA
thigh and leg	1	399	234	NA
wing	1	142	90	NA
Chinese Noodles	¼ cup	55	27	NA
Coleslaw	1 order	110	63	NA
Crescent Roll	1	287	162	NA
Danish				
Apple	1	249	108	NA
Cheese	1	271	108	NA
Cherry	1	271	126	NA
Egg and Biscuit Platter	1	394	243	NA
Bacon	1	435	270	NA
Ham	1	442	261	NA
Sausage	1	550	369	NA
French Fries				
large	1 order	357	162	NA
regular	1 order	268	126	NA
Hamburger	1	456	252	NA
RR Bar Burger	1	611	351	NA
Hot Chocolate	1	123	18	NA
Macaroni	1 order	186	99	NA
Pancake Platter (with syrup and butter)	1	452	135	NA
Bacon	1	493	162	NA
Ham	1	506	153	NA
Sausage	1	608	270	NA

FAST FOODS

FOOD	AMOUNT	CALORIES		
		TOTAL	FAT	SAT-FAT
Potato Salad	1	107	54	NA
Roast Beef Sandwich	1	317	90	NA
with cheese	1	424	171	NA
large	1	360	108	NA
with cheese	1	467	189	NA
Shake				
Chocolate	1	358	90	NA
Strawberry	1	315	90	NA
Vanilla	1	306	99	NA
Strawberry Shortcake	1 piece	447	171	NA
Sundae				
Caramel	1	293	72	NA
Strawberry	1	216	63	NA
Taco Bell				
Burritos				
Bean	1	447	126	18
Beef	1	493	189	72
Chicken	1	334	108	NA
Combo	1	407	144	45
Supreme	1	503	198	NA
Chilito	1	383	162	72
Cinnamon Twists	1 order	171	72	27
Guacamole	2 tbsp	34	18	0
MexiMelt				
Beef	1	266	135	72
Chicken	1	257	135	NA
Nacho Cheese Sauce	2 tbsp	103	72	27
Nachos	1 order	346	162	54
BellGrande	1 order	649	315	108
Supreme	1 order	367	243	45
Pintos 'n Cheese	1 order	190	81	36
Salsa	1 serving	18	0	0
Soft Taco	1	225	108	NA
Chicken	1	213	90	36
Supreme	1	272	144	72
Taco	1	183	99	45
Supreme	1	230	135	72
Taco Salad	1	905	549	171
without shell	1	680	279	126
Taco Sauce	1 serving	3	0	0
Tostada	1	243	99	36

FAST FOODS

FOOD	AMOUNT	CALORIES TOTAL	FAT	SAT-FAT
Wendy's				
Baked Potato, plain	1	250	0	0
Bacon and Cheese	1	510	153	36
Broccoli and Cheese	1	450	126	18
Cheese	1	550	216	72
Chili and Cheese	1	600	225	81
Sour Cream and Chives	1	500	207	84
Big Classic Sandwich	1	570	297	54
Breaded Chicken	1 fillet	220	90	18
Sandwich	1	450	180	36
Chicken Club Sandwich	1	520	225	54
Cheeseburger				
Double	1	590	297	128
Jr. Cheeseburger	1	320	117	45
Bacon	1	440	225	72
Deluxe	1	390	180	63
Kid's Meal	1	310	117	45
Chicken Nuggets	6	280	180	40
Chili				
large	1	290	81	36
small	1	190	54	18
Chocolate Chip Cookie	1	275	117	38
Chow Mein Noodles	¼ cup	74	36	5
Cole Slaw	½ cup	90	72	18
Country-Fried Steak Sandwich	1	460	234	63
Fish Sandwich	1	460	225	42
French Fries				
large	1 order	450	198	45
small	1 order	240	108	23
Frosty Dairy Dessert				
large	1	578	153	76
small	1	340	90	45
Fruit-Flavored Drink	12 fl oz	110	0	0
Grilled Chicken	1 fillet	100	27	9
Sandwich	1	290	63	9
Hamburger	1	350	135	54
with Everything	1	440	207	63
Double Hamburger	1	520	243	96
Jr. Hamburger	1	270	81	27
Kid's Meal	1 serving	270	81	27
Hot Chocolate	6 fl oz	100	27	9

FAST FOODS

FOOD	AMOUNT	CALORIES		
		TOTAL	FAT	SAT-FAT
Mexican Fiesta Superbar				
Cheese Sauce	4 tbsp	40	**36**	9
Picante Sauce	2 tbsp	10	**0**	0
Refried Beans	4 tbsp	70	**18**	8
Spanish Rice	4 tbsp	60	**9**	2
Taco Chips	8	160	**54**	9
Taco Sauce	2 tbsp	12	**0**	0
Taco Shells	1	50	**27**	6
Tortilla	1	100	**27**	4
Pasta Superbar				
Alfredo Sauce	4 tbsp	30	**9**	7
Fettuccine	½ cup	120	**36**	9
Garlic Toast	1 piece	70	**27**	9
Macaroni and Cheese	½ cup	130	**54**	27
Pasta Medley	4 tbsp	60	**18**	3
Rotini	4 tbsp	90	**18**	3
Spaghetti Meat Sauce	4 tbsp	45	**9**	6
Spaghetti Sauce	4 tbsp	30	**0**	0
Salad				
Caesar Side Salad	1	160	**54**	9
Chicken (salad bar)	¼ cup	120	**72**	14
Deluxe Garden, without dressing	1	110	**45**	9
Grilled Chicken, without dressing	1	200	**72**	9
Side, without dressing	1	60	**27**	<9
Taco, without dressing	1	640	**270**	108
Sunflower Seeds and Raisins	2 tbsp	140	**90**	67
Turkey Ham	¼ cup	35	**18**	4

FATS AND OILS

FOOD	AMOUNT	CALORIES		
		TOTAL	FAT	SAT-FAT
Animal Fats				
Beef tallow	1 tbsp	116	**116**	58
Butter				
regular	1 pat	36	**36**	23
	1 tbsp	100	**100**	65
	1 stick	813	**813**	515

FATS AND OILS

| FOOD | AMOUNT | CALORIES | | |
		TOTAL	FAT	SAT-FAT
Butter (*cont.*)				
whipped	1 tsp	23	**23**	12
	1 tbsp	67	**67**	38
Chicken fat	1 tbsp	115	**115**	34
Duck fat	1 tbsp	115	**115**	39
Goose fat	1 tbsp	115	**115**	32
Lard (pork)	1 tbsp	116	**116**	45
Mutton tallow	1 tbsp	116	**116**	55
Turkey fat	1 tbsp	115	**115**	34
Butter Substitutes				
Butter Buds Sprinkles	1 tsp (2 g)	8	**0**	0
Molly McButter	1 tsp (2 g)	5	**0**	0
Margarines				
Stick				
Fleischmann's	1 tbsp (14 g)	90	**90**	18
lower fat	1 tbsp (14 g)	40	**40**	0
Imperial	1 tbsp (14 g)	90	**90**	18
Land O Lakes				
Country Morning Blend	1 tbsp (14 g)	100	**100**	36
light	1 tbsp (14 g)	50	**50**	27
Spread with Sweet Cream	1 tbsp (14 g)	90	**90**	18
Move Over Butter	1 tbsp (14 g)	90	**90**	18
Promise	1 tbsp (14 g)	90	**90**	18
Shedd's Spread Country Crock				
Churn-Style	1 tbsp (14 g)	80	**80**	18
Spreadable Stick	1 tbsp (14 g)	80	**80**	14
Tub				
Fleischmann's	1 tbsp (14 g)	90	**90**	18
I Can't Believe It's Not Butter,				
light	1 tbsp (14 g)	70	**70**	14
Land O Lakes Spread with				
Sweet Cream	1 tbsp (14 g)	80	**80**	14
Move Over Butter	1 tbsp (10 g)	60	**60**	14
Parkay				
soft	1 tbsp (14 g)	100	**100**	18
spread	1 tbsp (14 g)	60	**60**	14
Promise	1 tbsp (14 g)	90	**90**	14
ultra	1 tbsp (14 g)	35	**35**	0
ultra-fat-free	1 tbsp (14 g)	5	**5**	0

FATS AND OILS

FOOD	AMOUNT	CALORIES		
		TOTAL	FAT	SAT-FAT
Shedd's Spread Country Crock	1 tbsp (14 g)	60	**60**	14
Churn-Style	1 tbsp (14 g)	60	**60**	14
Smart Beat, super light	1 tbsp (14 g)	20	**20**	0
Oils				
Canola	1 tbsp	120	**120**	9
Cocoa butter	1 tbsp	120	**120**	73
Coconut	1 tbsp	120	**120**	106
Corn	1 tbsp	120	**120**	15
Cottonseed	1 tbsp	120	**120**	32
Olive	1 tbsp	119	**119**	16
Palm	1 tbsp	120	**120**	60
Palm kernel	1 tbsp	120	**120**	100
Peanut	1 tbsp	119	**119**	21
Safflower	1 tbsp	120	**120**	11
Sesame	1 tbsp	120	**120**	17
Soybean	1 tbsp	120	**120**	18
Sunflower	1 tbsp	120	**120**	13
Walnut	1 tbsp	120	**120**	11
Salad Dressings and Spreads				
Bacon and Tomato (Kraft)	2 tbsp	140	**130**	23
Balsamic and Basil Vinaigrette				
(Ken's)	2 tbsp	110	**110**	14
Blue Cheese				
chunky (Wish-Bone)	2 tbsp	150	**140**	27
Free (Kraft)	2 tbsp	45	**0**	0
regular (Kraft)	2 tbsp	90	**70**	36
Caesar				
Gourmet (Good Seasons)	2 tbsp prep.	150	**140**	23
light (Ken's)	2 tbsp	70	**60**	5
regular (Ken's)	2 tbsp	140	**120**	18
Caesar Ranch (Kraft)	2 tbsp	140	**130**	23
Catalina				
Free (Kraft)	2 tbsp	45	**0**	0
regular (Kraft)	2 tbsp	140	**100**	18
Coleslaw Dressing				
Hidden Valley Ranch	2 tbsp	150	**140**	27
Kraft	2 tbsp	150	**110**	18
Cucumber and Chive, fat-free				
(Ken's)	2 tbsp	30	**0**	0
Cucumber Ranch (Kraft)	2 tbsp	60	**45**	9

FATS AND OILS

FOOD	AMOUNT	CALORIES TOTAL	CALORIES FAT	CALORIES SAT-FAT
French (Kraft)	2 tbsp	120	**100**	18
Free (Kraft)	2 tbsp	50	**0**	0
Garlic and Herb (Good Seasons)	2 tbsp prep.	140	**140**	20
Honey Dijon				
fat-free (Ken's)	2 tbsp	40	**0**	0
light (Hidden Valley)	2 tbsp	35	**0**	0
regular (Kraft)	2 tbsp	140	**120**	18
Italian				
Free (Kraft)	2 tbsp	10	**0**	0
light (Wish-Bone)	2 tbsp	15	**5**	0
regular (Good Seasons)	2 tbsp prep.	140	**140**	20
regular (Kraft)	2 tbsp	120	**110**	18
zesty (Good Seasons)	2 tbsp prep.	140	**140**	20
zesty (Kraft)	2 tbsp	110	**100**	14
Mayonnaise				
Hellman's				
light	1 tbsp (15 g)	50	**45**	9
regular	1 tbsp (15 g)	100	**100**	14
Kraft				
Free	1 tbsp (15 g)	10	**0**	0
light	1 tbsp (15 g)	50	**45**	9
regular	1 tbsp	100	**100**	18
Mayonnaise substitute				
Miracle Whip (Kraft)	1 tbsp	70	**60**	9
light	1 tbsp	40	**30**	9
Nacho Cheese Ranch (Hidden Valley)	2 tbsp	130	**120**	18
Oriental Sesame (Good Seasons)	2 tbsp prep.	150	**140**	23
Parmesan, creamy low-fat (Hidden Valley Ranch)	2 tbsp	30	**0**	0
Parmesan Pepper, light (Ken's)	2 tbsp	80	**60**	14
Peppercorn Free (Kraft)	2 tbsp	50	**0**	0
Pizza Ranch (Hidden Valley)	2 tbsp	140	**130**	18
Ranch				
Free (Kraft)	2 tbsp	50	**0**	0
light (Hidden Valley)	2 tbsp	80	**60**	9
original (Hidden Valley)	2 tbsp	140	**130**	18
regular (Kraft)	2 tbsp	170	**170**	27
super creamy (Hidden Valley Ranch)	2 tbsp	140	**130**	NA

FATS AND OILS

FOOD	AMOUNT	CALORIES		
		TOTAL	FAT	SAT-FAT
Raspberry Walnut, light (Ken's)	2 tbsp	80	**50**	0
Russian	2 tbsp	166	**160**	29
Salsa Zesty Garden (Kraft)	2 tbsp	70	**60**	9
Sun-Dried Tomato Vinaigrette, free (Ken's)	2 tbsp	15	**0**	0
Taco Ranch (Hidden Valley Ranch)	2 tbsp	130	**120**	18
Thousand Island				
Free (Kraft)	2 tbsp	45	**0**	0
regular (Kraft)	2 tbsp	110	**90**	14
Shortening				
Crisco	1 tbsp	110	**110**	27

FISH AND SHELLFISH

Unless otherwise noted, fish is baked, steamed, or broiled with *no added fat.* If fish is baked in butter or margarine and you are keeping track of total fat, for each teaspoon of butter or margarine you use, add 33 total calories to the total calories listed for each fish and 33 fat calories to the fat calories listed for each fish. If you are keeping track of saturated fat, for each teaspoon of butter you use, add 33 total calories to the total calories listed for each fish and 22 sat-fat calories to the sat-fat calories listed for each fish. For margarine, add 33 total calories to the total calories listed for each fish and 18 sat-fat calories to the sat-fat calories listed for each fish. *See also* **FROZEN, MICROWAVE, AND REFRIGERATED FOODS** and **FAST FOODS.**

*Remember that most of the following calorie figures are for **only 1 ounce** of seafood!*

FOOD	AMOUNT	CALORIES		
		TOTAL	FAT	SAT-FAT
Abalone				
raw	1 oz	30	**2**	0
cooked, fried	1 oz	54	**17**	4
Anchovy				
raw	1 oz	37	**12**	3
canned in oil, drained	1 oz	60	**25**	6
	5 anchovies (20 g)	42	**17**	4

FISH AND SHELLFISH

FOOD	AMOUNT	CALORIES		
		TOTAL	FAT	SAT-FAT
Bass				
freshwater, raw	1 oz	32	9	2
	1 fillet (79 g)	90	26	6
striped, raw	1 oz	27	6	1
	1 fillet (159 g)	154	33	7
Bluefish				
raw	1 oz	35	11	2
	1 fillet (150 g)	186	57	12
Burbot, raw	1 oz	25	2	0
	1 fillet (116 g)	104	8	2
Butterfish, raw	1 oz	41	20	NA
	1 fillet (32 g)	47	23	NA
Carp				
raw	1 oz	36	14	3
	1 fillet (218 g)	276	110	21
cooked, dry heat	1 oz	46	18	4
	1 fillet (170 g)	276	110	21
Catfish, channel				
breaded and fried	1 oz	65	34	8
	1 fillet (87 g)	199	104	26
raw	1 oz	33	11	3
	1 fillet (79 g)	92	30	7
Caviar, black and red	1 tbsp	40	26	15
	1 oz	71	45	27
Cisco (lake herring)				
raw	1 oz	28	5	1
	1 fillet (79 g)	78	14	3
smoked	1 oz	50	30	4
Clams				
raw, cherrystones or littlenecks	9 large or 20 small (180 g)	133	16	1
	1 oz	22	3	0
breaded and fried	1 oz	57	28	7
	20 small clams (188 g)	379	189	45
canned, drained solids	1 oz	42	5	0
	½ cup	118	14	1
cooked, moist heat	1 oz	42	5	0
	20 small clams (90 g)	133	16	2
fritters	1 fritter	124	54	NA

FISH AND SHELLFISH

FOOD	AMOUNT	CALORIES		
		TOTAL	FAT	SAT-FAT
Cod, Atlantic				
raw	1 oz	23	**2**	0
	1 fillet (231 g)	190	**14**	3
baked	1 oz	30	**2**	0
	1 fillet (180 g)	189	**14**	3
canned	1 oz	30	**2**	1
dried and salted	1 oz	81	**6**	0
Cod, Pacific, raw	1 oz	23	**2**	0
	1 fillet (116 g)	95	**7**	1
Crab				
Alaska king, steamed	1 oz	27	**4**	0
	1 leg (172 g)	129	**18**	2
Alaska king, imitation,				
made from surimi	1 oz	29	**3**	NA
Blue				
raw	1 oz	25	**3**	0
	1 crab (21 g)	18	**2**	0
cooked, moist heat	1 oz	27	**4**	1
canned	1 oz	28	**3**	0
	½ cup	67	**7**	2
Crab cakes	1 cake	93	**41**	8
	1 oz	44	**19**	4
Chesapeake Bay Deluxe				
Crab Cakes, frozen	1 oz	65	**41**	NA
Dungeness, raw	1 oz	24	**2**	0
Nutri Sea Crab Sticks	1 oz	29	**3**	NA
Nutri Sea King Crab	1 oz	31	**3**	NA
Sea Legs, Crabmeat Salad				
Style	1 oz	27	**3**	NA
Crayfish				
raw	1 oz	25	**3**	0
	8 crayfish (27 g)	24	**2**	0
steamed	1 oz	32	**3**	0
Croaker, Atlantic				
raw	1 oz	30	**8**	3
	1 fillet (79 g)	83	**22**	8
breaded and fried	1 oz	63	**32**	9
	1 fillet (87 g)	192	**99**	27
Cusk, raw	1 oz	25	**2**	NA
Cuttlefish, raw	1 oz	22	**2**	

FISH AND SHELLFISH

FOOD	AMOUNT	CALORIES		
		TOTAL	FAT	SAT-FAT
Dolphinfish, raw	1 oz	24	**2**	0
	1 fillet (204 g)	174	**13**	3
Drum, freshwater, raw	1 oz	34	**13**	3
	1 fillet (198 g)	236	**88**	20
Eel				
raw	1 oz	52	**30**	6
baked	1 oz	67	**38**	8
	1 fillet (159 g)	375	**214**	43
Flatfish (flounder or sole)				
raw	1 oz	26	**3**	1
	1 fillet (163 g)	149	**17**	4
baked or steamed	1 oz	33	**4**	1
	1 fillet (127 g)	148	**17**	4
Gefilte fish	1 piece	35	**7**	2
	1 oz	24	**4**	1
Grouper				
raw	1 oz	26	**3**	1
	1 fillet (259 g)	238	**24**	5
baked or steamed	1 oz	33	**3**	1
	1 fillet (202 g)	238	**24**	5
Haddock				
raw	1 oz	25	**2**	0
	1 fillet (193 g)	168	**12**	2
baked or steamed	1 oz	32	**2**	0
	1 fillet (150 g)	168	**12**	2
smoked	1 oz	33	**2**	0
Halibut, Atlantic and Pacific				
baked or steamed	1 oz	40	**7**	1
	½ fillet (159 g)	223	**42**	6
Herring, Atlantic				
raw	1 oz	45	**23**	5
	1 fillet (184 g)	291	**150**	34
baked or steamed	1 oz	57	**30**	7
canned	1 oz	59	**35**	7
in tomato sauce	1 herring (37 g)	97	**52**	10
pickled	1 oz	65	**39**	6
	1 herring	112	**68**	9
	1 piece (15 g)	33	**21**	3
smoked, kippered	1 oz	60	**33**	7
	1 fillet (40 g)	87	**45**	10
Herring, Pacific, raw	1 oz	55	**35**	8

FISH AND SHELLFISH

		CALORIES		
FOOD	AMOUNT	TOTAL	FAT	SAT-FAT
Lobster, northern				
raw	1 oz	26	2	0
	1 lobster (150 g)	136	12	NA
cooked, moist heat	1 oz	28	2	0
	1 cup	142	8	1
Newburg (with butter, eggs, sherry, cream)	1 cup	485	239	160
salad (with mayonnaise)	½ cup or 4 oz	286	149	NA
Lox (smoked salmon)	1 oz	33	11	2
Mackerel, Atlantic				
raw	1 oz	58	35	8
	1 fillet (112 g)	229	140	33
baked or steamed	1 oz	74	45	11
	1 fillet (88 g)	231	141	33
Mackerel, Jack, canned	1 cup	296	108	30
Mackerel, king, raw	1 oz	30	9	1
	½ fillet (198 g)	207	36	6
Mackerel, Pacific and Jack, raw	1 oz	44	20	6
	1 fillet (225 g)	353	160	46
Mackerel, Spanish				
raw	1 oz	39	16	5
	1 fillet (187 g)	260	106	31
baked or steamed	1 oz	45	16	5
	1 fillet (146 g)	230	83	24
Milkfish, raw	1 oz	42	17	NA
Monkfish, raw	1 oz	21	4	NA
Mullet, striped				
raw	1 oz	33	10	3
	1 fillet (119 g)	139	41	12
baked	1 oz	42	12	4
	1 fillet (93 g)	139	41	12
Mussels, blue				
raw	1 oz	24	6	1
	1 cup	129	30	6
Ocean perch, Atlantic				
raw	1 oz	27	4	1
	1 fillet (64 g)	60	9	1
baked	1 oz	34	5	1
	1 fillet (50 g)	60	9	1

FISH AND SHELLFISH

FOOD	AMOUNT	CALORIES		
		TOTAL	**FAT**	**SAT-FAT**
Ocean perch, Atlantic (*cont.*)				
breaded and fried	1 fillet	185	**99**	NA
Octopus, raw	1 oz	23	**3**	1
Oyster, eastern				
raw	6 medium (84 g)	58	**19**	5
	1 cup	170	**55**	14
breaded and fried	1 oz	56	**32**	8
	6 medium (88 g)	173	**100**	25
canned	1 oz	19	**6**	2
	½ cup	85	**28**	7
steamed	1 oz	39	**13**	3
	6 medium (42 g)	58	**19**	5
stew (2 parts milk, 1 part oyster)	1 cup	233	**139**	80
Oyster, Pacific, raw	1 oz	23	**6**	1
	1 medium (50 g)	41	**10**	2
Pike, northern				
raw	1 oz	25	**2**	0
	½ fillet (198 g)	175	**12**	2
baked	1 oz	32	**2**	0
	½ fillet (155 g)	176	**12**	2
Pike, walleye, raw	1 oz	26	**3**	1
	1 fillet (159 g)	147	**17**	4
Pollock, Atlantic, raw	1 oz	26	**2**	0
	½ fillet (193 g)	177	**17**	2
Pollock, walleye				
raw	1 oz	23	**2**	0
	1 fillet (77 g)	62	**6**	1
baked	1 oz	32	**3**	1
	1 fillet (60 g)	68	**6**	1
Pompano, Florida				
raw	1 oz	47	**24**	9
	1 fillet (112 g)	184	**95**	35
baked	1 oz	60	**31**	11
	1 fillet (88 g)	185	**96**	36
Pout, ocean, raw	1 oz	22	**2**	1
	½ fillet (176 g)	40	**14**	5

FISH AND SHELLFISH

FOOD	AMOUNT	CALORIES		
		TOTAL	FAT	SAT-FAT
Rockfish, Pacific				
raw	1 oz	27	**4**	1
	1 fillet (191 g)	180	**27**	6
baked	1 oz	34	**5**	1
	1 fillet (149 g)	180	**27**	6
Roughy, orange, raw	1 oz	36	**18**	0
Sablefish				
raw	1 oz	55	**39**	8
	½ fillet (193 g)	377	**266**	56
smoked	1 oz	72	**51**	10
Salmon, Atlantic, raw	1 oz	40	**16**	3
Salmon, chinook				
raw	1 oz	51	**27**	6
smoked	1 oz	33	**11**	2
Salmon, chum				
raw	1 oz	34	**10**	2
canned	1 oz	40	**14**	4
Salmon, coho				
raw	1 oz	41	**15**	3
Salmon, pink				
raw	1 oz	33	**9**	1
canned	1 oz	39	**15**	4
Salmon, sockeye				
raw	1 oz	48	**22**	4
canned, drained	1 oz	40	**14**	4
Salmon, smoked (lox)	1 oz	33	**11**	2
Sardines, Atlantic, canned in				
oil, drained	1 oz	59	**29**	3
	2 sardines (24 g)	50	**25**	3
	1 can (3¼ oz)	192	**95**	13
Sardines, Pacific, canned in				
tomato sauce, drained	1 oz	51	**31**	8
	1 sardine (38 g)	68	**41**	11
Scallops				
raw	1 oz	25	**2**	0
	2 large or 5 small (30 g)	26	**2**	0
breaded, fried	1 oz	61	**28**	6
	2 large (31 g)	67	**31**	7
steamed	1 oz	32	**4**	1

FISH AND SHELLFISH

FOOD	AMOUNT	CALORIES		
		TOTAL	FAT	SAT-FAT
Scup, raw	1 oz	30	7	NA
	1 fillet (64 g)	67	16	NA
Sea bass				
raw	1 oz	27	5	1
	1 fillet (129 g)	125	23	6
baked	1 oz	35	7	2
	1 fillet (101 g)	125	23	6
Sea trout, raw	1 oz	29	9	3
	1 fillet (238 g)	248	77	22
Shad				
raw	1 oz	56	35	NA
	1 fillet (184 g)	362	228	NA
baked	1 oz	57	29	NA
Shark				
raw	1 oz	37	11	2
batter-dipped and fried	1 oz	65	35	8
Sheepshead				
raw	1 oz	31	6	2
	1 fillet (238 g)	257	52	13
baked	1 oz	36	4	1
	1 fillet (186 g)	234	27	6
Shrimp				
raw	1 oz	30	4	1
	4 large (28 g)	30	4	1
breaded, fried	1 oz	69	31	5
	4 large (30 g)	73	33	6
canned	1 oz	34	5	1
	½ cup	77	11	2
cocktail (Sau-Sea)	½ cup	90	0	0
steamed	1 oz	28	3	1
	4 large (22 g)	22	2	1
Smelt, rainbow				
raw	1 oz	28	6	1
baked	1 oz	35	8	2
Snapper				
raw	1 oz	28	3	1
	1 fillet (218 g)	217	26	6
baked	1 oz	36	4	1
	1 fillet (170 g)	217	26	6
Sole (see Flatfish)				

FISH AND SHELLFISH

		CALORIES		
FOOD	AMOUNT	TOTAL	FAT	SAT-FAT
Spiny lobster, raw	1 oz	32	**4**	1
	1 lobster (209 g)	233	**28**	4
Spot, raw	1 oz	35	**12**	4
	1 fillet (64 g)	79	**28**	8
Squid				
raw	1 oz	26	**4**	1
fried	1 oz	50	**19**	5
Sturgeon				
raw	1 oz	30	**10**	2
baked	1 oz	38	**13**	3
smoked	1 oz	48	**11**	3
Sucker, white, raw	1 oz	26	**6**	1
	1 fillet (159 g)	147	**33**	6
Sunfish, pumpkinseed, raw	1 oz	25	**2**	0
	1 fillet (48 g)	43	**3**	0
Surimi	1 oz	28	**2**	0
Swordfish				
raw	1 oz	34	**10**	3
baked	1 oz	44	**13**	4
Tilefish				
raw	1 oz	27	**6**	1
	½ fillet (193 g)	184	**40**	8
baked	1 oz	42	**12**	2
	½ fillet (150 g)	220	**63**	12
Trout, rainbow				
raw	1 oz	33	**9**	2
	1 fillet (79 g)	93	**24**	5
baked	1 oz	43	**11**	2
	1 fillet (62 g)	94	**24**	5
Tuna				
raw	1 oz	41	**12**	3
baked	1 oz	52	**16**	4
canned, drained				
solid white in water	1 oz	37	**6**	2
chunk light in oil	1 oz	56	**21**	4
Tuna salad	½ cup	190	**85**	14
Turbot, European, raw	1 oz	27	**8**	NA
	½ fillet (204 g)	194	**54**	NA
Whelk				
raw	1 oz	39	**1**	0
steamed	1 oz	78	**2**	0

FISH AND SHELLFISH

FOOD	AMOUNT	CALORIES		
		TOTAL	FAT	SAT-FAT
Whitefish				
raw	1 oz	38	**15**	2
	1 fillet (198 g)	266	**104**	16
smoked	1 oz	30	**2**	1
Whiting				
raw	1 oz	26	**3**	1
	1 fillet (92 g)	83	**11**	2
baked	1 oz	33	**4**	1
	1 fillet (72 g)	83	**11**	2
Wolffish, Atlantic, raw	1 oz	27	**6**	1
	½ fillet (153 g)	147	**33**	5
Yellowtail, raw	1 oz	41	**13**	NA
	½ fillet (187 g)	273	**88**	NA

FROZEN, MICROWAVE, AND REFRIGERATED FOODS

FOOD	AMOUNT	CALORIES		
		TOTAL	FAT	SAT-FAT
Breakfast Foods				
Blintzes				
Ratner's				
Cheese	1 (71 g)	100	**5**	5
Cherry	1 (71 g)	110	**5**	5
Potato	1 (71 g)	120	**30**	18
Breakfast Burritos				
Great Starts				
Bacon (Swanson)	1 pkg (99 g)	250	**100**	36
Breakfast Sandwich				
Great Starts (Swanson)				
Egg, Canadian Bacon, and Cheese on a Muffin	1 pkg (116 g)	290	**140**	54
Pancakes with Sausage	1 pkg (170 g)	490	**230**	99
Sausage, Egg, and Cheese on a Biscuit	1 pkg (156 g)	490	**270**	108
Scrambled Eggs and Bacon with Home-Fried Potatoes	1 pkg (149 g)	290	**170**	81

FROZEN, MICROWAVE, AND
REFRIGERATED FOODS

		CALORIES		
FOOD	AMOUNT	TOTAL	FAT	SAT-FAT
Breakfast Sandwich				
Great Starts (Swanson) (*cont.*)				
Scrambled Eggs and				
Sausage with Hashed				
Brown Potatoes	1 pkg (177 g)	360	**230**	90
Morningstar Farms				
Breakfast Links	2 (45 g)	90	**50**	9
Breakfast Patties	1 (38 g)	90	**50**	14
Grillers	1 (64 g)	140	**65**	9
Weight Watchers				
English Muffin Sandwich	1 (113 g)	220	**60**	18
Croissants				
Original (Sara Lee)	1 (43 g)	170	**70**	27
Eggs				
Great Starts (Swanson)				
Scrambled Eggs and				
Bacon	1 pkg (149 g)	290	**170**	81
Scrambled Eggs and				
Home-Fried Potatoes	1 pkg (120 g)	200	**110**	72
Scrambled Eggs and				
Sausage	1 pkg (177 g)	360	**230**	90
French Toast, Frozen				
Aunt Jemima, all types	2 (118 g)	240	**50**	0
Breakfast Blast Mini Sticks				
(Swanson)	1 pkg (120)	310	**130**	36
Downyflake				
Cinnamon Swirl	2 (113 g)	270	**50**	14
Plain	2 (113 g)	260	**60**	14
Great Starts (Swanson)				
Cinnamon Swirl French				
Toast with Sausage	1 pkg (156 g)	440	**250**	108
French Toast Sticks	1 pkg (120 g)	320	**90**	45
French Toast with				
Sausage	1 pkg (156 g)	410	**230**	81
Muffins				
Blueberry (Sara Lee)	1 (64 g)	220	**100**	18
Pancakes, Frozen				
Aunt Jemima				
Buttermilk Pancake Batter	½ cup batter	260	**25**	9
Low-fat	3 (97 g)	130	**15**	0

FROZEN, MICROWAVE, AND
REFRIGERATED FOODS

		CALORIES		
FOOD	AMOUNT	TOTAL	FAT	SAT-FAT
Great Starts (Swanson)				
Silver Dollar	1 pkg (106 g)	340	**160**	81
with sausage	1 pkg (170 g)	490	**230**	99
Hungry Jack				
Blueberry	3 (116 g)	230	**30**	5
Buttermilk	3 (116 g)	240	**35**	9
Toaster Strudel				
Pillsbury, all flavors	1 (54 g)	180	**60**	14
Waffles, Frozen				
Aunt Jemima				
Blueberry	2 (71 g)	190	**60**	14
Buttermilk	2 (71 g)	170	**50**	14
Low-fat	2 (74 g)	160	**10**	0
Oatmeal	2 (84 g)	200	**70**	14
Original	2 (71 g)	180	**60**	14
Belgian Chef Belgian				
Waffles	2 (70 g)	140	**25**	5
Breakfast Blast 5 Waffle				
Sticks	1 pkg (78 g)	330	**150**	63
Downyflake				
Homestyle and Buttermilk	2 (68 g)	170	**35**	0
Eggo				
Blueberry, Buttermilk, or				
Homestyle	2 (78 g)	220	**70**	14
Common Sense Oat Bran	2 (78 g)	200	**60**	14
Fat-free	2 (58 g)	140	**0**	0
Minis, plain or blueberry	2 (85 g)	240	**70**	14
Special K	2 (58 g)	140	**0**	0
Nutri-Grain Eggo				
Multi-bran or Whole-grain	2 (78 g)	180	**50**	9

Dishes or Dinners
Amy's

Black Bean, Vegetable				
Enchilada	1 (135 g)	130	**40**	<9
Burrito, nondairy	1 (236 g)	250	**45**	23
Cheese Enchilada	1 (135 g)	210	**80**	0
Mexican Tamale Pie	1 (227 g)	220	**27**	0
Shepherd's Pie	1 (227 g)	160	**35**	0
Vegetable Lasagna	1 (269 g)	300	**90**	36

FROZEN, MICROWAVE, AND REFRIGERATED FOODS

FOOD	AMOUNT	CALORIES		
		TOTAL	FAT	SAT-FAT
Banquet				
Beef Pot Pie	1 (198 g)	330	140	63
Chicken Breast Patties	1 (70 g)	200	110	23
Chicken Breast Tenders	3 (85 g)	210	90	18
Chicken Nugget Meal	1 (191 g)	410	190	45
Chicken Nuggets	9 (84 g)	240	130	27
Chicken Patties	1 (70 g)	200	110	23
Chicken Pot Pie	1 (198 g)	350	160	63
Country Fried Chicken	3 oz (84 g)	270	160	45
Fried Chicken	3 oz (84 g)	270	160	45
Fried Chicken Meal	1 (255 g)	470	240	81
Mozzarella Cheese Nuggets	3 pieces (36 g)	110	50	23
Salisbury Steak Meal	1 (269 g)	310	150	63
Skinless Fried Chicken	3 oz (84 g)	210	120	27
Southern Chicken Chunks	19 nuggets (84 g)	230	140	27
Southern Fried Chicken	3 oz (84 g)	270	160	45
Spicy 'n Hot Fried Chicken	3 oz (84 g)	260	160	45
Turkey and Gravy	1 meal (262 g)	270	90	27
Turkey Pot Pie	1 (198 g)	370	180	72
Vegetable-Cheese Pot Pie	1 (198 g)	390	160	72
Banquet Extra Helping				
Southern Fried Chicken	1 meal (496 g)	750	330	81
Turkey and Gravy	1 meal (532 g)	560	180	45
Budget Gourmet				
Beef Cantonese	1 entree	280	70	27
Cheese Manicotti with Meat Sauce	1 entree	440	230	108
Cheese Tortellini	1 pkg	190	70	18
Chicken and Egg Noodles	1 entree	410	210	108
Chicken Marsala	1 entree	270	60	36
Chicken with Fettucini	1 entree	380	170	90
Escalloped Noodles and Turkey	1 entree	440	180	90
Fettucini Alfredo	1 entree	480	210	117
Italian Sausage Lasagna	1 entree	400	180	90
Linguini with Bay Shrimp and Clams Marinara	1 entree	300	100	54
Oriental Rice with Vegetables	1 pkg	220	110	45

FROZEN, MICROWAVE, AND
REFRIGERATED FOODS

		CALORIES		
FOOD	AMOUNT	TOTAL	FAT	SAT-FAT
Pepper Steak with Rice	1 entree	290	**70**	27
Rice Pilaf with Green Beans	1 pkg	230	**110**	27
Roast Sirloin Supreme	1 entree	300	**110**	63
Sirloin Cheddar Melt	1 entree	370	**190**	90
Sirloin Tips	1 entree	260	**130**	54
Swedish Meatballs	1 entree	550	**300**	144
Szechuan Vegetables and Chicken	1 entree	300	**80**	14
Three-Cheese Lasagna	1 entree	370	**140**	90
Wide Ribbon Pasta with Ricotta and Chunky Tomato Sauce	1 entree	420	**200**	72
Ziti in Marinara Sauce	1 pkg	220	**90**	36
Budget Gourmet Light & Healthy				
Chicken Oriental and Vegetable	1 entree	300	**60**	18
Chinese-Style Vegetables and Chicken	1 entree	290	**80**	14
Glazed Turkey	1 entree	250	**35**	18
Italian Style Vegetables and Chicken	1 entree	280	**60**	18
Lasagna with Meat Sauce	1 entree	250	**60**	27
Linguini with Scallops and Clams	1 entree	300	**90**	54
Macaroni and Cheese	1 entree	350	**70**	45
Mandarin Chicken	1 entree	250	**40**	9
Orange-Glazed Chicken Breast	1 entree	270	**25**	9
Oriental Beef	1 entree	290	**80**	45
Penne Pasta with Chunky Tomato Sauce and Italian Sausage	1 entree	330	**70**	23
Roast Chicken Breast with Herb Gravy	1 dinner	240	**60**	18
Sirloin of Beef in Herb Sauce	1 entree	280	**80**	36
Spaghetti with Chunky Tomato and Meat Sauce	1 entree	320	**70**	23
Special Recipe Sirloin of Beef	1 dinner	330	**70**	27

FROZEN, MICROWAVE, AND
REFRIGERATED FOODS

FOOD	AMOUNT	CALORIES		
		TOTAL	FAT	SAT-FAT
Budget Gourmet Light				
& Healthy (*cont.*)				
Stuffed Turkey Breast	1 dinner	260	**50**	18
Yankee Pot Roast	1 dinner	270	**60**	23
Celentano				
Cheese Ravioli	6 (182 g)	400	**80**	45
Manicotti with Sauce	1 (202 g)	320	**140**	63
Dinty Moore				
Beef Stew (canned)	1 cup	230	**120**	63
Beef Stew	1 cup	190	**90**	36
Chicken Stew	1 cup	180	**70**	18
Chicken and Dumplings	1 cup	190	**50**	14
Corned Beef Hash	1 cup	350	**200**	81
Don Miguel				
Bean and Cheese Burrito	1 (198 g)	420	**120**	54
Bean and Cheese				
Chimichanga	1 (198 g)	470	**160**	54
Beef and Cheese Burrito	1 (198 g)	390	**100**	36
Chicken and Cheese Burrito	1 (198 g)	410	**130**	36
Chicken Burrito	1 (198 g)	360	**70**	18
Gorton's				
Batter-Dipped Fish Portions	1 portion (70 g)	160	**90**	18
Crispy Fish Fillets in Batter	2 fillets (108 g)	280	**170**	45
Crispy Flounder	2 fillets (108 g)	290	**190**	36
Crispy Haddock	2 fillets (108 g)	270	**170**	36
Crunchy Breaded Fish Fillets	2 fillets (108 g)	270	**150**	45
Crunchy Breaded Fish Sticks	6 sticks (104 g)	250	**140**	36
Healthy Choice				
Beef and Peppers Cantonese	1 meal	270	**50**	23
Beef Broccoli Beijing	1 meal	330	**30**	9
Beef Burrito Ranchero	1 meal	300	**70**	23
Beef Macaroni	1 meal	200	**10**	5
Beef Pepper Steak Oriental	1 meal	250	**35**	14
Beef Tips	1 meal	260	**50**	18
Breast of Chicken	1 meal	280	**25**	9
Breast of Turkey	1 meal	280	**25**	9
Cacciatore Chicken	1 meal	260	**25**	5
Chicken Bangkok	1 meal	270	**30**	5

FROZEN, MICROWAVE, AND REFRIGERATED FOODS

		CALORIES		
FOOD	AMOUNT	TOTAL	FAT	SAT-FAT
Chicken Cantonese	1 meal	210	5	0
Chicken con Queso Burrito	1 meal	280	60	23
Chicken Dijon	1 meal	280	35	14
Chicken Fettuccine Alfredo	1 meal	250	30	9
Chicken Parmigiana	1 meal	300	15	5
Chicken Teriyaki	1 meal	270	20	5
Chicken and Vegetables Marsala	1 meal	220	10	0
Country Glazed Chicken	1 meal	200	15	5
Country Herb Chicken	1 meal	270	35	14
Country Inn Roast Turkey	1 meal	250	30	9
Country Roast Turkey	1 meal	220	35	9
Fettuccine Alfredo	1 meal	240	45	18
Fiesta Chicken Fajitas	1 meal	260	35	9
Garden Potato Casserole	1 meal	200	35	14
Ginger Chicken Hunan	1 meal	350	20	5
Honey Mustard Chicken	1 meal	260	20	0
Lemon Pepper Fish	1 meal	290	45	9
Macaroni and Cheese	1 meal	290	45	18
Mandarin Chicken	1 meal	280	20	0
Meat Loaf	1 meal	320	80	36
Mesquite Beef	1 meal	310	40	14
Mesquite Chicken BBQ	1 meal	320	20	5
Pasta Shells Marinara	1 meal	360	25	14
Salisbury Steak	1 meal	320	60	27
Sesame Chicken Shanghai	1 meal	310	45	9
Shrimp and Vegetables Maria	1 meal	260	15	5
Southwestern Glazed Chicken	1 meal	300	30	9
Spaghetti Bolognese	1 meal	260	25	9
Sweet and Sour Chicken	1 meal	310	45	9
Three-Cheese Manicotti	1 meal	310	80	45
Vegetable Pasta Italiano	1 meal	220	10	0
Yankee Pot Roast	1 meal	280	50	18
Hormel				
Chili, no beans	1 cup	360	230	90
Macaroni and Cheese	1 cup	270	100	54
Noodles and Chicken	1 cup	250	100	27
Kid Cuisine				
Chicken Nuggets	1 meal	440	150	41

FROZEN, MICROWAVE, AND REFRIGERATED FOODS

FOOD	AMOUNT	CALORIES		
		TOTAL	FAT	SAT-FAT
Kids Fun Feast (Swanson)				
Frazzlin' Fried Chicken	1 pkg	660	**320**	117
Frenzied Fish Sticks	1 pkg	360	**130**	45
Kid's Kitchen (Hormel)				
Beans and Weiners	1 cup	310	**110**	45
Beefy Mac	1 cup	190	**50**	23
Kosherific				
Fish Fillets	2 (109 g)	280	**140**	27
Lean Cuisine				
Angel Hair Pasta	1 pkg	210	**35**	9
Beef Pot Roast	1 pkg	210	**60**	14
Cheese Cannelloni	1 pkg	270	**70**	32
Cheese Ravioli	1 pkg	250	**70**	27
Chicken Chow Mein	1 pkg	210	**45**	9
Chicken Enchilada Suiza	1 pkg	290	**40**	18
Chicken Fettucini	1 pkg	270	**60**	23
Chicken à l'Orange	1 pkg	260	**20**	5
Chicken Parmesan	1 pkg	220	**40**	14
Chicken in Peanut Sauce	1 pkg	280	**60**	9
Chicken and Vegetables	1 pkg	240	**45**	9
Classic Cheese Lasagna	1 pkg	290	**60**	27
Deluxe Cheddar Potato	1 pkg	270	**90**	32
Fettucini Alfredo	1 pkg	270	**60**	27
Fettucini Primavera	1 pkg	260	**70**	23
Fiesta Chicken	1 pkg	240	**40**	9
Glazed Chicken	1 pkg	240	**60**	9
Honey Mustard Chicken	1 pkg	250	**40**	9
Lasagna with Meat	1 pkg	270	**50**	23
Macaroni and Beef	1 pkg	280	**70**	18
Meatloaf	1 pkg	270	**90**	36
Oriental Beef	1 pkg	250	**70**	27
Rigatoni	1 pkg	180	**35**	14
Spaghetti with Meat Sauce	1 pkg	290	**60**	14
Swedish Meatballs	1 pkg	290	**80**	27
Three-Bean Chili	1 pkg	210	**60**	18
Turkey	1 pkg	230	**50**	14
Zucchini Lasagna	1 pkg	240	**35**	14

FROZEN, MICROWAVE, AND
REFRIGERATED FOODS

FOOD	AMOUNT	CALORIES		
		TOTAL	FAT	SAT-FAT
Lean Cuisine Lunch				
Express				
Broccoli and Cheddar Cheese Sauce over Baked Potato	1 pkg	250	**80**	36
Cheese Lasagna Casserole	1 pkg	270	**60**	23
Chicken Fettucini	1 pkg	250	**60**	23
Macaroni and Cheese	1 pkg	240	**60**	27
Mandarin Chicken	1 pkg	270	**50**	9
Teriyaki Stir-Fry	1 pkg	260	**45**	9
Mama Lucia				
Italian-Style Meatballs	3 (84 g)	270	**190**	81
Matlaw's				
Stuffed Clams	1 clam (71 g)	120	**50**	5
Michelina's				
Creamed Sauce, Beef	1 pkg	360	**180**	54
Egg Noodles, Gravy, Swedish Meatballs	1 pkg	340	**130**	36
Fettuccine Alfredo	1 pkg	390	**130**	45
Lasagna with Meat Sauce	1 pkg	290	**90**	36
Macaroni and Cheese	1 pkg	370	**130**	54
Noodles Stroganoff	1 pkg	310	**150**	45
Penne Pollo	1 pkg	330	**130**	45
Risotto Parmesano	1 pkg	360	**180**	54
Spaghetti Bolognese	1 pkg	270	**70**	27
Spaghetti Marinara	1 pkg	250	**20**	9
Morton				
Macaroni and Cheese	1 cup	230	**35**	18
Mrs. Budd's				
White Meat Chicken Pie				
Fancy Vegetables	1 cup	310	**140**	45
Original Recipe	1 cup	330	**150**	45
Mrs. Paul's				
Breaded Fish Fillets	1 (113 g)	170	**25**	14
Deviled Crabs	1 cake (80 g)	180	**80**	27
Healthy Treasures	1 fillet (113 g)	170	**25**	14
Nancy's French Baked				
Quiche				
Broccoli Cheddar	1 (170 g)	490	**290**	144
Classic French	1 (170 g)	520	**330**	162
Florentine	1 (170 g)	480	**290**	144

FROZEN, MICROWAVE, AND REFRIGERATED FOODS

FOOD	AMOUNT	CALORIES TOTAL	FAT	SAT-FAT
Patio Burritos				
Beef and Bean	1	280	**60**	27
Beef and Bean Green Chili	1	260	**40**	14
Beef and Bean with Red Chili Peppers	1	270	**60**	18
Chicken	1	260	**35**	14
Perdue				
BBQ Chicken	1 breast (154 g)	220	**70**	23
	2 drumsticks (84 g)	110	**35**	9
	2 thighs (84 g)	180	**110**	32
Breaded Chicken Breast Nuggets	5 (84 g)	200	**110**	27
Breaded Chicken Breast Tenders	3 oz (84 g)	160	**60**	23
Ratner's				
Potato Pancakes (Latkes)	1 (43 g)	110	**60**	27
Rymel Menu Maker				
Beef, teriyaki	196 g	240	**90**	36
Chicken breasts, boneless without skin				
Breaded	1 (100 g)	130	**10**	0
Lemon Herb and Teriyaki	1 (100 g)	110	**10**	0
Teriyaki	1 (100 g)	110	**10**	0
Sea Pak				
Breaded Butterfly Shrimp	8 (112 g)	150	**10**	0
Clam Strips	1 pkg	410	**200**	36
Fantail Style Shrimp 'n Butter Batter	6 pieces	190	**80**	18
Jumbo Butterfly Shrimp	4 (84 g)	200	**80**	9
Popcorn Shrimp	15 (84 g)	210	**110**	18
Shrimp Fajitas	3 (340 g)	370	**60**	0
Shrimp Oriental Stir-Fry	½ pkg (269 g)	190	**25**	0
Shrimp Poppers	20 pieces (83 g)	210	**110**	18
Shrimp Primavera	½ pkg (284 g)	280	**70**	5
Tuna Steak	1 (170 g)	210	**50**	0
Spare the Rib				
Pork, no bones	5 oz	380	**260**	72
Stouffer's				
Baked Chicken Breast	1 pkg	270	**110**	27
Beef Pot Roast	1 pkg	270	**90**	27

FROZEN, MICROWAVE, AND REFRIGERATED FOODS

		CALORIES		
FOOD	AMOUNT	TOTAL	FAT	SAT-FAT
Cheese Tortellini in Alfredo Sauce	1 pkg	550	**300**	162
Chicken Breast Parmigiana	1 pkg	320	**100**	18
Chicken à la King	1 pkg	320	**90**	27
Chicken Monterey	1 pkg	410	**180**	81
Chicken Pie	1 pkg	520	**300**	72
Chili with Beans	1 pkg	270	**90**	36
Creamed Chicken	1 pkg	280	**180**	63
Creamed Chipped Beef	½ cup	160	**100**	27
Escalloped Chicken and Noodles	1 pkg	440	**260**	54
Fettucini Alfredo	1 pkg	480	**260**	153
Fish Filet	1 pkg	430	**190**	45
Four-Cheese Lasagna	1 pkg	410	**170**	90
Fried Chicken Breast	1 pkg	330	**150**	36
Green Pepper Steak	1 pkg	330	**80**	27
Lasagna with Meat and Sauce	1 pkg	360	**120**	45
Lasagna with Tomato Sauce and Italian Sausage	1 pkg	370	**160**	63
Macaroni and Beef	1 pkg	340	**110**	45
Macaroni and Cheese	1 cup	330	**150**	54
Meatloaf	1 pkg	390	**210**	72
Noodles Romanoff	1 pkg	490	**230**	54
Roast Turkey Breast	1 pkg	280	**100**	27
Salisbury Steak	1 pkg	370	**170**	54
Spaghetti with Meatballs	1 pkg	420	**130**	36
Spinach Soufflé	½ cup	150	**90**	18
Stuffed Peppers	1 pepper	180	**70**	9
Swedish Meatballs	1 pkg	440	**200**	72
Tuna Noodle Casserole	1 pkg	330	**130**	18
Turkey Tetrazzini	1 pkg	360	**170**	27
Veal Parmigiana	1 pkg	420	**170**	36
Vegetable Lasagna	1 pkg	370	**170**	45
Welsh Rarebit	¼ cup	120	**80**	36
Stouffer's Lunch Express				
Cheese Ravioli	1 pkg	310	**100**	36
Chicken Alfredo	1 pkg	360	**150**	54
Chicken Chow Mein	1 pkg	260	**35**	9
Fettucini Alfredo	1 pkg	460	**240**	135
Fettucini Primavera	1 pkg	420	**220**	108

FROZEN, MICROWAVE, AND REFRIGERATED FOODS

		CALORIES		
FOOD	AMOUNT	TOTAL	FAT	SAT-FAT
Stouffer's Lunch Express *(cont.)*				
Lasagna	1 pkg	350	**100**	45
Macaroni and Cheese	1 pkg	360	**170**	45
Rigatoni	1 pkg	340	**100**	23
Spaghetti with Meat Sauce	1 pkg	280	**70**	27
Swanson Dinners				
Chicken Pot Pie	1 pie	390	**200**	81
Fish 'n' Chips	1 pkg	500	**210**	135
Fried Chicken				
Dark portions	1 pkg	560	**250**	99
White portions	1 pkg	550	**230**	99
Salisbury Steak	1 pkg	610	**310**	153
Sirloin Beef Tips	1 pkg	450	**140**	54
Turkey (Mostly White Meat)	1 pkg	310	**70**	18
Turkey Pot Pie	1 pie	390	**190**	81
Veal Parmigiana	1 pkg	400	**160**	72
Yankee Pot Roast	1 pkg	270	**60**	36
Swanson Hungry Man				
Beef Pot Pie	1 pkg	620	**260**	126
Chicken Pot Pie	1 pkg	620	**320**	126
Fried Chicken (Mostly White Meat)	1 pkg	810	**360**	126
Sirloin Beef Tips	1 pkg	450	**140**	54
Turkey	1 pkg	490	**120**	54
Tyson				
Blackened Chicken	1 meal	270	**45**	9
Chicken Marsala	1 meal	180	**35**	9
Chicken Mesquite	1 meal	310	**70**	27
Chicken Picatta	1 meal	190	**25**	9
Chicken Supreme	1 meal	260	**180**	18
Grilled Chicken	1 meal	220	**25**	9
Grilled Italian-Style Chicken	1 meal	210	**35**	9
Honey Roasted Chicken	1 meal	220	**35**	9
Roasted Chicken	1 meal	240	**25**	9
Van de Kamp's				
Breaded Butterfly Shrimp	7 (112 g)	280	**120**	23
Breaded Fish Portions	3 portions (128 g)	330	**190**	27
Breaded Popcorn Shrimp	20 (112 g)	270	**110**	18
Breaded Shrimp	7 (112 g)	240	**90**	14

FROZEN, MICROWAVE, AND REFRIGERATED FOODS

FOOD	AMOUNT	CALORIES TOTAL	FAT	SAT-FAT
Weight Watchers				
Broccoli and Cheese Baked Potato	10 oz	230	60	18
Cheese Manicotti	1 meal	260	70	23
Cheese Tortellini	1 cup	290	35	18
Chicken Enchiladas Suiza	1 meal	230	60	14
Chicken Fettucini	1 meal	280	80	27
Fettucini Alfredo	1 cup	220	50	23
Garden Lasagna	1¼ cups	230	45	9
Grilled Chicken Suiza	1 entree	240	50	18
Grilled Salisbury Steak	1 entree	250	80	27
Italian Cheese Lasagna	1 meal	300	70	27
Lasagna with Meat Sauce	1 meal	270	50	18
Macaroni and Cheese	1¼ cups	260	50	18
Nacho Grande Chicken Enchiladas	1 pkg	290	70	23
Penne Pasta with Sun-dried Tomatoes	1 pkg	290	80	23
Spaghetti with Meat Sauce	1¼ cups	240	60	14
Stuffed Turkey Breast	1 entree	240	70	23
Swedish Meatballs	1 entree	280	70	27
Tex-Mex Chicken	1 entree	260	35	14
Three-Cheese Rotini	1¼ cups	270	80	27
Tuna Noodle Casserole	1¼ cups	240	60	23
Vegetable Primavera Baked Potato	1¼ cups	220	60	27
Weight Watchers Smart Ones				
Chicken Marsala	1 entree	110	5	0
Honey Mustard Chicken	1 pkg	140	10	5
Lasagna Florentine	1 pkg	190	10	5
Ravioli Florentine	1 pkg	170	10	0
Yu Sing				
Chicken Fried Rice	1 meal	250	45	18
Chicken Lo Mein	1 meal	230	40	18
Szechwan Shrimp with Rice	1 meal	210	35	9
Szechwan Vegetable with Rice	1 meal	220	25	9

FROZEN, MICROWAVE, AND REFRIGERATED FOODS

FOOD	AMOUNT	CALORIES		
		TOTAL	FAT	SAT-FAT
Egg Rolls				
Chung's				
Pork	2 (168 g)	400	**180**	45
Shrimp	2 (168 g)	360	**130**	23
Vegetable	2 (168 g)	380	**140**	23
White Meat Chicken	2 (168 g)	340	**100**	14
Lo-An				
Beef Steak Teriyaki	1 (78 g)	140	**35**	9
Chicken and Shrimp	1 (78 g)	140	**35**	9
Lobster	1 (78 g)	150	**35**	9
Shrimp	1 (78 g)	150	**45**	9
White Meat Chicken	1 (78 g)	140	**35**	9
Matlaw's				
Egg Roll Bites	2 pieces (28 g)	45	**5**	0
Pizzas				
Celeste				
Pizza Deluxe	¼ pizza (158 g)	350	**160**	54
Pizza-for-One				
Cheese	1 (184 g)	540	**230**	117
Four-Cheese				
Original	1 (198 g)	540	**270**	108
Zesty	1 (198 g)	530	**240**	117
Pepperoni	1 (191 g)	520	**240**	90
Suprema	1 (255 g)	580	**280**	90
Vegetable	1 (213 g)	480	**210**	72
Fox De Luxe				
Cheese	1 (198 g)	460	**100**	45
Hamburger	1 (198 g)	470	**130**	36
Pepperoni	1 (198 g)	530	**180**	54
Sausage	1 (198 g)	480	**150**	36
Sausage and Pepperoni	1 (198 g)	490	**160**	45
Healthy Choice French Bread Pizza				
Cheese	1 (158 g)	310	**35**	18
Pepperoni	1 (170 g)	360	**80**	36
Supreme	1 (180 g)	340	**50**	18
Heinz Mini Bagel Pizzas				
Cheese, Sausage, Pepperoni	4 (88 g)	200	**70**	23
Extra Cheese	4 (88 g)	190	**60**	18

FROZEN, MICROWAVE, AND REFRIGERATED FOODS

FOOD	AMOUNT	CALORIES		
		TOTAL	FAT	SAT-FAT
Jeno's				
Cheese	½ pizza (106 g)	250	**100**	32
Combination Sausage and				
Pepperoni	½ pizza (111 g)	290	**140**	36
Pepperoni	½ pizza (108 g)	280	**140**	32
Lean Cuisine French Bread Pizza				
Pepperoni	1 (148 g)	330	**70**	27
Macabee				
Cheese Bagel Pizza	1 (57 g)	150	**45**	23
McCain Ellio's				
Cheese	1 slice (75 g)	160	**45**	18
	⅓ pizza (151 g)	340	**100**	36
Healthy Slices	2 slices (168 g)	320	**45**	18
Stouffer's French Bread Pizza				
Cheese	1 (147 g)	350	**120**	45
Deluxe	1 (175 g)	440	**200**	72
Pepperoni	1 (159 g)	420	**180**	72
Sausage and Pepperoni	1 (177 g)	490	**220**	63
White	1 (144 g)	350	**120**	72
Totino's Party Pizza				
Cheese	½ pizza (139 g)	320	**130**	45
Combination	½ pizza (152 g)	380	**180**	45
Pepperoni	½ pizza (145 g)	380	**190**	45
Weight Watchers				
Deluxe Combo	1 (199 g)	330	**70**	36
Sandwiches				
Banquet Hot Sandwich Toppers				
Chicken à la King	1 bag	100	**40**	14
Creamed Chipped Beef	1 bag	100	**35**	14
Gravy and Salisbury Steak	1 bag	220	**140**	63
Gravy and Sliced Beef	1 bag	70	**20**	9
Gravy and Sliced Turkey	1 bag	90	**35**	14
Sloppy Joe	1 bag	140	**60**	27
Hormel Quick Meal Sandwich				
Bacon Cheeseburger	1 (142 g)	440	**200**	90
Barbecue Beef	1 (122 g)	360	**140**	54

FROZEN, MICROWAVE, AND REFRIGERATED FOODS

FOOD	AMOUNT	CALORIES		
		TOTAL	FAT	SAT-FAT
Hormel Quick Meal				
Sandwich (cont.)				
Cheeseburger	1 (136 g)	400	**180**	81
Grilled Chicken	1 (133 g)	300	**80**	27
Hot Pockets				
Pepperoni Pizza	1 (128 g)	350	**150**	72
Jimmie Dean				
Bacon, Egg, and Cheese				
on a Biscuit	1 (102 g)	300	**150**	54
Miniburgers with Cheese	2 (91 g)	270	**120**	81
Sausage, Egg, and Cheese				
on a Biscuit	1 (128 g)	390	**240**	90
Steak Biscuits	2 (94 g)	280	**90**	36
Ken & Roberts				
Veggie Burger	1 (71 g)	130	**10**	0
Morningstar Farms				
Garden Vege patties	1 (67 g)	110	**35**	5
Quaker Maid				
All-Beef Sandwich Steak	1 steak (56 g)	170	**130**	54
Philly Cheese Steak	1 (170 g)	400	**80**	36
Weight Watchers On-the-				
Go! Sandwiches				
Chicken, Broccoli, and				
Cheddar	1 sandwich	250	**50**	23
English Muffin with Ham				
and Cheese	1 sandwich	220	**60**	18
Grilled Chicken	1 sandwich	270	**50**	23
Honey Dijon Turkey Pretzel	1 sandwich	230	**35**	14
Reuben	1 sandwich	250	**50**	18
White Castle				
Cheeseburger	2 sandwiches	310	**160**	81
Hamburger	2 sandwiches	270	**130**	54
Vegetables				
Corn Soufflé (Stouffer's)	½ cup	170	**60**	18
Onions				
Onion Ringers (Ore Ida)	6 rings (88 g)	240	**130**	23
Onion Rings (Ore Ida)	4 pieces (86 g)	220	**110**	32
Potatoes				
Act II Microwave French				
Fries	1 box	240	**110**	23

FROZEN, MICROWAVE, AND
REFRIGERATED FOODS

		CALORIES		
FOOD	AMOUNT	TOTAL	FAT	SAT-FAT
Potatoes (*cont.*)				
Budget Gourmet				
Cheddared Potatoes	1 pkg	260	**150**	81
Cheddared Potatoes and				
Broccoli	1 pkg	170	**80**	54
McCain				
Crinkle-Cut French Fried				
Potatoes	3 oz	120	**30**	0
Spiral Fries	30 pieces (85 g)	160	**70**	14
Steak Fries	10 pieces (84 g)	110	**30**	9
Ultimate Crinkle Cut	12 pieces (85 g)	170	**60**	9
Ore Ida				
Country-Style Hash				
Browns	1 cup	60	**0**	0
Crispers	17 fries (84 g)	220	**110**	18
Dinner Fries	8 fries (84 g)	110	**30**	9
Fast Fries	23 fries (84 g)	140	**50**	18
Golden Crinkles	16 fries (84 g)	120	**35**	9
Golden Patties Shredded				
Potatoes	1 patty (71 g)	140	**70**	14
Golden Twirls	28 fries (84 g)	160	**60**	9
Hash Browns	¾ cup	70	**0**	0
Hot Tots	9 pieces (84 g)	150	**60**	14
Mashed Potatoes, butter				
flavor	½ cup	80	**20**	5
Onion Tater Tots	9 taters (84 g)	150	**60**	14
Potatoes O'Brien	¾ cup	60	**0**	0
Potato Wedges with skins	9 wedges (84 g)	110	**25**	9
Shoestrings	38 fries (84 g)	150	**50**	9
Shredded Potatoes	1 patty (71 g)	140	**70**	14
Shredded Potato Patties	2 patties (99 g)	190	**110**	18
Tater Tots	9 taters (84 g)	160	**70**	14
Toaster Hash Browns	2 patties (99 g)	190	**110**	18
Topped Baked Potatoes,				
Broccoli, and Cheese	½ potato (159 g)	150	**35**	14
Twice-Baked Potatoes				
Cheddar Cheese	1 potato (140 g)	200	**80**	27
Sour Cream and Chives	1 potato (140 g)	180	**60**	36
Zesties	12 fries (84 g)	160	**80**	14

FROZEN, MICROWAVE, AND REFRIGERATED FOODS

FOOD	AMOUNT	CALORIES		
		TOTAL	FAT	SAT-FAT
Potatoes (*cont.*)				
Stouffer's				
Potatoes au Gratin	½ cup	130	**60**	23
Spinach and Cheese				
Spanakopita (Apollo)	5 triangles	390	**200**	72
Spinach Soufflé (Stouffer's)	½ cup	150	**90**	18

FRUITS AND FRUIT JUICES

FOOD	AMOUNT	CALORIES		
		TOTAL	FAT	SAT-FAT
Apple				
fresh	1 (3/lb)	81	**0**	0
cooked, boiled				
canned, sweetened	½ cup slices	68	**0**	0
Apple juice	1 cup	116	**0**	0
Applesauce				
unsweetened	½ cup	53	**0**	0
sweetened	½ cup	97	**0**	0
Apricot	3 (12/lb)	51	**0**	0
dried, uncooked	10 halves	83	**0**	0
	1 cup halves	310	**0**	0
dried, cooked	1 cup halves	211	**0**	0
Avocado, fresh				
California	1	306	**270**	41
Florida	1	339	**243**	48
Banana, fresh	1	105	**5**	2
Blackberries, fresh	½ cup	37	**0**	0
Blueberries, fresh	1 cup	82	**0**	0
Boysenberries, canned, heavy syrup	½ cup	113	**0**	0
Cantaloupe, fresh	½ fruit	94	**0**	0
	1 cup cubes	57	**0**	0
Cherries, sour, fresh	1 cup with pits	51	**0**	0
canned, light syrup	½ cup	94	**0**	0
canned, heavy syrup	½ cup	116	**0**	0
Cherries, sweet, fresh	10	49	**0**	0
	1 cup	104	**0**	0
canned, light syrup	½ cup	85	**0**	0
canned, heavy syrup	½ cup	107	**0**	0

FRUITS AND FRUIT JUICES

FOOD	AMOUNT	CALORIES TOTAL	FAT	SAT-FAT
Cranberries, fresh	1 cup whole	46	0	0
Cranberry juice cocktail	1 cup	147	0	0
Cranberry sauce	½ cup	209	0	0
Dates, pitted	5–6 dates	120	0	0
	1 cup chopped	489	7	3
Figs, fresh	1 medium	37	0	0
	1 large	47	0	0
dried, uncooked	2	150	0	0
	1 cup	508	21	4
dried, cooked	1 cup	279	11	2
Fruit cocktail, canned				
juice pack	1 cup	113	0	0
light syrup pack	1 cup	110	0	0
heavy syrup pack	1 cup	186	0	0
Grapefruit, fresh	½ fruit	38	0	0
	1 cup sections	74	0	0
Grapefruit juice				
fresh	4 oz	47	0	0
canned, unsweetened	4 oz	47	0	0
canned, sweetened	4 oz	57	0	0
Grapes, fresh	10	15	0	0
	1 cup	58	0	0
Grape juice, canned or bottled	1 cup	155	0	0
Guava, fresh	1	45	0	0
Honeydew melon, fresh	1/10	46	0	0
	1 cup cubes	60	0	0
Kiwi, fresh	1 medium	46	0	0
	1 large	55	0	0
Kumquat, fresh	1	12	0	0
Lemon, fresh	1 medium	17	0	0
	1 large	25	0	0
Lemon juice	1 tbsp	4	0	0
	1 cup	60	0	0
Lime, fresh	1	20	0	0
Lime juice	1 tbsp	4	0	0
	1 cup	66	0	0
Mango, fresh	1	135	0	0
	1 cup slices	108	0	0
Mixed fruit, dried	11 oz	712	13	0
Mulberries, fresh	10	7	0	0
	1 cup	61	0	0

FRUITS AND FRUIT JUICES

FOOD	AMOUNT	CALORIES		
		TOTAL	FAT	SAT-FAT
Nectarine, fresh	1	67	**0**	0
	1 cup slices	68	**0**	0
Orange, fresh	1	60	**0**	0
Orange juice	1 cup	111	**0**	0
Papaya, fresh	1	117	**0**	0
	1 cup cubes	54	**0**	0
Peaches, fresh	1 (4/lb)	37	**0**	0
canned in juice	1 cup halves	109	**0**	0
canned in light syrup	1 cup halves	136	**0**	0
canned in heavy syrup	1 cup halves	190	**0**	0
dried, uncooked	10 halves	311	**9**	1
	1 cup halves	383	**11**	1
dried, cooked	1 cup halves	198	**6**	1
Pears, fresh	1	98	**0**	0
canned in juice	1 cup halves	123	**0**	0
canned in light syrup	1 cup halves	144	**0**	0
canned in heavy syrup	1 cup halves	188	**0**	0
dried, uncooked	10 halves	459	**10**	1
	1 cup halves	472	**10**	1
dried, cooked	1 cup halves	325	**7**	0
Pineapple, fresh	1 slice (¾″ thick)	42	**0**	0
	1 cup diced	77	**0**	0
canned in juice	1 cup chunks	150	**0**	0
canned in light syrup	1 cup	131	**0**	0
canned in heavy syrup	1 cup	199	**0**	0
Pineapple juice	1 cup	139	**0**	0
Plantain, fresh	1	218	**6**	NA
cooked	1 cup slices	179	**3**	NA
Plums, fresh	1	36	**0**	0
	1 cup slices	91	**0**	0
Prunes				
canned in heavy syrup	5	90	**0**	0
	1 cup	245	**0**	0
dried, uncooked	10	201	**0**	0
	1 cup	385	**7**	0
dried, cooked	1 cup	227	**4**	0
Prune juice	1 cup	181	**0**	0
Raisins, seedless	1 cup packed	494	**7**	0
Raspberries, fresh	1 cup	61	**0**	0
Rhubarb, fresh	1 cup diced	26	**0**	0

FRUITS AND FRUIT JUICES

FOOD	AMOUNT	CALORIES		
		TOTAL	FAT	SAT-FAT
Strawberries, fresh	1 cup	45	0	0
canned in heavy syrup	1 cup	234	0	0
Tangerine, fresh	1	37	0	0
	1 cup sections	86	0	0
Watermelon, fresh	1 cup diced	50	0	0

GRAINS AND PASTA

FOOD	AMOUNT	CALORIES		
		TOTAL	FAT	SAT-FAT
Bread				
Bagels				
Freshly baked, grocery				
Blueberry	1 (114 g)	310	10	5
Bran	1 (114 g)	310	15	5
Cinnamon Raisin	1 (114 g)	320	10	5
Combination	1 (114 g)	310	10	5
Garlic	1 (114 g)	300	10	0
Honey Wheat	1 (114 g)	310	15	5
Oat Bran	1 (114 g)	310	15	5
Onion	1 (114 g)	300	10	0
Plain	1 (114 g)	300	10	5
Poppy Seed	1 (114 g)	310	20	5
Pumpernickel	1 (114 g)	300	15	5
Raisin Bran	1 (114 g)	300	15	5
Rye	1 (114 g)	310	15	5
Sesame Seed	1 (114 g)	310	20	5
Water	1 (74 g)	210	5	0
Frozen				
Lender's				
Bagelettes	1 (25 g)	70	5	0
Big n'Crusty				
Cinnamon Raisin	1 (85 g)	240	20	0
Plain or Onion	1 (85 g)	220	15	0
Blueberry or Cinnamon				
Raisin	1 (71 g)	200	15	0
Egg, Onion, or Plain	1 (57 g)	160	10–15	0
Soft	1 (71 g)	210	30	5

GRAINS AND PASTA

FOOD	AMOUNT	CALORIES		
		TOTAL	FAT	SAT-FAT
Bagels				
Frozen (cont.)				
Sara Lee				
Cinnamon and Raisin	1 (80 g)	220	**5**	0
Oat Bran or Poppy Seed	1 (80 g)	210	**10**	0
Plain	1 (80 g)	210	**0**	0
Bialy	1 (110 g)	270	**15**	0
Biscuits (see also **FAST FOODS**)				
Pillsbury Ready-to-Bake				
Big Country				
Butter Tastin'	1 (34 g)	100	**35**	9
Country	3 (64 g)	150	**20**	0
1869 Brand Buttermilk	1 (31 g)	100	**45**	14
Grands!				
Butter Tastin'	1 (61 g)	200	**90**	9
Buttermilk	1 (61 g)	200	**90**	27
Cinnamon Raisin	1 (61 g)	200	**70**	18
Flaky	1 (61 g)	190	**80**	18
Southern-Style	1 (61 g)	200	**90**	23
Hungry Jack				
Biscuits	2 (57 g)	170	**60**	14
Butter Tastin' or				
Buttermilk	2 (57 g)	170	**70**	14
Tender Layer Buttermilk	3 (64 g)	160	**40**	9
Bran'nola	1 slice (38 g)	90	**20**	0
Country Oat	1 slice (38 g)	90	**25**	5
Bread Crumbs				
Cracker Meal (OTC)	¼ cup	110	**0**	0
Progresso Bread Crumbs				
Italian-Style	¼ cup	110	**15**	0
Plain	¼ cup	100	**15**	0
Shake 'n Bake				
Barbecue Chicken Glaze	⅛ packet (12 g)	45	**10**	0
Honey Mustard Chicken				
Glaze	¼ packet (25 g)	100	**20**	9
Pork Original Recipe	⅛ packet (11 g)	40	**0**	0
Tangy Honey Glaze	¼ packet (25 g)	90	**15**	5
Bread Mixes				
Bread Machine				
Dromedary				
Country White	½ inch (50 g)	140	**10**	5

GRAINS AND PASTA

FOOD	AMOUNT	CALORIES		
		TOTAL	FAT	SAT-FAT
Bread Mixes				
Bread Machine				
Dromedary (*cont.*)				
Italian Herb	½ inch (50 g)	140	20	14
Sourdough	½ inch (50 g)	140	15	9
Stoneground Wheat	½ inch (50 g)	140	15	9
Pillsbury				
Cracked Wheat	¹⁄₁₂ pkg (36 g)	130	20	0
Crusty White	¹⁄₁₂ pkg (36 g)	130	15	0
Hot Roll Mix (Pillsbury)	1 pan roll (28 g)	100	10	0
Quick Mix (Pillsbury)				
Apple Cinnamon	¹⁄₁₂ loaf (37 g mix)	140	10	0
Banana	¹⁄₁₂ loaf (33 g mix)	120	10	0
Bread Sticks				
Cheese (Angonoa's)	6 (28 g)	120	20	5
Italian	5 (28 g)	120	20	5
Italian (Angonoa's)	6 (28 g)	130	40	5
Mini Sesame Royale (Angonoa's)	24 (28 g)	130	35	5
Sesame	5 (28 g)	120	20	5
Sesame Royale	6 (28 g)	130	40	5
Soft (Bread du Jour)	1 (53 g)	130	10	0
Soft (Pillsbury)	1 (39 g)	110	25	5
Soft, Cheese	1 (28 g)	80	20	9
Bread Stuffing				
Arnold				
Sage and Onion	2 cups (67 g)	240	30	5
Seasoned	2 cups (67 g)	250	30	5
Kellogg's				
Croutettes Stuffing Mix	1 cup prep. (100 g)	240	120	18
Nabisco				
Cracker Meal	¼ cup (26 g)	100	0	0
Pepperidge Farm				
Corn Bread Stuffing	¾ cup (43 g)	170	20	0
Country Garden Herb Stuffing	½ cup (34 g)	150	10	9
Country-Style Stuffing	¾ cup (37 g)	140	15	0
Herb-Seasoned Stuffing	¾ cup (43 g)	170	15	0
Ritz Stuffing Mix	⅔ cup (38 g)	200	80	18

GRAINS AND PASTA

FOOD	AMOUNT	CALORIES TOTAL	FAT	SAT-FAT
Challah	1" slice (50 g)	160	35	9
Cocktail bread				
Rye or Pumpernickel	3 slices (31 g)	80	10	0
Cracked wheat (Pepperidge				
Farm)	1 slice (25 g)	70	10	0
Croissant				
Butter (Vie-de-France)	1 (56 g)	230	110	72
Croutons (Pepperidge Farm)	2 tbsp (7 g)	30	10	0
English muffin	1 (57 g)	120	10	0
Bran'nola (Arnold)	1 (66 g)	130	15	0
Raisin	1 (61 g)	140	10	0
Raisin (Sun Maid)	1 (68 g)	160	10	0
Flat Bread (JJ Flats)	1 piece (14 g)	50	10	0
French bread	2" slice	130	0	0
French loaf (Bread du Jour)	3" slice (56 g)	130	10	0
Crusty French loaf				
(Pillsbury)	⅕ loaf (62 g)	150	10	0

French toast (*see also* **FROZEN, MICROWAVE, AND REFRIGERATED FOODS)**

FOOD	AMOUNT	TOTAL	FAT	SAT-FAT
French toast	1 slice	140	70	40
Garlic bread	3½" slice (56 g)	190	80	14
with cheese	3½" slice (56 g)	180	60	14
Italian bread	1¼" slice (46 g)	130	10	0
Pepperidge Farm	⅑th loaf (50 g)	130	15	9
Italian Bread Shell (Boboli)	⅓ shell (57 g)	150	30	9
Italian Olive Bread	2 slices (50 g)	150	30	5
Muffins				
Almond Poppy Seed	2 mini (55 g)	180	50	9
Apple Walnut	1 (127 g)	400	100	18
Banana Walnut (Hostess)	5 mini (57 g)	260	140	18
Blueberry	1 (127 g)	400	140	32
Entenmann's	1 (57 g)	120	0	0
Hostess	5 mini (57 g)	240	120	18
Bran	1 (127 g)	390	90	23
Cinnamon Apple (Hostess)	5 mini (57 g)	260	140	23
Corn	1 (127 g)	400	110	18
	2 mini (55 g)	210	70	18
Corn Muffin Toasties	2 (65 g)	240	80	14
Oat Bran	1 (127 g)	390	90	23
Strawberry	1 (127 g)	400	110	23

GRAINS AND PASTA

FOOD	AMOUNT	CALORIES		
		TOTAL	FAT	SAT-FAT
Muffin Mixes				
Betty Crocker				
Wild blueberry	1 muffin (40 g)	170	50	<5
Gold Medal				
Golden Corn	1 muffin (31 g)	170	50	<5
Pillsbury				
Apple Cinnamon	1 muffin (38 g)	140	35	9
Banana Nut	1 muffin (37 g)	150	45	9
Twice the Blueberries	1 muffin (39 g)	140	35	9
Wild Blueberry	1 muffin (40 g)	170	50	9
Multi-Grain	1″ slice (50 g)	160	20	5
Oatmeal (Pepperidge Farm)	1 slice (25 g)	60	10	0
Soft (Pepperidge Farm)	1 slice (25 g)	60	5	0
Pita				
White	1 (6″ diam)	150	10	0
Whole-wheat	1 (6″ diam)	180	10	0
Pumpernickel	1 slice (32 g)	80	10	0
Raisin (Pepperidge Farm)	1 slice (28 g)	80	10	0
Rolls				
Cinnamon (Pillsbury)	1 (40 g)	140	45	14
Club (Pepperidge Farm)	1 (47 g)	120	10	5
Cornbread Twists (Pillsbury)	1 (41 g)	130	50	14
Dinner				
Arnold	2 (38 g)	110	25	5
Country-Style (Pepperidge Farm)	3 (57 g)	150	30	9
Crescent (Pillsbury)	2 (57 g)	200	100	23
Parker House (Pepperidge Farm)	3 (53 g)	150	40	14
Party (Pepperidge Farm)	5 (53 g)	170	40	14
Egg Twist	1 (47 g)	180	35	14
French (Pepperidge Farm)	½ (71 g)	180	20	5
Seven-Grain (Pepperidge Farm)	1 (38 g)	80	20	0
Hamburger	1 (43 g)	130	20	9
Potato (Martins)	1 (39 g)	110	20	0
Hard	1 (57 g)	160	10	5
Hoagie with Sesame Seeds (Pepperidge Farm)	1 (69 g)	200	40	23
Hot dog	1 (39 g)	110	20	5
Italian (Bread du Jour)	1 (35 g)	80	5	0

GRAINS AND PASTA

FOOD	AMOUNT	CALORIES		
		TOTAL	FAT	SAT-FAT
Rolls (cont.)				
Mix (Pillsbury)	1 pan roll			
	(28 g mix)	120	25	0
Oat Bran	1 (52 g)	140	20	5
Pumpernickel	1 (57 g)	160	20	0
Sub (La Parisienne)	⅗ 8″ roll (50 g)	130	0	0
Wheat	1 (57 g)	190	25	5
White	1 (6″ diam)	150	10	0
Whole-wheat	1 (6″ diam)	180	10	0
Rye				
Jewish	1 slice (32 g)	80	10	0
Seeded	1 slice (22 g)	55	8	3
Onion	1 slice (32 g)	80	10	0
Sunflower Seed	1 slice (50 g)	120	7	0
Seven-Grain (Dimplemeier)	1 slice (50 g)	120	18	0
Sicilian	¼ loaf (57 g)	150	15	0
Sourdough	1″ slice (50 g)	130	10	0
Boule (La Parisienne)	1 slice (57 g)	120	10	0
Tortillas				
Corn	1 (28 g)	60	0	0
Flour	1 (35 g)	110	25	0
Wheat Bread, Very Thin				
(Pepperidge Farm)	1 slice (15 g)	37	5	2
White	1 slice (25–27 g)	65–80	8–15	0
Light white	1 slice (22 g)	40	3	0
Whole-wheat				
Pepperidge Farm	1 slice (25 g)	60	10	0
Soft	1 slice (25 g)	60	5	0
Stroehmann	1 slice (36 g)	80	15	0
Wonder	1 slice (34 g)	80	15	0

Breakfast Cereals, Cold

If you are keeping track of total fat, add 73 fat calories per cup of whole milk, 42 per cup of 2% milk, 23 per cup of 1% milk, 4 per cup of skim milk. If you are keeping track of saturated fat, add 45 sat-fat calories per cup of whole milk, 27 per cup of 2% milk, 14 per cup of 1% milk, 0–3 per cup of skim milk.

All-Bran, original	½ cup	80	10	0
All-Bran, Extra Fiber	½ cup	50	10	0
Alpha-Bits	1 cup	130	5	0
Apple Cinnamon Squares	¾ cup	180	10	0

GRAINS AND PASTA

| FOOD | AMOUNT | CALORIES | | |
		TOTAL	FAT	SAT-FAT
Apple Raisin Crisp	1 cup	180	0	0
Apple Jacks	1 cup	110	0	0
Banana Nut Crunch	1 cup	250	50	9
Banana Nut Granola	½ cup	250	80	36
Basic 4	1 cup	210	30	0
Blueberry Morning	1¼ cups	230	30	5
Bran'nola	½ cup	200	25	5
Cap'n Crunch	¾ cup	110	15	0
Deep-Sea Crunch	1 cup	130	20	5
Peanut Butter Crunch	¾ cup	120	25	9
Cheerios	1 cup	110	15	0
Apple Cinnamon	¾ cup	120	25	0
Honey Nut Cheerios	1 cup	120	15	0
Multi-Grain Cheerios	1 cup	110	10	<5
Cinnamon Toast Crunch	¾ cup	130	30	5
Clusters	1 cup	220	40	5
Cocoa Krispies	¾ cup	110	0	0
Cocoa Pebbles	¾ cup	120	10	9
Cocoa Puffs	1 cup	120	10	0
Common Sense Oatbran	¾ cup	110	10	0
Complete Bran Flakes	1 cup	100	5	0
Cookie Crisp Chocolate Chip	1 cup	120	10	0
Corn Chex	1¼ cups	110	0	0
Corn Flakes	1 cup	110	0	0
Corn Pops	1 cup	110	0	0
Count Chocula	1 cup	120	10	0
Cracklin' Oat Bran	¾ cup	230	70	27
Crispix	1 cup	110	0	0
Crispy Wheats'n Raisins	1 cup	190	10	0
Double Chex	1¼ cups	120	0	0
Fiber One	½ cup	60	10	0
Froot Loops	1 cup	120	10	5
Frosted Bran	¾ cup	100	0	0
Frosted Flakes	¾ cup	120	0	0
Frosted Mini-Wheats	1 cup	190	10	0
Frosted Wheat Bites	1 cup	180	0	0
Fruit and Fibre Peaches, Raisins, and Almonds	1 cup	210	25	5
Fruity Pebbles	¾ cup	110	10	5
Golden Crisp	¾ cup	110	0	0
Golden Grahams	¾ cup	120	10	0

GRAINS AND PASTA

FOOD	AMOUNT	CALORIES		
		TOTAL	FAT	SAT-FAT
Graham Chex	1 cup	210	**15**	0
Granola, low-fat (Kellogg's)				
with raisins	⅔ cup	200	**30**	0
without raisins	½ cup	210	**30**	0
Grape Nuts	½ cup	200	**0**	0
Grape Nuts Flakes	¾ cup	100	**10**	0
Healthy Choice				
Multi-Grains Flakes	1 cup	110	**0**	0
Multi-Grains Raisins, Crunchy Oat				
Clusters, and Almonds	1¼ cups	200	**20**	0
Multi-Grains Squares	1¼ cups	190	**10**	0
Hidden Treasures	¾ cup	120	**15**	0
Honey Almond Delight	1 cup	230	**35**	0
Honey Bunches of Oats				
Honey Roasted	¾ cup	120	**15**	5
with Almonds	¾ cup	130	**30**	5
Honeycomb	1⅓ cups	110	**0**	0
Honey Graham Oh's	¾ cup	110	**20**	5
Just Right				
Crunchy Nugget	1 cup	210	**15**	0
Fruit and Nut	1 cup	200	**20**	0
Kenmei Rice Bran	¾ cup	110	**10**	0
Kix	1⅓ cups	120	**10**	0
Berry Berry	¾ cup	120	**10**	0
Life	¾ cup	120	**15**	0
Cinnamon	1 cup	190	**20**	0
Lucky Charms	1 cup	120	**10**	0
Muesli				
Cranberry with almonds or walnuts	¾ cup	220	**25**	0
Raspberry with almonds	¾ cup	220	**25**	0
Swiss (Familia)				
Granola	½ cup	210	**50**	9
No Added Sugar	½ cup	200	**30**	5
Original Recipe	½ cup	210	**30**	5
Puffed Wheat	½ cup	170	**45**	9
Müeslix				
Crispy Blend	⅔ cup	200	**25**	0
Golden Crunch	¾ cup	210	**50**	9
Multi Bran Chex	1¼ cups	220	**20**	0
Natural Bran Flakes	⅔ cup	90	**0**	0

GRAINS AND PASTA

| FOOD | AMOUNT | CALORIES | | |
		TOTAL	FAT	SAT-FAT
100% Natural	½ cup	190	25	9
Oats and Honey	½ cup	220	70	32
Oats, Honey, and Raisins	½ cup	220	70	32
Nut and Honey Crunch	⅔ cup	120	15	0
Nutri-Grain				
Almond Raisin	1¼ cups	200	25	0
Golden Wheat	¾ cup	100	5	0
Oat Squares	1 cup	220	25	5
Oatmeal Crisp				
with almonds	1 cup	230	50	5
with apples	1 cup	210	20	0
with raisins	1 cup	210	25	0
Product 19	1 cup	110	0	0
Puffed Rice	1 cup	50	0	0
Puffed Wheat	1¼ cups	50	0	0
Raisin Bran	1 cup	170	10	0
Raisin Nut Bran	1 cup	210	40	5
Raisin Squares	¾ cup	180	5	0
Reese's Peanut Butter Puffs	¾ cup	130	25	5
Rice Chex	1 cup	120	0	0
Rice Krispies	1¼ cups	110	0	0
Apple Cinnamon	¾ cup	110	0	0
Rice Krispies Treats	¾ cup	120	15	0
Shredded Wheat Spoon Size	1 cup	170	5	0
Shredded Wheat 'n Bran	1¼ cups	200	5	0
Smacks	¾ cup	110	5	0
Special K	1 cup	110	0	0
Sprinkle Spangle	1 cup	120	15	0
Toasted Oatmeal	¾ cup	120	10	0
Total	¾ cup	100	5	0
Corn Flakes	1⅓ cups	110	5	0
Raisin Bran	1 cup	180	15	0
Whole Grain	¾ cup	100	5	0
Triples	1 cup	120	10	0
Trix	1 cup	120	15	0
Wheat Chex	¾ cup	190	10	0
Wheaties	1 cup	110	10	0
Dunk-A-Balls	¾ cup	110	10	0
Honey Gold	¾ cup	110	5	0

Breakfast Cereals, Hot

If you are keeping track of total fat and you use butter or margarine, add 33
fat calories per teaspoon and 100 per tablespoon. If you use milk, add fat

GRAINS AND PASTA

FOOD	AMOUNT	CALORIES		
		TOTAL	FAT	SAT-FAT

calories depending on the type of milk (*see* **Breakfast Cereals, Cold**). If you are keeping track of saturated fat and you use butter, add 23 sat-fat calories per pat and 65 per tablespoon. If you use margarine, add 6 sat-fat calories per teaspoon and 18 per tablespoon. If you use milk, add sat-fat calories depending on the type of milk (*see* **Breakfast Cereals, Cold**).

FOOD	AMOUNT	TOTAL	FAT	SAT-FAT
Cream of Rice	1 oz dry	100	0	0
Cream of Wheat				
Mix 'n Eat, plain, cooked	1 pkt (1 oz)	100	0	0
regular, quick, instant,				
cooked	3 tbsp (33 g)	120	0	0
Farina (Pillsbury)	3 tbsp (28 g)	100	0	0
Grits (Quaker)	¼ cup	140	5	0
Instant				
Country Bacon	1 pkt (28 g)	100	5	0
Country Ham	1 pkt (28 g)	90	5	0
Original	1 pkt (28 g)	100	0	0
Real Butter	1 pkt (28 g)	100	15	0
Real Cheddar	1 pkt (28 g)	100	15	5
Sausage	1 pkt (28 g)	100	10	0
Malt-O-Meal, cooked	1 cup	120	0	0
Maypo	1 oz dry	100	9	NA
Oat Bran (Quaker)	½ cup	150	30	9
Oatmeal (Quaker)	½ cup dry	150	25	5
Ralston 100% Wheat	½ cup	130	10	0
Wheatena	⅓ cup	150	5	0
Flour				
All-Purpose (Pillsbury)	¼ cup	110	0	0
Bisquick, original (Betty				
Crocker)	⅓ cup	170	50	14
reduced-fat	⅓ cup	140	25	5
Brown rice	¼ cup	120	5	0
Buckwheat	¼ cup	100	10	0
Cake (Betty Crocker Softasilk)	¼ cup	100	0	0
Corn	1 cup	431	27	2
Cornmeal, yellow	¼ cup	120	10	0
Cornstarch	1 tbsp	29	0	0
Pastry	⅓ cup	100	5	0
Potato Starch	1 tbsp	30	0	0
Rye	¼ cup	100	5	0
Soy	½ cup	200	80	14

GRAINS AND PASTA

FOOD	AMOUNT	CALORIES TOTAL	FAT	SAT-FAT
White	¼ cup	100	0	0
Whole-wheat	¼ cup	130	5	0
Grains (Cereal Grasses)				
Barley, pearl, light, uncooked	1 cup	700	18	4
Buckwheat groats (Kasha)	¼ cup	170	15	0
Bulgur, uncooked	1 cup	600	3	0
Couscous (no added fat)	1 cup prep.	190	5	0
Rice				
Brown				
raw	1 cup	666	32	9
cooked	1 cup	218	9	3
White				
raw	1 cup	676	6	2
cooked	1 cup	264	0	0
Instant, prepared	1 cup	161	0	0
Wild				
raw	1 cup	571	2	0
cooked	1 cup	166	1	0

Pastas (see also FROZEN, MICROWAVE, AND REFRIGERATED FOODS)

FOOD	AMOUNT	TOTAL	FAT	SAT-FAT
Dry				
Macaroni, spaghetti, shells,				
noodles, etc.	2 oz	210	10	0
Barley egg	2 oz	220	25	9
Egg	2 oz	210	25	9
Spinach	2 oz	210	10	0
Whole-wheat	2 oz	210	15	0
Chow Mein Noodles				
Chung King	⅓ cup	140	65	9
Goodman's	⅔ cup	120	40	23
La Choy	½ cup	140	60	14
Refrigerated				
Celentano				
Broccoli Stuffed Shells	3 (280 g)	190	35	9
Contadina				
Angel's hair	1¼ cup	240	30	9
Fettucine	1¼ cups	250	30	9
Fettucine, cholesterol-free	1 cup	240	20	0
Linguine	1¼ cups	260	30	9
Ravioli, chicken and				
rosemary	1 cup	330	110	36

GRAINS AND PASTA

FOOD	AMOUNT	CALORIES		
		TOTAL	FAT	SAT-FAT
Refrigerated				
Contadina (*cont.*)				
Ravioli, garden vegetable	1 cup	240	**45**	27
Spinach tagliatelli	1¼ cups	270	**35**	9
Tortelloni, chicken and				
prosciutto	1¼ cups	360	**120**	36
Tortelloni, sausage and				
bell pepper	1 cup	330	**90**	36
DiGiorno				
Linguine	70 g	200	**10**	0
Tortelloni, mozzarella	1 cup	300	**80**	45
Mixed Pasta Dishes				
Fettuccine Alfredo	1 cup	880	**610**	377
Franco American				
Spaghetti with meatballs	1 cup	270	**90**	45
Hamburger Helper				
Beef Noodle	1 cup	240	**80**	31
Cheeseburger Macaroni	1 cup	300	**130**	50
Italian Rigatoni	1 cup	320	**110**	38
Lasagne	1 cup	310	**100**	34
Hormel				
Italian-Style Lasagna	1 bowl (284 g)	350	**72**	36
Macaroni and Cheese	1 cup	270	**100**	54
Noodles and Chicken				
(Hearty Helpings)	1 cup	250	**100**	27
Spaghetti	1 bowl (284 g)	240	**23**	14
Kid's Kitchen (Hormel)				
Cheezy Mac 'n Cheese	1 cup	260	**100**	54
Spaghetti and Franks	1 cup	270	**100**	45
Spaghetti and Mini				
Meatballs	1 cup	220	**60**	36
Kraft Pasta Dinners				
Deluxe	1 cup prep.	320	**90**	56
Dinomac and other kid				
dinners	1 cup prep.	410	**170**	40
Macaroni & Cheese				
Original and Mild White				
Cheddar	1 cup prep.	410	**170**	40
Legume (Vegetarian)				
Manicotti Florentine	1 pkg (312 g)	300	**70**	9

GRAINS AND PASTA

		CALORIES		
FOOD	AMOUNT	TOTAL	FAT	SAT-FAT
Lipton Pasta and Sauce				
Cheddar Broccoli	1 cup prep.	350	**110**	36
Rotini Primavera	1 cup prep.	320	**100**	36
Rice-A-Roni Noodle Roni				
Corkscrew Pasta	¾ cup prep.	420	**220**	60
Linguine Pasta with				
Parmesan Chicken	1 cup prep.	400	**150**	45
Rigatoni with Cheddar and				
Broccoli	1 cup prep.	400	**170**	45
Romano				
Tortelloni, cheese	142 g	310	**90**	45
Tortelloni, chicken	142 g	310	**80**	36
SpaghettiOs				
Meatballs	1 cup	260	**100**	45
Tuna Helper				
Cheesy Noodles	1 cup	290	**110**	25
Creamy Noodles	1 cup	300	**130**	32
Velveeta				
Rotini and Cheese	1 cup prep.	360	**130**	83
Shells and Cheese	1 cup prep.	410	**130**	79

Refrigerated Pasta Sauces: *see* **SAUCES, GRAVIES, AND DIPS.**

Miscellaneous
Pancakes (*see also* **FAST FOODS; FROZEN, MICROWAVE, AND REFRIGERATED FOODS;** and **RESTAURANT FOODS**)
Pancake Mix

Buttermilk (Hungry Jack)	3 4" pancakes	170	**15**	0
Extra Lights (Hungry Jack)	3 4" pancakes	180	**20**	5

Waffles: *see* **FAST FOODS; FROZEN, MICROWAVE, AND REFRIGERATED FOODS;** and **RESTAURANT FOODS.**

Wheat bran	1 cup	130	**25**	4
Wheat germ, toasted	1 tbsp	27	**7**	1
	1 cup	431	**109**	19

MEATS (BEEF, GAME, LAMB, PORK, AND VEAL)

The following cuts of beef are braised, roasted, or broiled, unless otherwise noted. *See also* **SAUSAGES AND LUNCHEON MEATS** for cold cuts made from beef and pork products and **FROZEN, MICROWAVE, AND REFRIGERATED FOODS.**

*Remember that most of the following calorie figures are for **only 1 ounce** of beef!*

| FOOD | AMOUNT | CALORIES | | |
		TOTAL	FAT	SAT-FAT
Beef				
Arm pot roast, braised				
lean and fat	1 oz	99	66	27
lean only	1 oz	68	25	11
Backribs	2 ribs (140 g)	370	220	99
Bottom round steak, braised				
lean and fat	1 oz	74	38	14
lean only	1 oz	67	25	9
Brisket flat half, braised				
lean and fat	1 oz	116	89	37
lean only	1 oz	74	40	17
Chuck steak, braised				
lean and fat	1 oz	108	78	32
lean only	1 oz	77	39	18
Club steak, broiled				
lean and fat	1 oz	129	104	50
lean only	1 oz	69	33	16
Flank steak, braised				
lean and fat	1 oz	73	39	18
lean only	1 oz	69	35	16
Ground beef, raw				
extra lean	1 oz	66	44	17
lean	1 oz	75	53	21
regular	1 oz	88	68	28
Ground beef, broiled, medium				
extra lean	1 oz	72	42	16
lean	1 oz	77	47	18
regular	1 oz	82	53	21
Ground beef, pan-fried, medium				
extra lean	1 oz	72	42	16
lean	1 oz	78	49	19
regular	1 oz	87	58	23
Porterhouse steak, broiled				
lean and fat	1 oz	85	54	22
lean only	1 oz	62	28	13

MEATS (BEEF, GAME, LAMB, PORK, AND VEAL)

| FOOD | AMOUNT | CALORIES | | |
		TOTAL	FAT	SAT-FAT
Rib roast				
lean and fat	1 oz	108	81	34
lean only	1 oz	68	35	17
Round, broiled				
lean and fat	1 oz	78	47	19
lean only	1 oz	55	20	7
Rump roast				
lean and fat	1 oz	98	70	33
lean only	1 oz	59	24	7
Shortribs, braised				
lean and fat	1 oz	133	107	45
lean only	1 oz	84	46	20
Sirloin steak, broiled				
lean and fat	1 oz	79	46	19
lean only	1 oz	59	22	12
T-bone steak, broiled				
lean and fat	1 oz	92	63	26
lean only	1 oz	61	26	11
Tenderloin steak, broiled				
lean and fat	1 oz	75	44	18
lean only	1 oz	58	24	9
Top round, broiled				
lean and fat	1 oz	60	22	8
lean only	1 oz	54	16	6

Beef Dishes, Mixed

Beef and vegetable stew	1 cup	220	99	40
Chili con carne, canned	1 cup	340	144	52
Lasagna	1/12 casserole	570	210	142
Spaghetti with meatballs and tomato sauce, canned	1 cup	260	90	22

Beef, Variety Meats and By-products

Brain, simmered	1 oz	45	32	7
Liver, braised	1 oz	46	12	5
Liver Pâté	1/2 cup	289	204	104
	1 tbsp	36	26	13
Tongue, simmered	1 oz	81	53	23
Tripe	1 oz	28	10	5

Game
*Remember that most of the following calorie figures are for **only 1 ounce** of game!*

Antelope, roasted	1 oz	42	7	2
Bear, simmered	1 oz	73	34	NA

MEATS (BEEF, GAME, LAMB, PORK, AND VEAL)

		CALORIES		
FOOD	AMOUNT	TOTAL	FAT	SAT-FAT
Beefalo, composite of cuts,				
roasted	1 oz	53	**16**	7
Bison, roasted	1 oz	41	**6**	2
Boar, wild, roasted	1 oz	45	**11**	3
Buffalo, water, roasted	1 oz	37	**5**	2
Caribou, roasted	1 oz	47	**11**	4
Deer, roasted	1 oz	45	**8**	3
Elk, roasted	1 oz	41	**5**	2
Goat, roasted	1 oz	41	**8**	2
Horse, roasted	1 oz	50	**15**	5
Moose, roasted	1 oz	38	**2**	1
Muskrat, roasted	1 oz	52	**23**	NA
Opossum, roasted	1 oz	63	**26**	NA
Rabbit				
domesticated, composite of				
cuts				
roasted	1 oz	44	**16**	5
stewed	1 oz	58	**21**	6
wild, stewed	1 oz	49	**9**	3
Raccoon, roasted	1 oz	72	**37**	NA
Squirrel, roasted	1 oz	39	**9**	1

Lamb

*Remember that most of the following calorie figures are for **only 1 ounce** of lamb!*

		CALORIES		
FOOD	AMOUNT	TOTAL	FAT	SAT-FAT
Cubed, for stew or kabob				
(leg and shoulder), lean				
only				
braised	1 oz	63	**22**	8
broiled	1 oz	53	**19**	7
Foreshank, braised				
lean and fat	1 oz	69	**34**	14
lean only	1 oz	53	**15**	6
Ground lamb				
broiled	1 oz	81	**50**	26
Leg, whole (shank and				
sirloin), roasted				
lean and fat	1 oz	73	**42**	18
lean only	1 oz	54	**20**	7
Leg, shank half, roasted				
lean and fat	1 oz	64	**32**	13
lean only	1 oz	51	**17**	6

MEATS (BEEF, GAME, LAMB, PORK, AND VEAL)

FOOD	AMOUNT	CALORIES TOTAL	FAT	SAT-FAT
Leg, sirloin half, roasted				
lean and fat	1 oz	83	53	23
lean only	1 oz	58	23	8
Loin, roasted				
lean and fat	1 oz	88	60	25
lean only	1 oz	57	25	9
Chop, with bone, broiled				
lean and fat	1 chop (3½ oz)	357	265	145
lean only	1 chop (3½ oz)	189	74	37
Rib, broiled or roasted				
lean and fat	1 oz	102	76	33
lean only	1 oz	67	34	12
Chop, with bone, broiled				
lean and fat	1 chop (3½ oz)	398	315	148
lean only	1 chop (3½ oz)	212	105	40
Shoulder, whole (arm and blade) braised				
lean and fat	1 oz	97	63	27
lean only	1 oz	80	40	16

Pork

*Remember that many of the following calorie figures are for **only 1 ounce** of pork!*

Loin				
whole, broiled				
lean and fat, with bone	1 oz	98	69	25
	1 chop (104 g)	284	202	73
lean only, with bone	1 oz	73	39	13
	1 chop (104 g)	169	91	31
blade, pan-fried				
lean and fat, with bone	1 oz	117	94	34
	1 chop (104 g)	368	296	107
lean only, with bone	1 oz	85	51	19
	1 chop (89 g)	177	111	39
center loin, pan-fried				
lean and fat, with bone	1 oz	106	78	28
	1 chop (112 g)	333	244	88
lean only, with bone	1 oz	75	41	14
	1 chop (112 g)	178	96	33
center rib, broiled				
lean and fat, with bone	1 oz	97	67	24
	1 chop (104 g)	264	183	66

MEATS (BEEF, GAME, LAMB, PORK, AND VEAL)

FOOD	AMOUNT	CALORIES		
		TOTAL	FAT	SAT-FAT
Pork loin				
center rib, broiled (*cont.*)				
lean only, with bone	1 oz	73	**38**	13
	1 chop (104 g)	162	**85**	29
sirloin, broiled				
lean and fat, with bone	1 oz	94	**64**	23
	1 chop (106 g)	278	**191**	69
lean only, with bone	1 oz	69	**35**	12
	1 chop (106 g)	165	**83**	29
tenderloin, roasted				
lean only	1 oz	47	**12**	4
top loin, broiled				
lean and fat, with bone	1 oz	102	**85**	26
	1 chop (104 g)	295	**211**	76
lean only, with bone	1 oz	73	**39**	13
	1 chop (104 g)	165	**86**	30
Shoulder				
whole, roasted				
lean and fat	1 oz	92	**65**	24
lean only	1 oz	69	**38**	13
arm picnic, roasted				
lean and fat	1 oz	94	**67**	24
lean only	1 oz	65	**32**	11
blade, Boston, roasted				
lean and fat	1 oz	91	**64**	23
lean only	1 oz	73	**43**	15
Spareribs, cooked				
lean and fat	1 oz	113	**77**	30

Pork Products, Cured (*see also* **SAUSAGES AND LUNCHEON MEATS**)

FOOD	AMOUNT	TOTAL	FAT	SAT-FAT
Bacon, cooked	1 strip	36	**28**	10
Breakfast strips, cooked	1 strip	52	**37**	13
Canadian bacon, grilled	1 slice	43	**18**	6
Ham, boneless				
Extra lean (5% fat)	1 slice (28 g)	41	**14**	5
Regular (11% fat)	1 slice (28 g)	52	**27**	9
Ham, canned				
Extra lean (4% fat)	1 slice (28 g)	39	**12**	4
Regular (13% fat)	1 slice (28 g)	64	**39**	13

MEATS (BEEF, GAME, LAMB, PORK, AND VEAL)

		CALORIES		
FOOD	AMOUNT	TOTAL	FAT	SAT-FAT
Ham, center slice				
Country-style				
Lean and fat	1 oz	57	**33**	12
Lean	1 oz	55	**21**	1
Salt pork, raw	1 oz	212	**205**	75
Pork, Variety Meats and By-products				
Backfat, raw	1 oz	230	**226**	226
Chitterlings, simmered	1 oz	86	**73**	37
Feet				
pickled	1 oz	58	**41**	14
simmered, with bone	1 oz	55	**32**	11
Liver pâté	2 oz (56 g)	200	**160**	54
Tongue, simmered	1 oz	81	**53**	23
Tripe	1 oz	28	**10**	5
Veal				
*Remember that the following calorie figures are for **only 1 ounce** of veal!*				
Breast, lean and fat, braised	1 oz	86	**54**	26
Cubed, for stew (leg and				
shoulder)				
lean only, braised	1 oz	53	**11**	3
Cutlet, lean and fat, braised	1 oz	62	**27**	12
Ground, broiled	1 oz	49	**19**	8
Leg				
top round, lean and fat,				
braised	1 oz	60	**16**	6
top round, lean, braised	1 oz	57	**13**	5
Loin				
lean and fat, braised	1 oz	81	**44**	16
lean only, braised	1 oz	64	**23**	7
lean and fat, roasted	1 oz	61	**31**	16
lean only, roasted	1 oz	50	**18**	7
Rib				
lean and fat, braised	1 oz	71	**32**	13
lean only, braised	1 oz	62	**20**	7
lean and fat, roasted	1 oz	65	**36**	14
lean only, roasted	1 oz	50	**19**	6
Shoulder				
arm, lean and fat, braised	1 oz	67	**26**	10
arm, lean only, braised	1 oz	57	**14**	4

MEATS (BEEF, GAME, LAMB, PORK, AND VEAL)

		CALORIES		
FOOD	AMOUNT	TOTAL	FAT	SAT-FAT
Veal shoulder (*cont.*)				
blade, lean and fat, braised	1 oz	64	**26**	9
blade, lean, braised	1 oz	56	**17**	5
Sirloin				
lean and fat, braised	1 oz	72	**34**	13
lean only, braised	1 oz	58	**17**	5

NUTS AND SEEDS

		CALORIES		
FOOD	AMOUNT	TOTAL	FAT	SAT-FAT
Nuts				
Almonds, shelled				
slivered	1 cup	795	**630**	60
whole, dry-roasted	1 oz (24 nuts)	167	**132**	13
Almond butter				
plain	1 tbsp	101	**85**	8
honey-cinnamon	1 tbsp	96	**75**	7
Almond paste	1 oz	127	**69**	7
	1 cup	1012	**556**	53
Beechnuts, dried	1 oz	164	**128**	15
Brazil nuts, shelled, dried	1 oz (8 med nuts)	186	**169**	41
Butternuts, dried	1 oz	174	**146**	3
Cashew nuts				
dry-roasted	1 oz (18 med nuts)	163	**118**	23
	1 cup	787	**572**	113
oil-roasted	1 oz (18 med nuts)	163	**123**	24
	1 cup	748	**564**	112
jumbo	12 nuts (30 g)	190	**130**	27
Cashew butter, plain	1 oz	167	**126**	25
	1 tbsp	94	**71**	14
Chestnuts, Chinese				
raw	1 oz	64	**3**	0
dried	1 oz	103	**5**	1
boiled and steamed	1 oz	44	**2**	0
roasted	1 oz	68	**3**	0

NUTS AND SEEDS

FOOD	AMOUNT	CALORIES		
		TOTAL	FAT	SAT-FAT
Chestnuts, European				
raw, unpeeled	1 oz	60	6	1
raw, peeled	1 oz	56	3	1
dried, unpeeled	1 oz	106	11	2
dried, peeled	1 oz	105	10	2
boiled and steamed	1 oz	37	4	1
roasted	1 oz (3 nuts)	70	6	1
	1 cup	350	28	5
Chestnuts, Japanese				
raw	1 oz	44	1	0
dried	1 oz	102	3	0
boiled and steamed	1 oz	16	1	0
roasted	1 oz	57	2	0
Coconut meat				
dried, creamed	1 oz	194	177	157
dried, sweetened, flaked	1 oz	135	82	73
	1 cup	351	214	190
dried, toasted	1 oz	168	120	107
fresh frozen with sugar	2 tbsp	45	25	18
fresh, shredded or grated	1 oz	101	86	76
	1 cup	283	241	214
Coconut cream				
fresh	1 tbsp	49	47	42
	1 cup	792	749	664
canned	1 tbsp	36	30	27
	1 cup	568	472	419
Coconut milk				
fresh	1 tbsp	35	32	29
	1 cup	552	515	457
canned	1 tbsp	30	29	26
	1 cup	445	434	385
frozen	1 tbsp	30	28	25
	1 cup	486	449	398
Filberts (hazelnuts)				
dried	1 oz	179	160	12
	1 cup, chopped	727	648	48
dry-roasted	1 oz	188	169	12
oil-roasted	1 oz	187	163	12
Hickory nuts, dried	1 oz	187	165	18
Macadamia nuts				
dried	1 oz	199	188	28

NUTS AND SEEDS

FOOD	AMOUNT	CALORIES		
		TOTAL	FAT	SAT-FAT
Macadamia nuts (*cont.*)				
oil-roasted	1 oz (24 halves)	204	**196**	29
	1 cup	962	**923**	139
Mixed nuts				
dry-roasted, with peanuts	1 oz	169	**131**	18
	1 cup	814	**634**	85
oil-roasted, with peanuts	1 oz	175	**144**	22
	1 cup	876	**720**	112
oil-roasted, without peanuts	1 oz	175	**144**	23
	1 cup	886	**728**	118
Peanuts, shelled				
dry-roasted	1 oz (35 kernels)	161	**126**	17
	1 cup	827	**646**	90
oil-roasted	1 oz (35 kernels)	165	**126**	18
	1 cup	841	**642**	89
Planters				
Hot Spicy (to heat)	37 pieces (28 g)	160	**120**	18
Snack Mix (to heat)	¼ cup	140	**70**	9
Sweet 'n Crunchy	18 pieces (28 g)	140	**60**	9
Peanut butter, smooth	2 tbsp	190	**148**	24
Peter Pan Smart Choice, reduced fat	2 tbsp	190	**110**	18
Pecans				
dried	1 oz	190	**173**	14
dry-roasted	1 oz (14 halves)	187	**165**	13
oil-roasted	1 oz	195	**182**	15
Pine nuts	1 oz	160	**144**	27
Pistachios				
dried	1 oz	164	**124**	16
dry-roasted	1 oz (47 kernels)	172	**135**	17
Walnuts, black, dried	1 oz (14 halves)	172	**145**	9
	1 cup	759	**637**	41
English or Persian, dried	1 oz (14 halves)	182	**158**	14
	1 cup	770	**668**	60
Walnut halves	⅓ cup	210	**190**	18
Walnut pieces	¼ cup	190	**170**	18

NUTS AND SEEDS

FOOD	AMOUNT	CALORIES		
		TOTAL	FAT	SAT-FAT
Seeds				
Poppy	1 tsp	15	11	NA
	1 tbsp	66	51	NA
Pumpkin and squash				
whole, roasted	1 oz	127	50	9
kernels, dried	1 oz	154	117	22
kernels, roasted	1 oz	148	108	20
Sesame, kernels, dried	1 tbsp	47	39	6
	1 cup	882	739	104
Sunflower				
in shell, roasted	1 oz	86	59	8
shelled	1 oz	80	59	8
dried	1 oz	162	127	13
dry-roasted	1 oz	165	127	13
	1 tbsp	48	34	7
	1 cup	745	574	60
oil-roasted	1 oz	175	147	15
	1 tbsp	47	44	5
toasted	1 oz	176	145	15
	1 tbsp	51	43	5
Tahini	1 tbsp	90	72	10
Watermelon, dried	1 oz	158	121	25

POULTRY

See also **SAUSAGES AND LUNCHEON MEATS** for cold cuts made from poultry products and **FROZEN, MICROWAVE, AND REFRIGERATED FOODS.**

*Remember that many of the following calorie figures are for **only 1 ounce** of poultry!*

FOOD	AMOUNT	CALORIES		
		TOTAL	FAT	SAT-FAT
Chicken				
Back				
meat and skin				
raw	½ back (99 g)	316	256	74
	1 oz	90	73	21
fried, batter-dipped	½ back (120 g)	397	237	63
	1 oz	94	56	15
fried, flour-coated	½ back (72 g)	238	134	36
	1 oz	94	53	14
roasted	½ back (53 g)	159	100	28
	1 oz	85	54	15

POULTRY

| FOOD | AMOUNT | CALORIES | | |
		TOTAL	FAT	SAT-FAT
Chicken back (*cont.*)				
meat only				
raw	½ back (51 g)	70	**27**	7
	1 oz	39	**15**	4
fried	½ back (58 g)	167	**80**	22
	1 oz	82	**39**	10
roasted	½ back (51 g)	70	**27**	7
	1 oz	39	**15**	4
Breast				
meat and skin				
raw	1 breast (145 g)	250	**121**	35
	1 oz	49	**24**	7
fried, batter-dipped	1 breast (140 g)	364	**166**	44
	1 oz	74	**34**	9
fried, flour-coated	1 breast (98 g)	218	**78**	22
	1 oz	63	**23**	6
roasted	1 breast (98 g)	193	**69**	19
	1 oz	56	**20**	6
meat only				
raw	1 breast (118 g)	129	**13**	4
	1 oz	31	**3**	1
fried	1 breast (86 g)	161	**36**	10
	1 oz	53	**12**	3
roasted	1 breast (86 g)	129	**13**	4
	1 oz	31	**3**	1
Drumstick				
meat and skin				
raw	1 drumstick (73 g)	117	**57**	16
	1 oz	46	**22**	6
fried, batter-dipped	1 drumstick (72 g)	193	**102**	27
	1 oz	76	**40**	10
fried, flour-coated	1 drumstick (49 g)	120	**60**	16
	1 oz	69	**35**	9
roasted	1 drumstick (52 g)	112	**52**	14
	1 oz	61	**28**	8
meat only				
raw	1 drumstick (62 g)	74	**19**	5
	1 oz	34	**9**	2

POULTRY

FOOD	AMOUNT	CALORIES		
		TOTAL	FAT	SAT-FAT
Drumstick (*cont.*)				
fried	1 drumstick			
	(42 g)	82	31	8
	1 oz	55	21	5
roasted	1 drumstick			
	(44 g)	74	19	5
	1 oz	34	9	2
Gizzard				
raw	1 gizzard (37 g)	44	14	4
	1 oz	33	11	3
simmered	1 cup	222	48	14
	1 oz	43	9	3
Ground				
Fresh (Perdue)	1 oz	48	30	9
Frozen (Longacre)	1 oz	55	30	9
Leg				
meat and skin				
raw	1 leg (167 g)	312	182	51
	1 oz	53	31	9
fried, batter-dipped	1 leg (158 g)	431	230	61
	1 oz	77	41	11
fried, flour-coated	1 leg (112 g)	285	145	39
	1 oz	72	37	10
roasted	1 leg (114 g)	265	138	38
	1 oz	66	34	9
meat only				
raw	1 leg (130 g)	156	45	11
	1 oz	34	10	2
fried	1 leg (94 g)	195	79	21
	1 oz	59	24	6
roasted	1 leg (95 g)	156	45	11
	1 oz	34	10	2
Liver				
chopped chicken livers	1 tbsp	28	17	4
raw	1 liver (32 g)	40	11	4
	1 oz	35	10	3
simmered	1 cup	219	69	23
	1 oz	44	14	5

POULTRY

FOOD	AMOUNT	CALORIES		
		TOTAL	FAT	SAT-FAT
Chicken neck				
meat and skin				
raw	1 neck (50 g)	148	118	33
	1 oz	84	67	18
fried, batter-dipped	1 neck (52 g)	172	110	29
	1 oz	94	60	16
fried, flour-coated	1 neck (36 g)	119	76	21
	1 oz	94	60	16
simmered	1 neck (38 g)	94	62	17
	1 oz	70	46	13
meat only				
raw	1 neck (20 g)	31	16	4
	1 oz	44	22	6
fried	1 neck (22 g)	50	23	6
	1 oz	65	30	8
simmered	1 neck (18 g)	32	13	3
	1 oz	44	21	5
Thigh				
meat and skin				
raw	1 thigh (94 g)	199	129	36
	1 oz	60	39	11
fried, batter-dipped	1 thigh (86 g)	238	128	34
	1 oz	78	42	11
fried, flour-coated	1 thigh (62 g)	162	84	23
	1 oz	74	38	11
roasted	1 thigh (62 g)	153	86	24
	1 oz	70	40	11
meat only				
raw	1 thigh (69 g)	82	24	6
	1 oz	34	10	3
fried	1 thigh (52 g)	113	48	13
	1 oz	62	26	7
roasted	1 thigh (52 g)	82	24	6
	1 oz	34	10	3
Wing				
meat and skin				
raw	1 wing (49 g)	109	70	20
	1 oz	63	41	11
fried, batter-dipped	1 wing (49 g)	159	96	26
	1 oz	92	56	15
fried, flour-coated	1 wing (32 g)	103	64	17
	1 oz	91	57	15

POULTRY

FOOD	AMOUNT	CALORIES		
		TOTAL	FAT	SAT-FAT
Wing				
meat and skin (*cont.*)				
roasted	1 wing (34 g)	99	**60**	17
	1 oz	82	**50**	14
meat only				
raw	1 wing (29 g)	36	**9**	2
	1 oz	36	**9**	2
fried	1 wing (20 g)	42	**16**	5
	1 oz	60	**23**	6
roasted	1 wing (21 g)	36	**9**	2
	1 oz	36	**9**	2
Chicken Dishes, Mixed (*see also* **FROZEN, MICROWAVE, AND REFRIGERATED FOODS.**)				
Chicken à la king	1 cup	470	**306**	116
Chicken and noodles	1 cup	365	**162**	46
Chicken potpie	⅓ pie	545	**279**	93
Duck, domesticated				
meat and skin				
raw	½ duck (634 g)	2561	**2245**	754
	1 oz	115	**100**	33
roasted	½ duck (382 g)	1287	**975**	332
	1 oz	96	**72**	25
meat only				
raw	½ duck (303 g)	399	**162**	63
	1 oz	37	**15**	6
roasted	½ duck (221 g)	399	**162**	63
	1 oz	37	**15**	6
liver, raw	1 liver (44 g)	60	**18**	6
	1 oz	39	**12**	4
Duck, wild				
meat and skin, raw	½ duck (270 g)	571	**369**	125
	1 oz	60	**39**	13
breast meat only, raw	1 breast (83 g)	102	**32**	10
	1 oz	35	**11**	3
Goose, domesticated				
meat and skin				
raw	½ goose (1319 g)	4893	**3991**	1161
	1 oz	105	**86**	25

POULTRY

FOOD	AMOUNT	CALORIES		
		TOTAL	FAT	SAT-FAT
Goose meat and skin (*cont.*)				
roasted	½ goose (774 g)	2362	**1527**	479
	1 oz	86	**56**	18
meat only				
raw	½ goose (766 g)	1237	**492**	192
	1 oz	46	**18**	7
roasted	½ goose (591 g)	1237	**492**	192
	1 oz	46	**18**	7
liver, raw	1 liver (94 g)	125	**36**	14
	1 oz	38	**11**	4
Pheasant				
meat and skin, raw	½ pheasant (400 g)	723	**335**	97
	1 oz	51	**24**	7
meat only, raw	½ pheasant (352 g)	470	**115**	39
	1 oz	38	**9**	3
breast meat only, raw	1 breast (182 g)	243	**53**	18
	1 oz	38	**8**	3
leg meat only, raw	1 leg (107 g)	143	**41**	14
	1 oz	38	**11**	4
Quail				
meat and skin, raw	1 quail (109 g)	210	**118**	33
	1 oz	54	**31**	9
meat only, raw	1 quail (92 g)	123	**38**	11
	1 oz	38	**12**	3
breast meat only, raw	1 breast (56 g)	69	**15**	4
	1 oz	35	**8**	2
Squab (pigeon)				
meat and skin, raw	1 squab (199 g)	584	**426**	151
	1 oz	83	**61**	21
meat only, raw	1 squab (168 g)	239	**113**	30
	1 oz	40	**19**	5
breast meat only, raw	1 breast (101 g)	135	**41**	11
	1 oz	38	**12**	3

POULTRY

FOOD	AMOUNT	CALORIES		
		TOTAL	FAT	SAT-FAT
Turkey				
Back				
meat and skin				
raw	½ back (183 g)	275	**120**	35
	1 oz	43	**18**	5
roasted	½ back (130 g)	265	**120**	35
	1 oz	58	**26**	8
meat only				
raw	½ back (150 g)	180	**47**	16
	1 oz	34	**9**	3
roasted	½ back (96 g)	180	**47**	16
	1 oz	34	**9**	3
Breast				
meat and skin				
raw	1 oz	35	**7**	2
roasted	1 oz	43	**8**	2
meat only				
raw	1 oz	31	**2**	1
roasted	1 oz	31	**2**	1
Cutlet, braised	1 oz	31	**2**	1
Ground				
Fresh				
Perdue	1 oz	40	**20**	6
Shady Brook	1 oz	43	**20**	6
Frozen				
Longacre	1 oz	53	**33**	7
Leg				
meat and skin				
raw	1 leg (349 g)	412	**112**	34
	1 oz	33	**9**	3
roasted	1 leg (245 g)	418	**119**	37
	1 oz	48	**14**	4
meat only				
raw	1 leg (329 g)	356	**70**	24
	1 oz	31	**6**	2
roasted	1 leg (224 g)	355	**70**	24
	1 oz	31	**6**	2
Wing				
meat and skin				
raw	1 wing (128 g)	203	**89**	24
	1 oz	45	**20**	5

POULTRY

FOOD	AMOUNT	CALORIES		
		TOTAL	FAT	SAT-FAT
Turkey wing				
meat and skin (*cont.*)				
roasted	1 wing (90 g)	186	**80**	22
	1 oz	59	**25**	7
meat only				
raw	1 wing (90 g)	96	**9**	3
	1 oz	30	**3**	1
roasted	1 wing (60 g)	96	**9**	3
	1 oz	30	**3**	1

RESTAURANT FOODS

FOOD	AMOUNT	CALORIES		
		TOTAL	FAT	SAT-FAT
Au Bon Pain				
Breads				
Bagels				
Cinnamon Raisin	1	280	**9**	<9
Plain, Onion, or Sesame	1	270	**9**	<9
Loaf				
Baguette	1	810	**18**	<9
Cheese	1	1670	**261**	81
Four Grain	1	1420	**99**	<9
Onion Herb	1	1430	**117**	<9
Parisienne	1	1490	**36**	<9
Muffins				
Blueberry	1	390	**99**	36
Bran	1	390	**99**	27
Carrot	1	450	**198**	45
Corn	1	460	**153**	27
Cranberry Walnut	1	350	**117**	18
Oat Bran Apple	1	400	**90**	18
Pumpkin	1	410	**144**	18
Whole Grain	1	440	**144**	18
Rolls				
Alpine	1	220	**27**	<9
Country Seed	1	220	**36**	<9
Hearth	1	250	**18**	<9
Petit Pain	1	220	**<9**	<9
Pumpernickel	1	210	**18**	<9
Rye	1	230	**18**	<9

RESTAURANT FOODS

FOOD	AMOUNT	CALORIES		
		TOTAL	FAT	SAT-FAT
Breads				
Rolls (*cont.*)				
3-Seed Raisin	1	250	36	<9
Vegetable	1	230	45	<9
Sandwich				
Braided Roll	1 roll	387	99	27
Croissant	1 roll	300	126	72
French	1 roll	320	<9	<9
Hearth	1 roll	370	27	<9
Multigrain	2 slices	391	27	9
Pita Pocket	1 pocket	80	<9	NA
Rye	2 slices	374	36	9
Cookies				
Chocolate Chip	1 serving	280	135	81
Chocolate Chunk Pecan	1 serving	290	153	54
Oatmeal Raisin	1 serving	250	81	27
Peanut Butter	1 serving	290	135	54
White Chocolate Chunk Pecan	1 serving	300	153	54
Croissants				
Dessert				
Almond	1	420	225	108
Apple	1	250	90	54
Blueberry Cheese	1	380	180	108
Chocolate	1	400	216	126
Cinnamon Raisin	1	390	117	72
Coconut Pecan	1	440	207	108
Hazelnut Chocolate	1	480	252	126
Plain	1	220	90	54
Strawberry or Raspberry Cheese	1	400	180	108
Sweet Cheese	1	420	207	126
Hot Filled				
Ham and Cheese	1	370	180	108
Spinach and Cheese	1	290	144	90
Turkey and Cheddar	1	410	198	117
Turkey and Havarti	1	410	189	117
Salads				
Chicken Tarragon Garden	1	310	135	18
Cracked Pepper Chicken Garden	1	100	18	<9
Garden, small	1	20	<9	<9

RESTAURANT FOODS

FOOD	AMOUNT	CALORIES		
		TOTAL	FAT	SAT-FAT
Salads (*cont.*)				
Garden, large	1	40	<9	<9
Grilled Chicken Garden	1	110	18	<9
Shrimp Garden	1	102	18	<9
Tuna Garden	1	350	225	36
Salad Dressings				
Balsamic Vinaigrette	2¼ oz	311	297	45
Champagne Vinaigrette	2¼ oz	251	234	36
County Blue Cheese	2¼ oz	325	279	54
Honey with Poppy Seed	2¼ oz	351	315	54
Low-Cal Italian	2¼ oz	68	54	<9
Olive Oil Caesar	2¼ oz	255	144	NA
Parmesan and Pepper	2¼ oz	235	189	45
Sesame French	2¼ oz	339	243	36
Tomato Basil	2¼ oz	66	<9	0
Sandwich Fillings				
Cheese				
Brie	1 serving	300	216	135
Cheddar	1 serving	110	81	45
Herb	1 serving	290	261	162
Provolone	1 serving	155	113	66
Swiss	1 serving	330	216	135
Meat				
Albacore Tuna Salad	1 serving	310	216	36
Bacon	1 serving	140	108	36
Chicken Tarragon	1 serving	270	135	18
Country Ham	1 serving	150	63	27
Cracked Pepper Chicken	1 serving	120	18	<9
Grilled Chicken	1 serving	130	36	<9
Roast Beef	1 serving	180	72	36
Smoked Turkey	1 serving	100	9	<9
Soups (*see also* **SOUPS,** *Homemade or Restaurant*)				
Beef Barley	1 cup	74	18	<9
	1 bowl	112	23	9
Chicken Noodle	1 cup	79	9	<9
	1 bowl	119	15	<9
Clam Chowder	1 cup	289	162	81
	1 bowl	433	243	126
Cream of Broccoli	1 cup	201	153	72
	1 bowl	302	234	108
Garden Vegetarian	1 cup	29	<9	<9
	1 bowl	44	<9	<9

RESTAURANT FOODS

FOOD	AMOUNT	TOTAL	CALORIES FAT	SAT-FAT
Soups (*cont.*)				
Minestrone	1 cup	105	**9**	<9
	1 bowl	158	**15**	<9
Split Pea	1 cup	176	**9**	<9
	1 bowl	264	**15**	<9
Tomato Florentine	1 cup	61	**9**	<9
	1 bowl	92	**15**	<9
Vegetarian Chili	1 cup	139	**27**	<9
	1 bowl	208	**36**	<9

Chinese Restaurant

FOOD	AMOUNT	TOTAL	FAT	SAT-FAT
Barbecued pork (not fried)	1 whole dish	1374	**986**	355
Barbecued spareribs	1 whole dish	1863	**1232**	480
Beef with vegetables	1 whole dish	1572	**1068**	263
Chicken with cashews	1 whole dish	1765	**1075**	186
Chicken with vegetables	1 whole dish	1224	**652**	102
Chinese Noodle soup	1 serving	265	**81**	NA
Egg roll	1	152	**103**	30
Hot and sour soup	1 serving	165	**72**	NA
Hunan shrimp (not fried)	1 whole dish	1068	**755**	100
Kung pao beef	1 whole dish	2458	**1706**	444
Kung pao chicken	1 whole dish	1806	**1134**	158
Kung pao shrimp	1 whole dish	1068	**755**	115
Moo shu pork	1 whole dish	1383	**1053**	258
Orange beef	1 whole dish	1710	**1216**	342
Pork with vegetables	1 whole dish	1574	**1219**	338
Sweet and sour pork	1 whole dish	1845	**1509**	389
Sweet and sour shrimp	1 whole dish	1069	**805**	130
Szechuan pork	1 whole dish	1694	**1339**	356
Velvet corn soup	1 serving	115	**27**	NA
Wonton soup	1 serving	283	**108**	NA

International House of Pancakes (IHOP)

FOOD	AMOUNT	TOTAL	FAT	SAT-FAT
Pancakes				
Buttermilk	1 (56 g)	108	**28**	6
Buckwheat	1 (63 g)	134	**45**	11
Country Griddle	1 (63 g)	134	**34**	9
Egg	1 (56 g)	102	**45**	11
Harvest Grain 'n Nut	1 (63 g)	160	**74**	12
Foods prepared with Eggstro'dnaire				
Broccoli and Mushroom Omelette	1	310	**62**	NA

RESTAURANT FOODS

FOOD	AMOUNT	CALORIES		
		TOTAL	FAT	SAT-FAT
Foods prepared with Eggstro'dnaire (*cont.*)				
Breakfast Burrito	1	456	**109**	NA
Chicken Fajita Burrito	1	523	**89**	NA
French Toast	1 piece	99	**18**	NA
Waffles				
Regular	1 (112 g)	305	**133**	30
Belgian				
Regular	1 (168 g)	408	**177**	100
Harvest Grain 'n Nut	1 (168 g)	445	**251**	107
Italian Restaurant				
Appetizers				
Antipasto	1½ lbs	629	**423**	132
Entrees				
Eggplant Parmigiana with spaghetti	2½ cups	1208	**558**	145
Fettuccine Alfredo	2½ cups	1498	**873**	434
Lasagna	2 cups	958	**477**	192
Linguine with red clam sauce	3 cups	892	**207**	36
Linguine with white clam sauce	3 cups	907	**261**	45
Spaghetti with meat sauce	3 cups	918	**225**	92
Spaghetti with meatballs	3½ cups	1155	**351**	92
Spaghetti with sausage	2½ cups	1043	**351**	94
Spaghetti with tomato sauce	3½ cups	849	**153**	34
Veal Parmigiana with spaghetti	1½ cups	1064	**396**	128
Side Dishes				
Fried calamari	3 cups	1037	**630**	83
Garlic bread	8 oz	822	**360**	90
Spaghetti with tomato sauce	1½ cups	409	**72**	16
Mexican Restaurant				
Appetizers				
Beef and cheese nachos with sour cream and guacamole	1 serving	1362	**801**	250
Cheese quesadilla with sour cream and guacamole	1 serving	900	**531**	220
Cheese Nachos	1 serving	807	**500**	225

RESTAURANT FOODS

FOOD	AMOUNT	CALORIES		
		TOTAL	FAT	SAT-FAT
Entrees				
Beef burrito	1 serving	833	**360**	121
with beans, rice, sour cream, and guacamole	1 serving	1639	**711**	248
Beef chimichanga	1 serving	802	**423**	113
with beans, rice, sour cream, and guacamole	1 serving	1607	**774**	241
Beef enchilada	1 serving	324	**171**	67
two enchiladas with beans and rice	1 serving	1253	**522**	140
Chicken fajitas and flour tortillas	1 serving	839	**216**	54
with beans, rice, sour cream, and guacamole	1 serving	1661	**567**	173
Chile rellenos	1 serving	487	**342**	45
two chile rellenos with beans and rice	1 serving	1578	**864**	173
Chicken enchilada	1 serving	329	**162**	103
two enchiladas with beans and rice	1 serving	1264	**513**	270
Chicken taco	1 serving	219	**99**	27
two tacos with beans and rice	1 serving	1042	**378**	119
Taco salad				
with sour cream and guacamole	1 serving	1099	**639**	177
Side Dishes				
Rice	¾ cup	229	**34**	5
Refried beans	¾ cup	375	**146**	60
Tortilla chips	50 chips	645	**432**	81
Swiss Chalet				
Apple pie	1 serving	413	**171**	36
Back rib	½ rib	405	**234**	81
	full rib	810	**468**	162
Caesar Salad Appetizer	1 serving	345	**171**	18
Caesar Salad Entree	1 serving	454	**342**	36
Chicken				
white (with skin)	¼ chicken	381	**198**	36
white (skinless)	¼ chicken	225	**72**	18
dark (with skin)	¼ chicken	313	**153**	45
dark (skinless)	¼ chicken	232	**90**	27

RESTAURANT FOODS

FOOD	AMOUNT	CALORIES		
		TOTAL	FAT	SAT-FAT
Chicken (with skin)	½ chicken	694	**351**	81
Chicken Pot Pie	1 pie	494	**216**	45
Chicken Salad and Roll	1 serving	466	**198**	36
Roll	1 roll	116	**9**	0

SALAD BAR FOODS

FOOD	AMOUNT	CALORIES		
		TOTAL	FAT	SAT-FAT
Bacon bits	1 tbsp	105	**30**	0
Baked beans	½ cup	160	**36**	<9
Breadsticks, sesame	2	20	**<9**	NA
Cheese, shredded Cheddar	2 tbsp	110	**81**	54
Cheese nachos	2 tbsp	70	**45**	NA
Chow mein noodles	½ cup	140	**60**	14
Cole slaw	½ cup	180	**108**	20
Cottage cheese (4% fat)	½ cup	110	**43**	23
Croutons	2 tbsp	30	**10**	0
Puddings				
Bread pudding	½ cup	170	**36**	NA
Chocolate mousse	½ cup	160	**45**	NA
Chocolate pudding	½ cup	140	**27**	NA
Lemon mousse	½ cup	160	**45**	NA
Rice pudding	½ cup	135	**18**	NA
Vanilla pudding	½ cup	140	**27**	NA
Salads				
Macaroni	½ cup	280	**162**	NA
Pasta				
with broccoli	½ cup	150	**81**	NA
chicken	½ cup	215	**144**	NA
fiesta	½ cup	190	**90**	NA
seafood	½ cup	245	**171**	NA
tuna	½ cup	240	**153**	NA
Polynesian	½ cup	160	**45**	NA
Potato	½ cup	135	**45**	14
Red skin potato	½ cup	150	**72**	14
Three-bean	½ cup	130	**18**	NA
Tuna	½ cup	190	**85**	NA

SALAD BAR FOODS

FOOD	AMOUNT	CALORIES TOTAL	FAT	SAT-FAT
Salad dressings	1 tbsp	60–90	50–72	9–18
	4 tbsp	240–360	200–288	36–72
Soup, prepared from canned soup (*see also* **SOUPS**, *Homemade or Restaurant*)				
Bean and ham	¾ cup	145	**36**	NA
Beef barley	¾ cup	95	**18**	NA
Beef stew	¾ cup	85	**9**	NA
Chicken corn noodle	¾ cup	85	**9**	NA
Chicken rice	¾ cup	85	**9**	NA
Chili con carne with beans	¾ cup	170	**45**	NA
Clam chowder, New England–style	¾ cup	180	**45**	NA
Crab	¾ cup	55	**18**	NA
Cream of broccoli	¾ cup	95	**45**	NA
Sunflower seeds	1 tbsp	48	**34**	7
Tofu	½ cup	90	**36**	7
Tortilla chips	1 oz	140	**54**	9
Turkey, diced	2 tbsp	60	**45**	NA
Toppings for Home-Prepared Salads				
Bac·Os (Betty Crocker)	1 tbsp	30	**10**	0
Bac'n Pieces (McCormick)	1½ tbsp	30	**10**	0
Real Bacon Bits (Hormel)	1 tbsp	90	**45**	9
Salad Crispins, Mini Croutons (Hidden Valley)	1 tbsp	35	**10**	0

SAUCES, GRAVIES, AND DIPS

FOOD	AMOUNT	CALORIES TOTAL	FAT	SAT-FAT
Sauces				
Barbecue				
Masterpiece	2 tbsp	40–60	**0**	0
Honey Dijon	2 tbsp	50	**10**	0
Open Pit	2 tbsp	50	**5**	0
Bearnaise	1 tbsp	53	**48**	29
	½ cup	423	**383**	232
Browning and Seasoning	1 tbsp	15	**0**	0
Cheese	1 tbsp	31	**21**	14
	½ cup	250	**170**	110

SAUCES, GRAVIES, AND DIPS

FOOD	AMOUNT	CALORIES TOTAL	FAT	SAT-FAT
Clam, white	½ cup	120	**80**	14
Cooking sauces				
Uncle Ben's				
Sauce for Beef with Mushrooms	½ cup	70	**10**	0
Sauce for Country Chicken	½ cup	130	**80**	45
Sauce for Pepper Steak	½ cup	70	**15**	0
Sweet and Sour	½ cup	120	**0**	0
Campbell's Simmer Chef				
Creamy Mushroom and Herb	½ cup	110	**80**	18
Golden Honey Mustard	½ cup	150	**20**	0
Hearty Onion and Mushroom	½ cup	50	**10**	0
Old Country Cacciatore	½ cup	110	**35**	9
Oriental Sweet and Sour	½ cup	110	**10**	0
Cream	1 tbsp	28	**22**	14
	½ cup	225	**175**	110
Curry Cream	1 tbsp	40	**31**	20
	½ cup	317	**250**	160
Hollandaise	1 tbsp	82	**80**	47
	½ cup	660	**627**	377
Horseradish (Kraft)	1 tbsp	20	**15**	0
Louis	1 tbsp	63	**60**	14
	½ cup	504	**480**	112
Nacho Cheese (Kaukauna)	2 tbsp	90	**60**	18
Pasta, refrigerated				
Contadina				
Alfredo (light)	½ cup	190	**120**	63
Pesto with Basil	¼ cup	310	**270**	45
Pesto with Sun-dried Tomatoes	¼ cup	250	**220**	36
DiGiorno				
Alfredo	¼ cup	220	**200**	126
Marinara	½ cup	100	**40**	9
Romano				
Alfredo	3½ oz	140	**90**	54
Soy	1 tbsp	11	**0**	0
Spaghetti				
Healthy Choice				
Traditional	½ cup	50	**5**	5

SAUCES, GRAVIES, AND DIPS

FOOD	AMOUNT	TOTAL	FAT	SAT-FAT
Spaghetti (*cont.*)				
Prego				
Flavored with Meat	½ cup	160	**50**	14
Garden Combination	½ cup	90	**10**	5
Marinara	½ cup	110	**50**	14
Mushroom and Diced Onion	½ cup	120	**35**	14
Mushroom and Diced Tomato	½ cup	110	**35**	9
Mushroom and Extra Spices	½ cup	120	**35**	9
Mushroom and Green Pepper	½ cup	100	**35**	9
Onion and Garlic	½ cup	120	**9**	9
Three Cheese	½ cup	100	**20**	5
Tomato, Onion, and Garlic	½ cup	120	**55**	14
Traditional	½ cup	150	**50**	18
Ragú				
All Chunky Garden Style	½ cup	120	**40**	5
Garlic and Basil	½ cup	90	**25**	0
Light Garden Harvest	½ cup	50	**0**	0
Light Pasta Sauce	½ cup	60	**15**	0
Vegetable Primavera	½ cup	110	**35**	5
Tartar				
fat-free (Kraft)	2 tbsp	25	**0**	0
regular (Hellman's)	1 tbsp	70	**70**	9
Tomato, canned	1 cup	74	**0**	0
White	1 tbsp	24	**17**	11
	½ cup	195	**138**	88
Worcestershire	1 tbsp	0	**0**	0
Gravies				
Beef, canned	½ cup	62	**25**	13
Franco-American Chicken	¼ cup	45	**35**	9
Heinz				
Classic Chicken	¼ cup	30	**15**	0
Fat-Free, all	¼ cup	15	**0**	0
Rich Mushroom	¼ cup	20	**5**	0
Roasted Turkey	¼ cup	25	**10**	0
Savory Brown	¼ cup	25	**10**	0
Zesty Brown	¼ cup	20	**5**	0

SAUCES, GRAVIES, AND DIPS

FOOD	AMOUNT	CALORIES		
		TOTAL	FAT	SAT-FAT
Dips				
Bean (Fritos)	2 tbsp (35 g)	40	**10**	5
Cheddar Cheese, mild (Herr's)	2 tbsp (30 g)	45	**25**	14
Jalapeño (Frito-Lay)	2 tbsp (34 g)	50	**30**	9
Jalapeño (Herr's)	2 tbsp (30 g)	30	**25**	9
French Onion				
Bacon (Lucerne)	2 tbsp	60	**45**	23
Frito-Lay's	2 tbsp (33 g)	60	**45**	27
Green Onion (Lucerne)	2 tbsp	50	**45**	18
Guacamole	2 tbsp	50	**30**	5
Hummus with tahini	2 tbsp	57	**30**	0
Salsa				
Chunky (Herr's)	2 tbsp (31 g)	12	**0**	0
Chunky (Utz)	2 tbsp (30 g)	60	**0**	0
Dip (Pace)	2 tbsp (31.8 g)	10	**0**	0
Dip (Tostistos)	2 tbsp (33 g)	15	**0**	0
Mexican (Kaukauna)	2 tbsp (28 g)	15	**0**	0
Mild (Rojo's)	2 tbsp (29 g)	10	**0**	0
Salsa and Cream Cheese				
(Kaukauna)	2 tbsp (28 g)	70	**50**	27
Salsa con Queso (Tostistos)	2 tbsp (34 g)	40	**20**	5
Southwest, mild (Safeway)	2 tbsp (28 g)	10	**0**	0

SAUSAGES AND LUNCHEON MEATS

FOOD	AMOUNT	CALORIES		
		TOTAL	FAT	SAT-FAT
Bacon	2 slices (11 g)	60	**45**	18
Hickory-smoked				
(Smithfield)	2 slices (15 g)	90	**70**	27
Thick-sliced (Gwaltney)	1 slice (8 g)	45	**35**	9
Turkey (Louis Rich)	1 slice (14 g)	30	**20**	5
Barbecue loaf, pork, beef	28 g	49	**23**	8
	1 slice (22 g)	40	**18**	7
Beerwurst, beer salami				
beef	28 g	92	**75**	31
	1 slice (22 g)	75	**61**	25
pork	28 g	67	**48**	16
	1 slice (22 g)	55	**39**	13

SAUSAGES AND LUNCHEON MEATS

FOOD	AMOUNT	CALORIES		
		TOTAL	FAT	SAT-FAT
Berliner, pork, beef	28 g	65	**44**	15
	1 slice (22 g)	53	**36**	13
Bockwurst, raw	28 g	87	**70**	26
	1 link (64 g)	200	**161**	59
Bologna				
Beef (Oscar Mayer)	1 slice (28 g)	90	**70**	36
Chicken (Gwaltney)	1 slice (32 g)	80	**60**	36
Chicken, pork, and beef				
(Thorn Apple)	1 slice (37 g)	120	**90**	18
Pork	1 slice (28 g)	70	**51**	18
Pork and beef (Oscar				
Mayer)	1 slice (28 g)	90	**70**	27
Pork, chicken, and beef				
(Oscar Mayer)	1 slice (28 g)	90	**70**	27
Light	1 slice (28 g)	60	**35**	14
Pork and turkey (Gwaltney)	1 slice (38 g)	120	**100**	36
Turkey (Louis Rich)	1 slice (28 g)	50	**35**	9
Bratwurst, pork, beef	28 g	92	**71**	25
	1 link (70 g)	226	**175**	63
Bratwurst, pork, cooked	28 g	85	**66**	24
	1 link (84 g)	256	**198**	71
Braunschweiger, pork	28 g	102	**82**	28
	1 slice (17 g)	65	**52**	18
Breakfast strips, beef, cured				
cooked	1 slice (11 g)	51	**35**	15
Cheese dog	1 frank (45 g)	150	**120**	45
Chicken breast				
Deli Thin				
Fat-free (Oscar Mayer)	4 slices (52 g)	40	**0**	0
Oven-roasted (Louis Rich)	5 slices (55 g)	60	**15**	5
Chicken roll, white meat				
(Tyson)	3 slices (55 g)	90	**50**	18
Chipped beef	28 g	50	**20**	9
Corned beef brisket				
Cooked	28 g	71	**48**	16
Loaf, jellied	1 slice (28 g)	43	**16**	7
Thorn Apple Valley	84 g	190	**150**	63
Cured beef				
Oven-roasted (Hillshire				
Farms)	6 slices (57 g)	50	**5**	0
Dried beef, cured (beef jerky)	28 g	47	**10**	4

SAUSAGES AND LUNCHEON MEATS

FOOD	AMOUNT	CALORIES		
		TOTAL	FAT	SAT-FAT
Dutch brand loaf, pork, beef	1 slice (28 g)	68	**45**	16
Frankfurter				
Beef	1 frank (57 g)	190	**150**	63
Healthy Choice Low-Fat				
Beef Franks	1 frank (50 g)	60	**15**	5
Quarter-pound (Hebrew				
National)	1 frank (114 g)	350	**300**	108
Chicken (Wampler-				
LongAcre)	1 frank (56 g)	120	**100**	27
Pork and Turkey (Oscar				
Mayer)	1 frank (45 g)	150	**120**	45
Pork, Turkey, and Beef				
Light (Oscar Mayer)	1 frank (57 g)	110	**80**	27
Healthy Choice	1 frank (57 g)	70	**15**	5
Turkey				
Louis Rich	1 frank (57 g)	110	**70**	23
Extra Lean (Jennie-O)	1 frank (45 g)	45	**20**	5
Ham (*see also* **MEATS**, *Pork*				
Products, Cured)				
Baked (Oscar Mayer)	3 slices (63 g)	60	**10**	5
Boiled (Oscar Mayer)	3 slices (63 g)	70	**15**	5
Chopped	28 g	68	**48**	16
	1 slice (21 g)	50	**36**	12
Cured (Hormel)	85 g	100	**45**	14
Danish (Plumrose)	2 slices (56 g)	65	**25**	9
Deli Thin				
Baked Ham	4 slices (52 g)	50	**10**	0
Honey Ham	4 slices (52 g)	50	**15**	5
Minced	28 g	75	**53**	18
	1 slice (21 g)	55	**39**	14
Salad spread	28 g	61	**40**	13
	1 tbsp	32	**21**	7
Smoked				
Esskay	85 g	120	**50**	18
Hickory-Smoked	3 slices (89 g)	160	**100**	36
Oscar Mayer	3 slices (63 g)	60	**20**	9
Smok-a-Roma	57 g	120	**70**	27
Turkey ham (*see* Turkey cold				
cuts)				
Ham and cheese loaf or roll	1 slice (28 g)	73	**52**	19
Ham and cheese spread	28 g	69	**47**	22
	1 tbsp	37	**25**	12

SAUSAGES AND LUNCHEON MEATS

FOOD	AMOUNT	CALORIES		
		TOTAL	FAT	SAT-FAT
Headcheese, pork	1 slice (28 g)	60	**40**	13
Honey loaf, pork, beef	1 slice (28 g)	36	**11**	4
Honey roll sausage, beef	28 g	52	**27**	10
	1 slice (22 g)	42	**22**	8
Kielbasa, pork, beef (Eckrich)	28 g	90	**75**	27
	1 slice (25 g)	81	**64**	23
Knockwurst, beef (Hebrew National)	1 link (85 g)	260	**210**	81
Lebanon bologna, beef	28 g	64	**38**	16
	1 slice (22 g)	52	**31**	13
Liver cheese, pork	28 g	86	**65**	23
Liver pudding, pork	45 g	170	**110**	9
Liverwurst (Braunschweiger)				
Jones	1 slice (56 g)	150	**110**	36
Oscar Mayer	1 slice (56 g)	190	**160**	54
Luncheon meat				
beef, loaved	1 slice (28 g)	87	**67**	29
beef, thin-sliced	28 g	35	**8**	3
	5 slices (21 g)	26	**6**	2
pork, beef	1 slice (28 g)	100	**82**	30
pork, canned	28 g	95	**77**	28
	1 slice (21 g)	70	**57**	20
Luxury loaf, pork	1 slice (28 g)	40	**12**	4
Mortadella, beef, pork	28 g	88	**65**	24
	1 slice (14 g)	47	**34**	13
Mother's loaf, pork	28 g	80	**57**	20
	1 slice (21 g)	59	**42**	15
Olive loaf	1 slice (28 g)	70	**45**	15
Pastrami				
beef	1 slice (28 g)	99	**74**	27
turkey	1 slice (28 g)	40	**16**	9
Pâte				
Chicken liver	1 tbsp	26	**15**	4
Goose liver	28 g	131	**112**	NA
	1 tbsp	60	**51**	NA
Pork	28 g	100	**80**	27
Peppered beef (Carl Buddig)	71 g	100	**45**	18
Peppered loaf, pork, beef	1 slice (28 g)	42	**16**	6
Pepperoni (Hormel)	15 slices (28 g)	140	**120**	54
	1 sausage (252 g)	1248	**993**	364

SAUSAGES AND LUNCHEON MEATS

FOOD	AMOUNT	CALORIES		
		TOTAL	FAT	SAT-FAT
Pickle and pimento loaf (Oscar Mayer)	1 slice (28 g)	70	**50**	18
Picnic loaf, pork, beef	1 slice (28 g)	66	**42**	15
Pork cracklins (fried pork fat with skin)	½ oz (14 g)	80	**50**	9
Potted meat	¼ cup (58 g)	110	**80**	27
Salami				
Beef (Hebrew National)	56 g	170	**130**	54
Cotto (Oscar Mayer)	2 slices (46 g)	100	**80**	32
Dry or hard, pork	28 g	115	**86**	30
Sandwich spread, pork, beef	28 g	67	**44**	15
	1 tbsp	35	**23**	8
Sausage				
Beef (Jones Dairy Farm)	2 links (45 g)	170	**140**	NA
Biscuits (Jimmy Dean)	2 (96 g)	330	**190**	63
Blood	28 g	107	**88**	34
	1 slice (25 g)	95	**78**	30
Ham (Smithfield)	48 g	180	**140**	54
Italian, cooked, pork	28 g	92	**66**	23
	1 link (5/lb)	216	**155**	55
	1 link (4/lb)	268	**192**	68
Italian Turkey (Shady Brook Farms)	1 link (64 g)	100	**45**	14
Liver, liverwurst, pork	28 g	93	**73**	27
	1 slice (17 g)	59	**46**	17
Luncheon, pork and beef	28 g	74	**53**	19
	1 slice (22 g)	60	**43**	16
New England brand, pork, beef	28 g	46	**19**	6
	1 slice (22 g)	37	**16**	5
Polish, pork	28 g	92	**73**	26
	1 sausage (8 oz)	739	**587**	211
Pork				
Bob Evans	2 patties, pan-fried (53 g)	230	**180**	63
Country	28 g	120	**100**	36
Hot				
Gwaltney	39 g	150	**130**	45
Jamestown	36 g	170	**140**	45
Links (Parks)	2 links (42 g)	170	**150**	54
Smoked	1 link (85 g)	290	**230**	81

SAUSAGES AND LUNCHEON MEATS

| FOOD | AMOUNT | CALORIES | | |
		TOTAL	FAT	SAT-FAT
Sausage (*cont.*)				
Pork and beef, cooked	1 patty (28 g)	112	**92**	33
	1 link (13 g)	52	**33**	15
Smoked link				
pork	28 g	110	**81**	29
	1 link (67 g)	265	**194**	69
	1 link (16 g)	62	**46**	16
pork and beef	28 g	95	**77**	27
	1 link (67 g)	229	**186**	65
	1 link (16 g)	54	**44**	15
Summer, beef	3 slices (57 g)	180	**140**	63
Vienna (Hormel)	28 g	70	**60**	36
Scrapple (Parks)	¼" slice (55 g)	110	**60**	23
Tongue, beef				
raw	28 g	63	**41**	18
simmered	28 g	80	**53**	23
Tripe, beef, raw	28 g	28	**10**	5
Turkey breast, processed				
Oven-Roasted (Oscar Mayer)	3 slices (63 g)	70	**15**	0
Fat-Free Deli Thin (Oscar Mayer)	4 slices (52 g)	40	**0**	0
Smoked white (Louis Rich)	1 slice (28 g)	30	**10**	0
Turkey cold cuts				
Bacon (Louis Rich)	1 slice (14 g)	30	**20**	5
Bologna (Louis Rich)	1 slice (28 g)	50	**35**	9
Ham				
Chopped	1 slice (28 g)	40	**20**	9
Jennie-O	56 g	80	**40**	7
Louis Rich	1 slice (28 g)	35	**10**	0
Pastrami	1 slice (28 g)	40	**16**	9
Salami (Louis Rich)	1 slice (28 g)	45	**25**	9
Cotted Salami (Louis Rich)	1 slice (28 g)	90	**50**	18
Turkey roll				
Light and dark meat	1 slice (28 g)	42	**18**	5
Light meat	1 slice (28 g)	42	**18**	5

SNACK FOODS

FOOD	AMOUNT	CALORIES		
		TOTAL	FAT	SAT-FAT
Breadsticks				
Grissini-style, garlic (Stella D'oro)	3 (15 g)	60	**0**	0
Thin Bread Sticks (Pepperidge Farm)				
Cheddar Cheese	7 (16 g)	70	**25**	9
Chips and Crisps				
Bagel Chips				
New York Style	31 g	140	**30**	5
Planet	55 g	150	**0**	0
Bugles				
Crisp-baked	1½ cups	130	**25**	5
Original	1⅓ cups	160	**80**	72
Cheese Curls (Weight Watchers)	1 pkg (14 g)	70	**25**	9
Cheese Puffs Super Cheese (Safeway)	30 pieces (28 g)	160	**100**	9
Cheese Corn Curls	25 pieces (30 g)	150	**70**	18
Cheese Twists	1 cup (30 g)	150	**100**	18
Cheetos	21 pieces (28 g)	150	**80**	18
Cheez'n Breadsticks (Kraft)	1 unit (32 g)	130	**60**	36
Cheez'n Crackers (Kraft)	1 unit (31 g)	130	**70**	36
Corn Chips	20 chips (30 g)	170	**80**	14
Durkee French Fried Onions	½ cup (28 g)	180	**120**	36
Fritos	32 chips (28 g)	160	**90**	14
Scoops	10 chips (28 g)	150	**80**	14
Jax (Bachman)	25 pieces (30 g)	150	**70**	9
Crunchy	⅔ cup	170	**110**	18
PB'n Grahamsticks (Kraft)	1 unit (32 g)	170	**90**	23
Pop Chips (Betty Crocker)	1½ cups	130	**30**	5
Pita Chips (Shra-Lins)	1 serving (14 g)	60	**18**	9
Potato Chips				
Lay's	18 chips (28 g)	150	**90**	23
Bar-B-Q	15 chips (28 g)	150	**90**	18
Sour Cream and Onion	22 chips (28 g)	150	**90**	23
Wavy Lay's Au-Gratin	13 chips (28 g)	150	**90**	23
Mr. Phipps				
Sour Cream 'n Onion	22 chips (28 g)	130	**35**	5
Pringles				
Original	14 crisps (28 g)	160	**90**	23
Right Crisps	16 crisps (28 g)	140	**60**	18
Sour Cream and Onion	14 crisps (28 g)	160	**90**	23

SNACK FOODS

FOOD	AMOUNT	CALORIES		
		TOTAL	FAT	SAT-FAT
Potato Chips (*cont.*)				
Ruffles (Frito-Lay)	12 chips (28 g)	150	**90**	27
Cheddar and Sour Cream	13 chips (28 g)	160	**90**	23
Ranch	13 chips (28 g)	150	**80**	23
Safeway				
Barbecue Ripple Chips	18 chips (28 g)	140	**90**	23
Utz	20 chips (28 g)	150	**80**	18
Bar-B-Q Ripple Cut	20 chips (28 g)	150	**80**	18
Grandma Utz's				
Handcooked	20 chips (28 g)	150	**80**	27
Kettle Classics Crunchy	20 chips (28 g)	150	**80**	14
Ripple Cut	20 chips (28 g)	150	**80**	18
Sour Cream and Onion				
Ripple Cut	20 chips (28 g)	160	**90**	27
Potato Sticks (Durkee)	¾ cup	160	**90**	14
Pretzel Chips (Mr. Phipps)				
Original	16 chips (28 g)	120	**20**	0
Fat-free	16 chips (28 g)	100	**0**	0
Tortilla Chips				
Doritos	15 chips (28 g)	140	**60**	9
Guiltless Gourmet	22 chips (28 g)	110	**15**	0
Mr. Phipps				
Tortilla Crisps, original	29 crisps (30 g)	130	**40**	5
Tortilla Crisps, nacho				
cheese	28 crisps (31 g)	140	**40**	9
Safeway Tortilla Chips				
Blue corn	14 chips (28 g)	140	**60**	14
Extra cheese	13 chips (28 g)	140	**60**	14
White corn	7 chips (28 g)	140	**60**	14
Yellow and white corn	8 chips (28 g)	140	**70**	9
Tostitos	6 chips (28 g)	130	**50**	9
Utz	17 chips (28 g)	140	**60**	9
Nacho Tortilla	17 chips (28 g)	140	**60**	9
Crackers				
Austin				
Cheese Crackers on Cheese	6 (39 g)	210	**100**	27
Cheese Crackers and Peanut				
Butter	6 (39 g)	210	**90**	23
Toasty Crackers and Peanut				
Butter	6 (39 g)	210	**90**	23
Delicious				
Crispy Bacon	11 (30 g)	150	**60**	14

SNACK FOODS

| FOOD | AMOUNT | CALORIES | | |
		TOTAL	FAT	SAT-FAT
Delicious crackers (*cont.*)				
Hearty Wheat	13 (31 g)	140	**50**	14
Real Cheddar Cheese	11 (30 g)	140	**50**	14
Sesame Wheat	13 (31 g)	150	**60**	14
Snack	9 (31 g)	150	**60**	14
Tangy Onion	11 (30 g)	140	**50**	14
Devonsheer				
Melba Rounds				
Garlic	5 (15 g)	60	**10**	0
Honey bran	5 (15 g)	50	**0**	0
Onion	5 (15 g)	50	**0**	0
Plain	5 (15 g)	50	**0**	0
Sesame	5 (15 g)	60	**20**	5
12 Grain	5 (15 g)	50	**0**	0
Vegetable	5 (15 g)	50	**0**	0
Melba Toast				
Plain	3 (14 g)	50	**0**	0
Sesame	3 (14 g)	50	**10**	0
Rye	3 (14 g)	50	**0**	0
Keebler				
Club				
Garlic Bread	4 (14 g)	60	**15**	5
Original	4 (14 g)	70	**25**	9
Cracker Paks				
Club and Cheddar	1 pkg (36 g)	190	**100**	23
Toast and Peanut Butter	1 pkg (39 g)	190	**80**	18
Munch 'ems				
Cheddar	28 (30 g)	140	**50**	9
Ranch	28 (30 g)	130	**45**	9
Seasoned Original	28 (30 g)	130	**45**	9
Sour Cream and Onion	28 (30 g)	140	**50**	9
Toasteds Complements				
Buttercrisp	9 (29 g)	140	**60**	14
Onion	9 (29 g)	140	**50**	9
Rye	9 (29 g)	140	**60**	9
Sesame	9 (29 g)	140	**60**	9
Wheat	9 (29 g)	140	**60**	14
Reduced Fat	10 (28 g)	120	**30**	9
Town House				
Original	5 (16 g)	80	**40**	9
Reduced-fat	5 (16 g)	70	**20**	5

SNACK FOODS

FOOD	AMOUNT	CALORIES		
		TOTAL	FAT	SAT-FAT
Keebler crackers (*cont.*)				
Wheatables				
Ranch	26 (30 g)	150	**70**	18
All other flavors	26 (30 g)	150	**60**	18
Zesta Saltines				
Fat-free	5 (14 g)	50	**0**	0
Original	5 (15 g)	60	**15**	5
Lu				
Milk Lunch New England				
Biscuits	4 (32 g)	140	**35**	9
Manischewitz crackers				
Matzo				
American	1 board (28 g)	110	**15**	5
Premium Gold Unsalted				
Tops	1 sheet (31 g)	140	**40**	23
Snack Bits	15 bits (28 g)	130	**35**	23
Mrs. Wright's (Safeway)				
Cheddar Cheese Snack	28 (30 g)	150	**60**	18
Chicken Flavored Snack	11 (31 g)	160	**80**	18
Garden Vegetable	13 (31 g)	150	**60**	14
Onion Snack	11 (31 g)	140	**50**	14
Oyster and Soup	21 (30 g)	120	**30**	0
Saltine	5 (15 g)	60	**15**	5
Sesame Cheddar Snack	13 (31 g)	150	**60**	14
Sesame Snack	9 (31 g)	160	**60**	18
Sesame Wheat Snack	13 (31 g)	150	**60**	14
Snack	10 (15 g)	70	**20**	9
Unsalted Tops	5 (15 g)	60	**15**	5
Wheat Snack	13 (31 g)	140	**50**	14
Wheatstone	8 (28 g)	130	**50**	14
Nabisco				
Better Cheddars	22 (30 g)	150	**70**	18
Reduced-fat	24 (30 g)	140	**50**	14
Bugs Bunny Graham Snacks				
Chocolate	13 (30 g)	140	**40**	9
Cinnamon	13 (30 g)	140	**35**	5
Cheese Nips	29 (30 g)	150	**60**	14
Cheese Tid-Bit	32 (30 g)	150	**70**	14
Chicken in a Biskit	14 (30 g)	160	**80**	14
Garden Crisps	15 (30 g)	130	**30**	5

SNACK FOODS

| FOOD | AMOUNT | CALORIES | | |
		TOTAL	FAT	SAT-FAT
Nabisco crackers (*cont.*)				
Harvest Crisps				
5-Grain	13 (31 g)	130	30	5
Nabs				
Cheese Crackers with				
Peanut Butter	1 pkg (40 g)	200	100	18
Toasted, with Peanut				
Butter	1 pkg (40 g)	200	100	18
Oysterettes	19 (15 g)	60	20	5
Premium Saltines				
Fat-Free	5 (15 g)	60	0	0
Low-Sodium	5 (14 g)	60	10	0
Original	5 (14 g)	60	15	0
Unsalted Tops	5 (14 g)	60	15	0
with Multi-Grain	5 (14 g)	60	15	0
Rice crackers	½ cup (30 g)	110	0	0
Ritz crackers	5 (16 g)	80	35	5
Ritz Bits				
Mini Ritz	48 (30 g)	160	80	14
Peanut Butter				
Sandwiches	14 (31 g)	160	80	14
Cheese Ritz with Peanut				
Butter	1 pkg (40 g)	210	110	23
with Real Cheese	1 pkg (40 g)	210	110	27
Whole-Wheat	5 (15 g)	70	20	0
SnackWell's (see listing after Ry-Krisp)				
Sociables	7 (15 g)	80	35	5
Swiss Cheese	15 (29 g)	140	60	14
Teddy Grahams				
Cinnamon	24 pieces (30 g)	140	40	9
Honey	24 pieces (30 g)	140	40	9
Toasted Oat Thins	18 (30 g)	140	50	9
Triscuit Wafers	7 wafers (31 g)	140	45	9
Deli-style Rye	7 wafers (32 g)	140	45	9
Garden Herb	6 wafers (28 g)	130	40	9
Reduced Fat	7 wafers (32 g)	120	30	5
Wheat 'n Bran	7 wafers (32 g)	140	45	9
Uneeda Biscuits Unsalted				
Tops	2 (15 g)	60	15	0
Vegetable Thins	14 (31 g)	160	80	14

SNACK FOODS

FOOD	AMOUNT	CALORIES		
		TOTAL	FAT	SAT-FAT
Nabisco crackers (*cont.*)				
Waverly	5 (15 g)	70	30	9
Wheat Thins				
Multigrain	17 (30 g)	130	35	5
Original	16 (29 g)	140	50	9
Reduced Fat	18 (31 g)	130	35	5
Wheatsworth Stone Ground				
Wheat	5 (16 g)	80	30	5
Pepperidge Farm				
Swirled Bread Crisps, garlic				
and butter	1 oz (28 g)	140	50	9
Distinctive				
Butter Thins	4 (15 g)	70	25	9
Hearty Wheat	3 (16 g)	80	30	0
Quartet	3 (13 g)	60	20	0
Symphony	4 (17 g)	80	30	5
Three Cracker	3 (14 g)	70	20	0
Goldfish				
Cheddar Cheese	55 (30 g)	140	50	14
Original	55 (30 g)	140	60	18
Parmesan Cheese	60 (30 g)	140	50	14
Pizza	55 (30 g)	140	60	14
Real Vanilla	19 (30 g)	150	60	23
Reduced sodium cheddar				
cheese	60 (30 g)	150	60	14
Sesame Snack Sticks				
Sesame	9 (31 g)	150	50	5
Three-Cheese	9 (31 g)	140	45	18
Quaker				
Honey Nut Mini Rice Cakes	5 (14 g)	50	0	0
Rice Cakes	1 cake	35	0	0
Ry-Krisp				
Natural	2 (15 g)	60	0	0
SnackWell's (Nabisco)				
Cheese	38 (30 g)	130	20	5
Cinnamon Graham Snacks	20 (30 g)	110	0	0
Classic Golden	6 (14 g)	60	10	0
Cracked Pepper	7 (15 g)	60	0	0
Wheat	5 (15 g)	60	0	0
Sunshine				
Cheez-It	27 (30 g)	160	80	18
Hot and Spicy	26 (30 g)	160	80	14
White Cheddar	26 (30 g)	160	80	18

SNACK FOODS

FOOD	AMOUNT	CALORIES		
		TOTAL	FAT	SAT-FAT
Sunshine (*cont.*)				
Hi-Ho, all flavors	9 (31 g)	160	**80**	14
Krispy Saltines				
Mild Cheddar	5 (15 g)	60	**20**	5
Original	5 (14 g)	60	**10**	0
Soup and Oyster	17 (15 g)	60	**15**	0
Fruit Snacks				
Fruit by the Foot	1 roll (21 g)	80	**15**	0
Fruit Gushers	1 pouch (14 g)	90	**10**	0
Fruit Jammers	1 pouch (28 g)	100	**10**	5
Fruit Roll-ups	1 roll (14 g)	50	**5**	0
Troll	1 pouch (28 g)	90	**0**	0
Trolls in Trouble	1 pouch (28 g)	80	**15**	5
Weight Watchers	1 pkg (14 g)	50	**0**	0
Granola Bars				
Carnation Breakfast Bars				
Chewy Chocolate Chip	1 bar (36 g)	150	**50**	23
Chewy Peanut Butter	1 bar (36 g)	140	**45**	18
Kellogg's				
Chewy Granola Chocolate				
Chunk	1 bar (28 g)	110	**20**	5
Low-Fat Granola Bar	1 bar (21 g)	80	**15**	0
Nutrigrain Cereal Bar				
Oat and Fruit	1 bar (37 g)	140	**35**	9
Kudos				
Chocolate Chip	1 bar (28 g)	130	**45**	23
Chocolate Chunk with nuts	1 bar (20 g)	90	**30**	9
Honey Nut	1 bar (20 g)	90	**30**	9
Nutty Fudge	1 bar (28 g)	130	**50**	23
Nature Valley Low-fat Chewy	1 bar (28 g)	110	**20**	0
Quaker Chewy				
Apple Berry	1 bar (28 g)	120	**35**	9
Chocolate Chip	1 bar (28 g)	120	**30**	14
Peanut Butter and				
Chocolate Chip	1 bar (28 g)	120	**40**	14
S'mores	1 bar (28 g)	120	**35**	14
Trail Mix	1 bar (28 g)	120	**45**	9
Quaker Low-fat, all flavors	1 bar (21 g)	80	**15**	0

SNACK FOODS

FOOD	AMOUNT	CALORIES		
		TOTAL	FAT	SAT-FAT
Sunfelt				
Almond	1 bar (28 g)	130	**60**	18
Chocolate Chip	1 bar (35 g)	160	**60**	27
Oatmeal Raisin or Raisin	1 bar (35 g)	150	**50**	18
Oats and Honey	1 bar (28 g)	120	**45**	18
Lunch Packs				
Lunch 'n Munch (Hillshire Farm)				
Smoked Turkey Breast	1 pkg (128 g)	400	**320**	81
Lunchables (Oscar Mayer)				
Delux Variety Pack				
Turkey and Ham with cheese	1 pkg (145 g)	360	**180**	99
Chicken and Turkey with cheese	1 pkg (145 g)	380	**190**	90
Fun Pack				
Bologna	1 pkg (318 g)	530	**260**	126
Ham	1 pkg (318 g)	450	**180**	90
Turkey	1 pkg (318 g)	430	**170**	81
Ham and Cheddar	1 pkg (128 g)	340	**180**	99
Lean Turkey and Cheddar	1 pkg (128 g)	360	**200**	99
With dessert				
Chicken and Monterey Jack	1 pkg (176 g)	378	**160**	81
Popcorn				
Air-popped, no added fat	1 cup popped	30	**0**	0
Commercially Popped				
Bachman All Natural				
Air-Popped	2¾ cups	170	**100**	9
Cheese Popcorn	3 cups	160	**80**	9
with white Cheddar cheese	2½ cups	160	**80**	9
Boston's				
Caramel Popcorn	⅔ cup	120	**20**	0
Lite Popcorn	4 cups	140	**50**	5
Crunch 'n Munch Buttery Toffee				
Popcorn with Peanuts	⅔ cup	140	**35**	9
Fiddle Faddle Caramel				
Popcorn with peanuts	¾ cup	140	**50**	27
Smartfood, Butter-flavored	3 cups	150	**80**	18

SNACK FOODS

FOOD	AMOUNT	CALORIES		
		TOTAL	FAT	SAT-FAT
Popcorn, commercially popped (*cont.*)				
Utz				
Butter	2 cups	160	**110**	18
Caramel Corn Clusters	1¼ cups	160	**20**	0
Cheese	2 cups	120	**80**	14
White Cheddar Cheese	2 cups	150	**70**	14
Weight Watchers (Smart Snackers)				
Butter	1 pkg (19 g)	90	**20**	0
Butter Toffee	1 pkg (26 g)	110	**25**	9
Caramel	1 pkg (26 g)	110	**10**	9
White Cheddar Cheese	1 pkg (19 g)	100	**35**	0
Microwave				
Jolly Time Light	5 cups popped	120	**50**	9
Newman's Own Oldstyle				
Picture Show	3½ cups popped	170	**100**	18
Orville Redenbacher's				
Butter, snack-size	1 bag (50 g)	210	**130**	18
Natural	1 cup popped	30	**18**	0
Reden Budders	2 tbsp (36 g)	150	**90**	23
Smart Pop, butter	3 tbsp (45 g)	100	**15**	0
Pop·Secret				
Original Butter	4 cups popped	170	**110**	27
Buttery Burst	4 cups popped	170	**100**	27
Video Club Generic				
Butter Flavor Light	5 c	170	**60**	9
Natural	4½ c	200	**110**	23
Movie Theater				
Popped in coconut oil	kids (5 cups)	300	**180**	126
	sm (7 cups)	398	**243**	171
	med (11 cups)	647	**387**	279
	med (16 cups)	901	**540**	387
	lg (20 cups)	1161	**693**	495
Popped in coconut oil with butter topping	kid's (5 cups)	472	**333**	198
	sm (7 cups)	632	**450**	261
	med (11 cups)	910	**639**	369
	med (16 cups)	1221	**873**	504
	lg (20 cups)	1642	**1134**	657

SNACK FOODS

FOOD	AMOUNT	CALORIES		
		TOTAL	FAT	SAT-FAT
Popped in Canola shortening	sm (7 cups)	361	**198**	63
	med (11 cups)	627	**342**	108
	lg (16 cups)	850	**468**	144
Pop-Tarts				
Kellogg's				
Apple cinnamon	1 tart (52 g)	210	**50**	9
Blueberry	1 tart (52 g)	210	**60**	9
Brown sugar cinnamon	1 tart (50 g)	220	**80**	9
Chocolate fudge	1 tart (52 g)	200	**40**	9
Frosted blueberry or cherry	1 tart (52 g)	200	**50**	9
Frosted brown sugar cinnamon	1 tart (50 g)	210	**70**	9
Frosted choc vanilla creme	1 tart (52 g)	200	**50**	9
Frosted chocolate fudge	1 tart (52 g)	200	**40**	9
Frosted strawberry	1 tart (52 g)	200	**40**	9
Nutri-Grain, all flavors	1 bar (37 g)	140	**35**	5–9
S'Mores	1 tart (52 g)	200	**50**	5
Strawberry	1 tart (52 g)	210	**50**	9
Pretzels				
Buttermilk Ranch Pretzels (Snyders of Hanover)	⅓ cup	130	**45**	9
Cheez'n Pretzels	1 unit (24 g)	110	**50**	36
Hard (Wege)	1 pretzel (30 g)	110	**10**	0
Honey Mustard Pretzel Bits	11 pieces (28 g)	140	**70**	9
Honey Mustard and Onion				
Snyders of Hanover	⅓ cup	130	**95**	0
Utz	⅓ cup	80	**50**	9
Nibs	½ cup	110	**15**	0
Oat bran (Weight Watchers)	1 pkg (42 g)	170	**25**	0
Party Mix	25 pieces (30 g)	150	**70**	9
Petites	18 (30 g)	120	**10**	10
Sourdough Hard (Snyders of Hanover)	1 pretzel (28 g)	111	**0**	0
Cheddar Cheese	1 pretzel (28 g)	160	**70**	9
Stix (Snyders of Hanover)	32 sticks	100	**10**	0
Thin (Rold Gold)	10 (28 g)	110	**0**	0
Wheel (Utz)	20 (28 g)	110	**9**	0

SNACK FOODS

FOOD	AMOUNT	CALORIES		
		TOTAL	FAT	SAT-FAT
Snack Mixes				
Cheerios Snack Mix				
Cheddar Cheese	¾ cup	130	**45**	9
Original	¾ cup	130	**45**	9
Chex Mix (Ralston)				
Traditional	⅔ cup	150	**45**	9
Zesty Ranch	½ cup	130	**40**	9
Doo Dads Snack Mix	½ cup	150	**60**	9
Fiesta Fun Mix	½ cup	300	**180**	27
Gold Fish (Pepperidge Farm)				
Honey Mustard	½ cup	180	**90**	14
Nutty Deluxe	½ cup	180	**80**	14
Original	½ cup	170	**70**	14
Roasted Peanuts	½ cup	170	**70**	14
Seasoned	½ cup	170	**70**	9
Zesty Cheddar	½ cup	180	**90**	14
Party Mix				
Oriental	½ cup	300	**180**	27
Pastamore	½ cup	260	**100**	18
Sesame Walnut	½ cup	300	**180**	27
Smokehouse	½ cup	260	**160**	18
Swiss Mix	½ cup	380	**160**	72
Trail Mix	½ cup	300	**160**	27
Deluxe Super	½ cup	300	**120**	45
Tropical	½ cup	300	**120**	72
Vending Machine Foods (Lance)				
Cakes				
Brownies	1¾ oz/pkg	200	**81**	9
Dunking Sticks	5½ oz/pkg	380	**180**	54
Fig Cake	2⅛ oz/pkg	210	**27**	9
Oatmeal Cake	2 oz/pkg	240	**99**	27
Raisin Cake	2 oz/pkg	230	**90**	27
Candy				
Chocolaty Peanut Bar	2 oz/pkg	320	**162**	54
Peanut Bar	1¾ oz/pkg	260	**126**	27
Chips, etc.				
Cheese Balls	1⅛ oz/pkg	190	**117**	27
Corn Chips				
BBQ	1¾ oz/pkg	260	**144**	36
Plain	1¾ oz/pkg	270	**153**	27

SNACK FOODS

| FOOD | AMOUNT | CALORIES | | |
		TOTAL	FAT	SAT-FAT
Crunchy Cheese Twists	1½ oz/pkg	260	**144**	36
Gold-n-Chee	1⅜ oz/pkg	180	**81**	18
6-pak tray	6 oz/pkg	780	**432**	54
Jalapeno Cheese Tortilla Chips	1⅛ oz/pkg	160	**72**	18
Nacho Tortilla Chips	1⅛ oz/pkg	160	**72**	18
Popcorn				
Cheese	⅞ oz/pkg	130	**72**	9
Plain	1 oz/pkg	160	**90**	18
Pork Skins				
BBQ	½ oz/pkg	80	**45**	18
Plain	½ oz/pkg	80	**45**	18
Potato Chips				
BBQ	1⅛ oz/pkg	190	**108**	27
Cajun-style	2 oz/pkg	320	**180**	36
Plain	1⅛ oz/pkg	190	**135**	36
Sour Cream and Onion	1⅛ oz/pkg	190	**108**	27
Pretzel Twists	1½ oz/pkg	150	**9**	0
Cookies				
Apple-Cinnamon	2 oz/pkg	240	**72**	18
Apple-Oatmeal	1.65 oz/pkg	190	**63**	18
Blueberry	2 oz/pkg	240	**72**	18
Bonnie Sandwich	1³⁄₁₆ oz/pkg	160	**63**	18
Choc-O-Lunch	1⁵⁄₁₆ oz/pkg	180	**63**	18
	4½ oz/pkg	585	**203**	41
Choc-O-Mint	1¼ oz/pkg	180	**90**	27
Coated Graham	1⁵⁄₁₆ oz/pkg	200	**90**	36
Fig Bar	1½ oz/pkg	150	**18**	9
Fudge–Chocolate Chip	2 oz/pkg	260	**90**	36
Malt	1¼ oz/pkg	190	**99**	18
Nekot	1½ oz/pkg	210	**90**	18
Nut-O-Lunch	4½ oz/pkg	630	**243**	81
Oatmeal Cookies	2 oz/pkg	260	**90**	18
Peanut Butter Creme-Filled	1¾ oz/pkg	240	**90**	27
Soft Chocolate Chip	2 oz/pkg	260	**90**	36
Strawberry	2 oz/pkg	240	**72**	18
Van-O-Lunch	1⁵⁄₁₆ oz/pkg	180	**63**	18
	4½ oz/pkg	630	**162**	41
Crackers				
Captain's Wafers with Cream				
Cheese and Chives	1⁵⁄₁₆ oz/pkg	170	**81**	18

SNACK FOODS

FOOD	AMOUNT	CALORIES		
		TOTAL	FAT	SAT-FAT
Cheese-on-Wheat	1⁵⁄₁₆ oz/pkg	180	**81**	18
Lanchee	1¼ oz/pkg	180	**99**	18
Nip-Chee	1⁵⁄₁₆ oz/pkg	130	**81**	18
Peanut Butter Wheat	1⁵⁄₁₆ oz/pkg	190	**99**	18
Rye-Chee	1⁷⁄₁₆ oz/pkg	190	**81**	18
Spicy Gold-n-Chee	10 oz/pkg	1400	**540**	180
Thin Wheat Snacks	10 oz/pkg	1600	**720**	180
Toastchee	1⅜ oz/pkg	190	**99**	18
Toasty	1¼ oz/pkg	180	**90**	18
Nuts				
Cashews	1⅛ oz/pkg	190	**135**	27
long tube	2½ oz/pkg	400	**288**	54
Peanuts				
Honey-toasted	1⅜ oz/pkg	230	**153**	27
Roasted (shell)	1¾ oz/pkg	190	**135**	27
Salted	1⅛ oz/pkg	190	**135**	27
tube	3 oz/pkg	480	**360**	72
Pistachios	1⅛ oz/pkg	180	**126**	18
Pie				
Pecan Pie	3 oz/pkg	350	**135**	27

SOUPS

If you are keeping track of total fat calories and your soup is made with whole milk, add 100 fat calories and 206 total calories per can. With 2% milk, add 58 fat calories and 166 total calories per can. If you are keeping track of saturated fat and your soup is made with whole milk, add 62 sat-fat calories and 206 total calories per can. With 2% milk, add 37 sat-fat calories and 166 total calories per can.

FOOD	AMOUNT	CALORIES		
		TOTAL	FAT	SAT-FAT
Canned				
Condensed, prepared with water				
Campbell				
Bean with Bacon	1 cup prep.	180	**45**	18
Beef Broth	1 cup prep.	15	**0**	0
Beef Noodle	1 cup prep.	70	**25**	9

SOUPS

FOOD	AMOUNT	CALORIES		
		TOTAL	FAT	SAT-FAT
Campbell (*cont.*)				
Broccoli Cheese	1 cup prep.	110	60	27
Cheddar Cheese	1 cup prep.	150	90	45
Chicken Alphabet	1 cup prep.	80	20	9
Chicken Broth	1 cup prep.	30	20	5
Chicken and Dumplings	1 cup prep.	80	25	9
Chicken Gumbo	1 cup prep.	60	15	5
Chicken Noodle	1 cup prep.	70	25	9
Chicken NoodleO's	1 cup prep.	80	25	9
Chicken and Stars	1 cup prep.	70	20	5
Chicken with Rice	1 cup prep.	70	25	9
Chicken Vegetable	1 cup prep.	80	20	5
Chicken Won Ton	1 cup prep.	45	10	0
Consomme Beef	1 cup prep.	25	0	0
Cream of Asparagus	1 cup prep.	110	60	18
Cream of Celery	1 cup prep.	110	60	23
Cream of Chicken	1 cup prep.	130	70	27
Cream of Mushroom	1 cup prep.	110	60	23
Cream of Mushroom (Healthy Request)	1 cup prep.	70	30	9
Cream of Potato	1 cup prep.	90	25	14
Cream of Shrimp	1 cup prep.	100	60	18
Creamy Chicken Mushroom	1 cup prep.	130	80	23
Double Noodle	1 cup prep.	100	25	9
French Onion	1 cup prep.	70	25	0
Golden Mushroom	1 cup prep.	80	25	9
Green Pea	1 cup prep.	180	25	9
Homestyle Chicken Noodle	1 cup prep.	70	25	14
Italian Tomato	1 cup prep.	100	5	0
Manhattan Clam Chowder	1 cup prep.	70	20	5
Minestrone	1 cup prep.	90	20	9
New England Clam Chowder	1 cup prep.	90	25	5
Old-Fashioned Tomato Rice	1 cup prep.	120	20	5
Old-Fashioned Vegetable	1 cup prep.	70	25	5
Split Pea with Ham and Bacon	1 cup prep.	180	30	18
Tomato (Healthy Request)	1 cup prep.	90	20	5
Tomato Bisque	1 cup prep.	130	25	14
Turkey Noodle	1 cup prep.	80	25	9
Turkey Vegetable	1 cup prep.	80	25	9
Vegetable	1 cup prep.	90	15	5

SOUPS

FOOD	AMOUNT	CALORIES		
		TOTAL	FAT	SAT-FAT
Campbell (*cont.*)				
Vegetable Beef	1 cup prep.	80	**20**	9
Vegetarian Vegetable	1 cup prep.	90	**20**	0
Pepperidge Farm				
Gazpacho	⅔ cup	70	**20**	0
Ready to Serve				
Campbell's				
Chunky				
Beef	10¾ oz	200	**50**	18
Chicken Mushroom				
Chowder	1 cup	210	**110**	36
Hearty Vegetable with				
Pasta	1 cup	130	**25**	5
New England Clam				
Chowder	10¾ oz	300	**160**	63
Sirloin Burger	1 cup	190	**80**	32
Vegetable	10¾ oz	160	**35**	9
Healthy Request				
Chicken Broth	1 cup	20	**0**	0
Hearty Chicken Vegetable	1 cup	120	**20**	9
Home Cookin'				
Bean and Ham	1 cup	160	**25**	9
Chicken Noodle	10¾ oz	130	**30**	14
Old-Fashioned				
Vegetable Beef	1 cup	150	**45**	14
Progresso Pasta Soups				
Hearty Penne in Chicken				
Broth	1 cup	70	**10**	0
Hearty Vegetable and Rotini	1 cup	110	**10**	0
Dehydrated				
Knorr's				
Black Bean	1 pkg (53 g)	200	**10**	0
Chicken Flavor Vegetable	1 pkg (30 g)	100	**0**	0
Hearty Lentil	1 pkg (57 g)	220	**0**	0
Navy Bean	1 pkg (38 g)	140	**0**	0
Potato Leek	1 pkg (34 g)	120	**0**	0

SOUPS

FOOD	AMOUNT	CALORIES		
		TOTAL	FAT	SAT-FAT
Nissin Top Ramen				
Cup Noodles Ramen Noodle Soup				
Chicken flavor	1 pkg (64 g)	300	**110**	54
Oodles of Noodles, all flavors	½ pkg (43 g)	200	**70**	36
Soup Starter (Borden)				
Beef Vegetable	⅛ pkg (28 g dry)	90	**5**	0
Chicken Noodle	⅛ pkg (24 g dry)	80	**5**	0
The Spice Hunter				
Hunan Noodle	1 pkg (29 g)	110	**10**	0
Szechwan Noodle	1 pkg (33 g)	130	**5**	0
Homemade or Restaurant				
Cream of Mushroom	1 cup	170	**155**	98
French Onion	1 cup	350	**125**	65
Gazpacho	1 cup	111	**80**	11
New England Clam Chowder	1 cup	230	**145**	65
Vichyssoise	1 cup	315	**210**	140
Mix				
Matzo Ball	2 tbsp	80	**0**	0

SWEETS

FOOD	AMOUNT	CALORIES		
		TOTAL	FAT	SAT-FAT
Brownies				
Fudge (Little Debbie)	2 (61 g)	270	**120**	23
Low-fat (Hostess)	1 (40 g)	140	**25**	5
Nonfat (Entenmann's)	1 (40 g)	110	**0**	0
with Nuts	1 (40 g)	180	**80**	18
without Nuts	1 (40 g)	160	**60**	18
Brownie mixes				
Betty Crocker				
Fudge	1 (34 g)	200	**80**	16
White Chocolate Swirl	1 (33 g)	180	**70**	25
Duncan Hines				
Chocolate Lover's	1 (31 g)	160	**60**	11

SWEETS

FOOD	AMOUNT	CALORIES		
		TOTAL	FAT	SAT-FAT
Pillsbury				
Cream Cheese Swirl	1 (30 g)	190	**80**	23
Fudge	1 (30 g)	200	**80**	14
Hot Fudge	1 (31 g)	160	**60**	18
Buns				
Breakfast	1 (55 g)	170	**25**	9
Butterfly	1 (55 g)	190	**35**	9
Cinnamon Raisin				
(Entenmann's)	1 (61 g)	160	**0**	0
Honey (Morton)	1 (64 g)	250	**90**	23
Hot Cross	1	168	**56**	16
Rum	1 (55 g)	190	**45**	9
Sticky	1 (55 g)	210	**70**	14
Entenmann's	1 (71 g)	270	**100**	18
Cakes (Bakery, Homemade, and Restaurant)				
Almond Danish coffee cake	⅛ cake (57 g)	230	**100**	18
Almond poppy seed loaf	⅕ cake (80 g)	330	**130**	23
Angel food	1/12 cake	125	**0**	0
Angel food loaf	2″ slice (55 g)	150	**5**	0
Angel food ring	⅙ cake (47 g)	130	**5**	0
Apple Danish coffee cake	⅛ cake (57 g)	160	**60**	18
Baked Alaska	1/12	263	**112**	60
Banana nut loaf	2″ slice (76 g)	270	**120**	27
Bavarian chocolate	2 × 2″ square (80 g)	340	**180**	63
Black Forest	1 slice (80 g) (7″ diam.)	330	**170**	41
Blueberry cheese coffee cake	⅛ cake (57 g)	170	**70**	18
Boston cream	⅙ cake (113 g)	320	**120**	27
Carrot	1 slice (80 g) (7″ diam.)	300	**130**	36
Cheesecake	1/12 cake	280	**162**	89
Blueberry-topped	⅙ cake (113 g)	350	**180**	81
French	4″ wedge (125 g)	370	**200**	54
Cherry pudding	⅛ cake (74 g)	290	**130**	23
Chocolate crunch ring	⅛ cake (71 g)	310	**140**	36
Chocolate fudge	1 slice (80 g) (7″ diam.)	300	**140**	32
Chocolate marble loaf	⅕ cake (80 g)	340	**150**	32

SWEETS

FOOD	AMOUNT	CALORIES		
		TOTAL	FAT	SAT-FAT
Chocolate sheet cake				
with vanilla icing	1 slice (80 g)	320	**160**	36
Cinnamon sticks	1 stick (57 g)	200	**60**	14
Cupcake	1 (80 g)	340	**140**	36
Devil's food fudge	⅙ cake (85 g)	340	**140**	36
Devil's food layer with white	2½" wedge			
icing	(80 g)	360	**170**	45
Fruitcake	1 slice (125 g)	470	**171**	32
German chocolate	⅟₁₆ cake			
	(10" diam.)	521	**277**	27
Golden coconut	1 slice (80 g)			
	(7" diam.)	320	**160**	36
Hazelnut torte	⅟₁₆ torte	315	**187**	56
Ladyfingers	12 (85 g)	280	**35**	14
Lemon crunch ring	⅛ cake (71 g)	270	**110**	23
Lemon Supreme	1 slice (80 g)			
	(7" diam.)	320	**160**	36
Pecan cinnamon ring	⅛ cake (71 g)	300	**130**	23
Pecan twirls sweet rolls	2 twirls (56 g)	220	**80**	9
Pound	2" slice (80 g)	300	**140**	45
Strawberry cheese Danish				
coffee cake	⅛ cake (57 g)	170	**80**	18
Yellow layer				
with chocolate icing	2½" wedge			
	(80 g)	320	**140**	36
with white icing	2½" wedge			
	(80 g)	350	**170**	45

Cakes and Snack Cakes, by Brand Name
Entenmann's
All Butter Pound Loaf	¼ cake (85 g)	330	**130**	81
Apple Puffs	1 puff (85 g)	260	**110**	27
Assorted Rugelach	1 piece (21 g)	100	**60**	41
Cheese Coffee Cake	⅑ cake (54 g)	190	**70**	42
Cheese Crumb Babka	⅟₁₀ danish (57 g)	220	**90**	42
Cheese-Filled Crumb Coffee				
Cake	⅛ cake (57 g)	210	**90**	36
Cinnamon Filbert Ring	⅙ danish (61 g)	270	**150**	27
Cinnamon Rugelach	1 piece (21 g)	100	**60**	32
Crumb Coffee Cake	⅟₁₀ cake (57 g)	250	**110**	27

SWEETS

FOOD	AMOUNT	CALORIES TOTAL	CALORIES FAT	CALORIES SAT-FAT
Entenmann's Fat-and-Cholesterol-Free				
Apple Spice	⅕ cake (79 g)	200	**0**	0
Banana Crunch	⅕ cake (85 g)	220	**0**	0
Banana Loaf	⅙ cake (76 g)	190	**0**	0
Blueberry Crunch	⅙ cake (76 g)	180	**0**	0
Chocolate Crunch	⅕ cake (79 g)	210	**0**	0
Chocolate Loaf	⅕ cake (85 g)	210	**0**	0
Golden Chocolatey Chip Loaf	⅕ cake (85 g)	220	**0**	0
Golden Loaf	¼ cake (85 g)	220	**0**	0
Lemon Twist	⅛ danish (53 g)	130	**0**	0
Marble Loaf	⅙ cake (71 g)	200	**0**	0
Mocha Iced Chocolate	⅙ cake (85 g)	200	**0**	0
Pineapple Crunch	⅙ cake (76 g)	190	**0**	0
Raspberry Cheese Pastry	⅑ cake (54 g)	140	**0**	0
Raspberry Twist	⅛ danish (53 g)	140	**0**	0
Hostess				
Blueberry Muffin Loaf	1 muffin (108 g)	440	**170**	27
Cinnamon Crumb, low-fat	2 cakes (51 g)	150	**10**	0
Cup Cakes with Creamy Filling	2 cakes (91 g)	330	**100**	45
Cup Cakes, reduced-fat	2 cakes (77 g)	240	**25**	5
HoHos	3 cakes (85 g)	370	**160**	108
Suzy Q's	1 cake (58 g)	220	**80**	36
Twinkies	2 cakes (77 g)	280	**80**	27
Little Debbie				
Apple Delights	1 cake (35 g)	140	**40**	14
Apple Streusel Coffee Cake	2 cakes (57 g)	220	**70**	9
Chocolate Chip Snack Cake	2 cakes (68 g)	290	**130**	27
Creme-Filled Snack Cake	2 cakes (71 g)	300	**130**	23
Devil Square	1 wrap (62 g)	260	**110**	27
Fudge Round	1 cake (34 g)	140	**50**	9
Marshmallow Pie	1 pie (39 g)	160	**50**	27
Marshmallow Supreme	1 cake (32 g)	130	**45**	9
Oatmeal Creme Pie	1 pie (38 g)	170	**70**	14
Oatmeal Light	1 wrap (38 g)	140	**50**	9
Strawberry Shortcake Roll	1 roll (61 g)	230	**70**	14
Swiss Cake Roll	2 cakes (61 g)	250	**110**	27
Zebra Cake	2 cakes (74 g)	320	**150**	27

SWEETS

FOOD	AMOUNT	CALORIES		
		TOTAL	FAT	SAT-FAT
Pepperidge Farm				
Chocolate Fudge	⅙ cake (80 g)	300	**140**	45
Chocolate Mousse	⅛ cake (73 g)	250	**100**	27
Classic Carrot	⅛ cake (80 g)	350	**190**	36
Devil's Food	⅙ cake (80 g)	290	**122**	45
Sara Lee				
All Butter Pound Cake	⅙ cake (76 g)	310	**150**	81
Butter Streusel Coffee Cake	⅙ cake (54 g)	220	**110**	54
Crumb Coffee Cake	⅛ cake (57 g)	220	**80**	14
Double Chocolate Layer	⅛ cake (79 g)	260	**110**	99
Flaky Coconut Layer	⅛ cake (81 g)	280	**130**	108
French Cheesecake	⅙ cake (111 g)	350	**190**	127
Original Cream Cheesecake	¼ cake (121 g)	350	**160**	81
Pecan Coffee Cake	⅙ cake (54 g)	220	**110**	54
Strawberry French Cheesecake	⅙ cake (123 g)	320	**130**	81
Strawberry Shortcake	⅛ cake (71 g)	180	**70**	45
Tastykake				
Butterscotch Krimpets	3 cakes (85 g)	320	**70**	18
Chocolate Cupcakes	2 cakes (60 g)	220	**60**	14
Chocolate Junior Yellow Layer	1 cake (94 g)	360	**120**	23
Chocolate Kandy Kakes	4 cakes (76 g)	360	**150**	90
Creme-Filled Chocolate Cupcake	2 cakes (64 g)	200	**25**	9
Butter Cream–Iced	2 cakes (64 g)	250	**70**	18
Chocolate-Iced	2 cakes (64 g)	250	**70**	18
Creme-Filled Koffee Kake	2 cakes (57 g)	240	**80**	18
Fudge Bar	1 bar (43 g)	170	**60**	9
Koffee Kake	1 cake (71 g)	270	**80**	14
Oatmeal Raisin Bar	1 bar (43 g)	190	**60**	14
Peanut Butter Kandy Kake	4 cakes (76 g)	370	**170**	81
Tasty Minis, Creme-Filled Chocolate Cupcakes				
Butter Creme–Iced	4 cakes (57 g)	240	**80**	18
Chocolate-Iced	4 cakes (57 g)	240	**80**	18
Koffee Kake	4 cakes (51 g)	210	**80**	14
Vanilla Cupcake, Chocolate-Iced	4 cakes (57 g)	220	**70**	14
Weight Watchers				
Double Fudge	1 dessert (78 g)	190	**40**	9

SWEETS

FOOD	AMOUNT	CALORIES		
		TOTAL	FAT	SAT-FAT
Cake Mixes				
Angel food	¹⁄₁₂ cake	140	**0**	0
Betty Crocker				
Peanut Butter–Chocolate Swirl	¹⁄₁₂ cake	240	**90**	23
Duncan Hines				
Butter Recipe	¹⁄₁₀ cake	320	**140**	63
Caramel, Raspberry, White, Yellow, Fudge Marble, or Spice	¹⁄₁₂ cake	250	**100**	23
Devil's Food	¹⁄₁₂ cake	290	**130**	27
Pillsbury				
Banana Bread	¹⁄₁₂ loaf	170	**50**	9
Blueberry Bread	¹⁄₁₂ loaf	180	**60**	0
Butter Recipe	¹⁄₁₂ cake	260	**110**	54
Chocolate Caramel Nut	¹⁄₁₆ cake	290	**170**	36
Date Bread	¹⁄₁₂ loaf	160	**25**	0
Devil's Food	¹⁄₁₂ cake	270	**130**	27
Double Hot Fudge	¹⁄₁₆ cake	310	**150**	63
Funfetti	¹⁄₁₂ cake	240	**80**	18
Lemon	¹⁄₁₀ cake	310	**120**	27
Strawberry Cream Cheese	¹⁄₁₆ cake	300	**150**	41
Yellow	¹⁄₁₂ cake	260	**110**	27
Candy				
Almond Joy	1 pkg (49 g)	240	**120**	81
Andes				
Creme de Menthe Thins	8 pieces (38 g)	200	**110**	90
Toasted Coconut Thins	8 pieces (38 g)	210	**120**	99
Baby Ruth	1 bar (59.5 g)	280	**110**	63
Fun size	2 bars (42 g)	200	**80**	45
Butterfinger, fun size	2 bars (42 g)	200	**70**	36
Caramels				
Chocolate (Riesen)	5 pieces (40 g)	180	**60**	27
Creams (Goetze's)	3 pieces (36 g)	135	**30**	9
Plain				
Brach's	4 pieces (37 g)	150	**35**	9
Kraft	5 pieces (41 g)	170	**30**	9
Carob peanut clusters	1 piece (28 g)	150	**90**	36
Carob raisins	40 pieces (41 g)	160	**45**	36
Chocolate-covered peanuts	15 pieces (40 g)	220	**120**	54
Chocolate-covered peanut clusters	3 pieces (43 g)	230	**130**	63

SWEETS

| FOOD | AMOUNT | CALORIES | | |
		TOTAL	FAT	SAT-FAT
Chocolate-covered fudge mix	14 pieces (40 g)	190	70	36
Chocolate Mint Pattie (Brach)	3 pieces (36 g)	140	26	18
Dots	12 pieces (43 g)	150	0	0
Fondant (mints, candy corn, other)	1 oz	105	0	0
French burnt peanuts	28 pieces (40 g)	190	80	9
Good and Plenty	33 pieces (40 g)	130	0	0
Gumdrops	1 oz	100	0	0
Gummi Bears	10 pieces (40 g)	140	0	0
Halvah (Joyva)				
Chocolate-covered	½ bar (57 g)	380	210	45
Chocolate-flavored	½ bar (57 g)	390	230	36
Marble	½ bar (57 g)	390	230	36
Hard	1 oz	110	0	0
Heath Sensations	⅓ bag (43 g)	220	120	63
Hershey's Chocolate				
Cookies 'n' Mint	1 bar (43 g)	230	110	54
Hugs	8 pieces (38 g)	210	110	72
Kisses	8 pieces (39 g)	210	110	72
with almonds	8 pieces (38 g)	210	120	63
Milk Chocolate	1 bar (43 g)	230	120	81
with Almonds	1 bar (41 g)	230	130	63
Miniatures	5 pieces (42 g)	230	130	72
Hot Tamales	19 pieces (40 g)	150	0	0
Jellybeans	1 oz	105	0	0
Jordan almonds	13 pieces (42 g)	200	70	9
Jujy Fruits	15 pieces (40 g)	160	0	0
Kit Kat	1 bar (42 g)	220	110	72
Licorice sticks	4 pieces (37 g)	120	0	0
M & M's				
Peanut	1 bag (49.3 g)	250	120	45
Plain	1 bag (47.9 g)	230	90	54
Semi-Sweet Mini	1 tbsp (14 g)	70	35	18
Malted Milk Balls	17 pieces (40 g)	180	60	60
Marshmallows (Kraft)	5 pieces (34 g)	110	0	0
Mighty Malts	10 pieces (42 g)	200	60	60
Milk Chocolate–Covered Jots	39 pieces (40 g)	190	60	36
Milk Chocolate Peanut Jots	17 pieces (40 g)	200	90	27
Milk Duds	13 pieces (40 g)	170	50	36
Milky Way	1 bar (61 g)	280	100	45
Mr. Goodbar	1 bar (42 g)	280	160	63
Mounds Bar	1 bar (53 g)	250	120	99

SWEETS

FOOD	AMOUNT	CALORIES		
		TOTAL	FAT	SAT-FAT
Necco Mints	2 pieces (6 g)	24	0	0
Nerds	1 box (11 g)	40	0	0
Nestlé				
Crunch, fun size	4 bars (39 g)	200	90	54
Milk Chocolate Giant Bar	¼ bar (35 g)	190	100	54
Nonpareils (dark chocolate)	17 pieces (41 g)	200	80	54
Pastel Mints (Petite)	¼ cup	210	100	18
Payday	1 bar (52 g)	240	110	90
Peanut brittle	40 g	180	40	9
Peanut Butter Cups (Estee)	5 candies (38 g)	200	110	63
Peanut Chews (Goldenberg's)	3 pieces (37 g)	180	80	18
Planters				
Chocolate Crisp, bite-size	13 pieces (30 g)	140	60	18
Peanut Butter Chocolate	4 pieces (42 g)	230	130	45
Peanut Butter Crisp	12 pieces (31 g)	150	70	14
Raisinets (Nestlé)	¼ cup	200	70	36
Raisins, chocolate-covered	34 pieces (40 g)	170	60	45
Reese's				
Miniatures	5 pieces (39 g)	210	110	45
NutRageous	1 bar (45 g)	250	140	36
Peanut Butter Cup	2 cups	240	130	54
Rolo	1 package (54 g)	260	110	81
Skittles (all flavors)	¼ cup	170	15	0
	1 bag (61.5 g)	250	25	5
Snickers	1 bar (59 g)	280	120	45
Peanut Butter	1 bar (57 g)	310	180	63
3 Musketeers	1 bar (60.4 g)	260	70	36
Fun size	2 bars (33.2 g)	140	40	23
Tootsie Roll				
Midgie	6 pieces (40 g)	160	25	5
Pop	1 pop (17 g)	60	0	0
Snack Bar	2 bars (28 g)	110	20	0
Whitman's				
Bars				
Cookies-n-Cream	1 bar (28 g)	150	80	63
Super Extra Crispy	1 bar (21 g)	120	60	27
Super Extra Dark	1 bar (28 g)	140	80	54
Super Extra Milk	1 bar (28 g)	160	90	45
Sampler				
Assorted Chocolates	3 pieces (40 g)	200	100	54
Assorted Creams	3 pieces (40 g)	180	70	45

SWEETS

FOOD	AMOUNT	CALORIES		
		TOTAL	FAT	SAT-FAT
Whitman's				
Sampler (*cont.*)				
Dark Chocolate	3 pieces (40 g)	200	90	54
Milk Chocolate	3 pieces (40 g)	200	90	54
Nut, Chewy, and Crisp	3 pieces (40 g)	200	110	54
Whoppers Malted Milk Balls	7 pieces (45 g)	210	80	63
Yogurt-covered				
Almond	11 pieces (42 g)	210	120	63
Peanut	17 pieces (41 g)	210	120	54
Pretzel	⅓ cup	140	45	36
Raisin	30 pieces (41 g)	180	60	45
York Peppermint Pattie	1 bar (42 g)	170	35	23
	3 pieces (41 g)	170	35	23
Cookies and Bars				
Assorted				
Biscotti	1 piece (30 g)	270	20	5
Mundle Bread	2 pieces (30 g)	140	50	14
Archway cookies				
Apple-Filled Oatmeal	1 (28 g)	110	30	5
Apple n' Raisin	1 (30 g)	130	40	9
Chocolate Chip and Toffee	1 (29 g)	140	60	14
Coconut Macaroon	1 (23 g)	90	45	36
Frosty Lemon	1 (28 g)	120	45	9
Fruit Bar	1 (28 g)	90	0	0
Gingersnap	5 (30 g)	130	40	9
Granola	2 (28 g)	100	0	0
Lemon Snap	5 (30 g)	150	70	14
Oatmeal	1 (27 g)	110	25	9
Date-Filled	1 (28 g)	110	35	9
Iced	1 (28 g)	120	45	9
Raisin	1 (28 g)	100	0	0
Ruth's Golden	1 (28 g)	120	40	9
Old-Fashioned Molasses	1 (27 g)	120	30	9
Raspberry-Filled	1 (28 g)	110	40	9
Rocky Road	1 (28 g)	130	60	14
Delicious cookies				
Animal Cracker	9 (28 g)	130	45	14
Assorted Sandwiches	2 (26 g)	120	45	18
Assorted Sugar Wafers	4 (29 g)	160	80	18
Banana Rama	2 (25 g)	120	40	18
Butter Thin	10 (29 g)	110	45	18

SWEETS

FOOD	AMOUNT	CALORIES		
		TOTAL	FAT	SAT-FAT
Delicious cookies (*cont.*)				
Chocolate Chip Thin	10 (29 g)	110	**45**	18
Coconut Bar	3 (28 g)	140	**60**	27
Coconut Sandwich	3 (33 g)	150	**50**	27
Cookie Legend				
Chocolate Chip	3 (31 g)	150	**60**	18
Fudge Graham	2 (25 g)	120	**50**	36
Fudge Mint	4 (28 g)	140	**60**	36
Pecan Shortbread	2 (36 g)	180	**90**	14
Duplex Sandwich	2 (26 g)	120	**45**	18
English Toffee made with				
Heath	2 (30 g)	145	**72**	18
Fig Bar	2 (36 g)	115	**35**	9
Ginger Snap	4 (29 g)	130	**30**	5
Graham				
Cinnamon	2 (27 g)	130	**45**	5
Honey Graham	2 (27 g)	120	**30**	9
Land O Lakes Frosted Butter	2 (35 g)	180	**90**	9
Lemon Sandwich	3 (33 g)	150	**50**	27
Musselman's Apple Sauce				
Oatmeal	2 (32 g)	130	**35**	9
Oatmeal	2 (28 g)	120	**45**	9
Iced	2 (28 g)	120	**40**	9
Peanut Butter Sandwich	3 (33 g)	155	**50**	27
Shortbread	5 (30 g)	140	**50**	27
Skippy and Welch's Peanut				
Butter and Jelly Sandwich	1 (26 g)	120	**60**	14
Strawberry Sandwich	3 (33 g)	150	**50**	27
Sugar	2 (28 g)	130	**40**	9
Vanilla Sandwich	2 (26 g)	120	**45**	18
Vanilla Wafer	8 (28 g)	110	**15**	9
Entenmann's cookies				
Chocolate Chip	3 (30 g)	140	**60**	18
Entenmann's Fat-and-				
Cholesterol-Free				
Chocolate Brownie	2 (24 g)	80	**0**	0
Estee cookies				
Chocolate Chip	4 (31 g)	150	**60**	18
Chocolate Sandwich	3 (34 g)	160	**50**	14
Oatmeal Raisin	4 (34 g)	130	**40**	9
Peanut Butter Sandwich	3 (34 g)	160	**60**	9

SWEETS

FOOD	AMOUNT	CALORIES		
		TOTAL	FAT	SAT-FAT
Vanilla	4 (28 g)	140	**50**	9
Vanilla Sandwich	3 (34 g)	160	**50**	9
Famous Amos cookies				
Chocolate Chip	4 (30 g)	130	**50**	18
Fifty 50 cookies				
Chocolate Chip	4 (32 g)	170	**90**	27
Frookie cookies				
Apple Cinnamon Oat Bran	2 (21 g)	100	**35**	5
Chocolate Chip	2 (21 g)	90	**45**	5
Dream Cream				
Strawberry Yogurt Cream Wafer	2 (15 g)	70	**36**	18
Vanilla Yogurt Cream Wafer	2 (15 g)	70	**36**	18
Fig Fruits	2 (30 g)	110	**18**	0
Honey Graham	2 (30 g)	110	**25**	5
Oatmeal Raisin	2 (21 g)	90	**30**	5
Keebler cookies				
Chocolate Chip				
Chips Deluxe	1 (16 g)	80	**40**	14
Chips Deluxe Bakery Crisp	3 (36 g)	180	**80**	27
Chocolate Lover's	1 (17 g)	90	**40**	23
Rainbow Chips Deluxe	1 (16 g)	80	**35**	18
Soft Batch	1 (16 g)	80	**35**	9
Chocolate Fudge Sandwich	1 (17 g)	80	**35**	9
Coconut Chocolate Drop	1 (16 g)	80	**45**	18
Elfin Delight				
Caramel Apple Oatmeal	1 (18 g)	70	**15**	9
Chocolate Sandwich				
with Fudge Creme	3 (34 g)	150	**30**	9
with Vanilla Creme	3 (34 g)	150	**30**	9
Creme Sandwich	3 (35 g)	150	**30**	9
E. L. Fudge				
Butter-Flavored Chocolate Sandwich	3 (34 g)	170	**70**	18
Chocolate Sandwich with Vanilla Creme Filling	3 (35 g)	170	**70**	18
Fudge Sandwich	3 (34 g)	160	**60**	18
Fudge Vanilla Creme	1 (17 g)	80	**30**	9
French Vanilla Creme	1 (17 g)	80	**30**	9

SWEETS

FOOD	AMOUNT	TOTAL	FAT	SAT-FAT
		CALORIES		
Keebler cookies (*cont.*)				
Fudge 'n Caramel	2 (24 g)	120	**50**	36
Fudge Stick	3 (29 g)	150	**70**	41
Fudge Stripe	3 (32 g)	160	**70**	41
Graham crackers				
Chocolate	8 (31 g)	140	**50**	14
Cinnamon Crisp	8 (30 g)	140	**40**	9
Cinnamon Crisp (low-fat)	8 (28 g)	110	**10**	5
Deluxe Fudge-Covered	3 (28 g)	140	**60**	41
Honey	8 (31 g)	150	**50**	14
Honey (low-fat)	9 (31 g)	120	**15**	5
Grasshopper	4 (30 g)	150	**60**	45
PB Fudgebutter	2 (24 g)	130	**70**	36
Pecan Sandie	1 (16 g)	80	**45**	9
Sweet Spot	1 pkg (23 g)	120	**50**	27
Toffee Sandie	2 (26 g)	130	**70**	18
Vanilla Wafer	8 (31 g)	150	**60**	18
Little Debbie cookies				
Figaroo	2 (43 g)	160	**35**	5
Fudge Macaroo	1 (29 g)	140	**70**	36
Lemon Stix	1 (44 g)	220	**90**	23
Nutty Bar	2 (57 g)	290	**150**	27
Oatmeal Light	1 (38 g)	140	**50**	9
Peanut Butter Bar	2 (54 g)	270	**130**	23
Peanut Butter Natural	1 wrap (44 g)	230	**120**	18
Star Crunch	1 (31 g)	140	**60**	9
Supreme	1 (32 g)	130	**45**	9
Lu cookies				
The Little Schoolboy	2 (25 g)	130	**60**	27
Le Petit-Beurre	4 (33 g)	150	**35**	18
Mrs. Wright's cookies				
Animal	6 (28 g)	130	**45**	14
Chocolate Chip	2 (31 g)	160	**70**	27
Chocolate Devil's Food	2 (34 g)	120	**10**	0
Creme Wafer	5 (28 g)	140	**60**	14
Devil's Food Sandwich				
Creme	2 (30 g)	140	**50**	9
Dutch Apple Bar	2 (35 g)	120	**15**	5
Fig Bar	2 (35 g)	120	**30**	9
Whole-Wheat	2 (35 g)	120	**30**	9

SWEETS

FOOD	AMOUNT	CALORIES		
		TOTAL	FAT	SAT-FAT
Ginger Lotta Snap	6 (30 g)	130	35	9
Graham				
Fudge	1 (24 g)	120	50	36
Honey Graham	4 (28 g)	130	30	0
Lemon Sandwich Creme	2 (30 g)	130	40	9
Oatmeal	2 (26 g)	130	50	14
Striped Shortbread	2 (27 g)	140	70	36
Sugar	2 (28 g)	140	60	18
Vanilla Sandwich Creme	2 (30 g)	140	60	18
Murray cookies				
Assortment	5 (27 g)	120	45	14
Butter	8 (30 g)	130	40	9
Duplex Creme	3 (28 g)	130	60	14
Lemon Creme	3 (28 g)	130	60	14
Sugar Wafer	6 (33 g)	130	20	0
Vanilla Creme	3 (28 g)	130	60	14
Vanilla Wafer	8 (28 g)	120	25	9
Nabisco cookies				
Apple Newtons, fat-free	2 (29 g)	100	0	0
Barnum's Animal Cracker	12 (31 g)	140	35	5
Biscos Sugar Wafer	3 (28 g)	140	60	14
Brown Edge Wafer	5 (29 g)	140	50	14
Cameo Creme Sandwich	2 (28 g)	130	40	9
Chips Ahoy!	3 (32 g)	160	70	23
Chewy	3 (36 g)	170	70	23
Chunky	1 (17 g)	80	40	27
reduced-fat	3 (32 g)	150	50	14
Sprinkled	3 (36 g)	170	70	23
Chocolate Teddy Graham	24 (30 g)	140	40	9
Cranberry Newtons, fat-free	2 (29 g)	100	0	0
Famous Chocolate Wafer	5 (32 g)	140	35	14
Fig Newton	2 (31 g)	110	25	9
fat-free	2 (29 g)	100	0	0
Fudge-Striped Shortbread	3 (32 g)	160	70	14
Ginger Snap	4 (28 g)	120	25	5
Grahams				
Cinnamon	5 (32 g)	140	25	5
Honey	4 (28 g)	120	25	5
Fudge-Covered	3 (28 g)	140	60	14
Lorna Doone Shortbread	4 (29 g)	140	60	9
Mallomars	2 (26 g)	120	45	27

SWEETS

| FOOD | AMOUNT | CALORIES | | |
		TOTAL	FAT	SAT-FAT
Nabisco cookies (*cont.*)				
Marshmallow Twirl	1 (30 g)	130	**50**	14
Mystic Mint Sandwich	1 (17 g)	90	**35**	9
Nilla Wafers	8 (32 g)	140	**40**	9
Nutter Butter				
Bites	10 (30 g)	150	**60**	14
Peanut Creme Patties	5 (31 g)	160	**80**	14
Peanut Butter Sandwich	2 (28 g)	130	**50**	9
Oatmeal	1 (17 g)	80	**30**	5
Iced Oatmeal	1 (17 g)	80	**25**	5
Oreos				
Chocolate Sandwich	3 (33 g)	160	**60**	14
Double Stuf Chocolate				
Sandwich	2 (28 g)	140	**60**	14
Fudge-Covered	1 (21 g)	110	**50**	14
Mini Oreo	9 (30 g)	140	**60**	14
White Fudge–Covered	1 (21 g)	110	**50**	14
Pinwheels	1 (30 g)	130	**45**	23
Raspberry Newton, fat-free	1 (20 g)	70	**0**	0
Social Tea Biscuit	6 (28 g)	120	**30**	5
SnackWell's (*see listing after* **Safeway Select Cookies**)				
Strawberry Newton	1 (20 g)	70	**0**	0
Vanilla Sandwich	3 (35 g)	170	**70**	18
Pepperidge Farm cookies				
Beacon Hill	1 (26 g)	130	**60**	18
Bordeaux	4 (28 g)	130	**50**	23
Milk Chocolate	3 (32 g)	160	**80**	32
Brussels	3 (30 g)	150	**60**	27
Charleston	1 (26 g)	130	**60**	23
Chesapeake Chocolate				
Chunk Pecan	1 (26 g)	140	**70**	14
Chessmen	3 (26 g)	120	**45**	27
Chocolate Chip	3 (28 g)	140	**60**	23
Dessert Favorite	3 (33 g)	170	**80**	27
Fruitful				
Apricot Raspberry Cup	3 (32 g)	140	**50**	18
Cherry Cobbler	1 (17 g)	70	**25**	9
Peach Tart	2 (30 g)	120	**25**	9
Raspberry Tart	2 (30 g)	120	**25**	9
Strawberry Cup	3 (32 g)	140	**50**	18
Geneva	3 (31 g)	160	**80**	32
Ice Cream Favorite	5 (33 g)	180	**90**	23

SWEETS

FOOD	AMOUNT	TOTAL	FAT	SAT-FAT
			CALORIES	
Lido	1 (17 g)	90	40	14
Milano	3 (34 g)	180	90	41
Double Chocolate	2 (28 g)	150	70	27
Hazelnut	2 (25 g)	130	70	18
Milk Chocolate	3 (35 g)	180	90	32
Mint	2 (26 g)	140	70	32
Orange	2 (26 g)	140	70	23
Nantucket Chocolate Crunch	1 (26 g)	130	60	27
Old-Fashioned				
Brownie Chocolate Nut	3 (30 g)	160	80	27
Chocolate Chip	3 (28 g)	140	60	23
Ginger Man	4 (27 g)	120	35	9
Lemon Nut Crunch	3 (31 g)	170	80	18
Oatmeal Raisin	3 (34 g)	160	60	14
Shortbread	2 (26 g)	140	70	23
Sugar	3 (30 g)	140	60	14
Party Favorites Assortment	3 (32 g)	170	80	27
Santa Fe Oatmeal Raisin	1 (26 g)	120	40	9
Sausalito Milk Chocolate Macademia	1 (26 g)	140	70	18
Soft-Baked				
Chocolate Chunk	1 (26 g)	130	50	23
Milk Chocolate Macademia	1 (26 g)	130	60	23
Oatmeal Raisin	1 (26 g)	110	40	9
Tahoe White Chunk Macademia	1 (26 g)	130	70	27
Rippin' Good cookies				
Assorted Creme Wafers	3 (28 g)	140	60	14
Chocolate Chip	3 (32 g)	150	60	18
Chocolate Chip Sandwich	2 (31 g)	150	60	18
Coconut Bar	3 (26 g)	130	50	23
Cookie Jar Assortment	3 (33 g)	150	60	18
Duplex Sandwich	3 (34 g)	160	50	14
Frosted Fudgie	3 (32 g)	140	50	14
Granola and Peanut Butter Sandwich	2 (31 g)	150	60	23
Holly Jolly Wafer	4 (33 g)	170	80	45
Iced Spice	3 (32 g)	130	25	5
Lemon Crisp	3 (32 g)	160	70	14

SWEETS

FOOD	AMOUNT	CALORIES TOTAL	FAT	SAT-FAT
Rippin' Good cookies (*cont.*)				
Macaroon Sandwich	2 (31 g)	150	**60**	23
Mini Bits Striped Daintie	13 (30 g)	140	**50**	27
Oatmeal	3 (32 g)	150	**50**	14
Iced	3 (36 g)	150	**40**	9
Striped	2 (28 g)	150	**70**	36
Peanut Butter Sandwich	2 (31 g)	150	**50**	14
Sugar	3 (32 g)	150	**60**	14
Toffee 'n Creme Sandwich	2 (31 g)	150	**60**	14
Vanilla Sandwich	3 (34 g)	160	**50**	14
Safeway Select cookies				
Biscotti				
Chocolate dipped in				
Dark Chocolate	2 (38 g)	170	**80**	36
White Chocolate	2 (38 g)	170	**80**	36
The Original	2 (38 g)	150	**60**	23
dipped in Dark				
Chocolate	2 (38 g)	170	**70**	36
Very Chocolate	2 (32 g)	160	**70**	14
Very Peanut Butter				
Chocolate Chip Oatmeal	2 (32 g)	160	**80**	14
Very Raisin Oatmeal	2 (32 g)	150	**50**	14
SnackWell's Cookies				
(Nabisco)				
Chocolate Chip	13 (29 g)	130	**30**	14
Chocolate Sandwich	2 (25 g)	100	**20**	5
Creme Sandwich	2 (26 g)	110	**20**	5
Double Fudge Cookie Cake				
Fat-free	1 (16 g)	50	**0**	0
Oatmeal Raisin	2 (27 g)	110	**25**	0
Stella D'Oro cookies				
Fruit Delight	1 (23 g)	70	**0**	0
Fruit Slice	1 (17 g)	50	**0**	0
Sunshine cookies				
Almond Crescent	4 (31 g)	150	**50**	15
Fig Bar	2 (28 g)	110	**25**	5
Ginger Snap	7 (29 g)	130	**40**	9
Golden Fruit				
Apple Biscuit	1 (20 g)	70	**10**	0

SWEETS

| FOOD | AMOUNT | CALORIES | | |
		TOTAL	FAT	SAT-FAT
Golden Fruit (*cont.*)				
Cranberry Biscuit	1 (20 g)	70	**10**	0
Raisin Biscuit	1 (20 g)	70	**10**	0
Graham				
Cinnamon	2 (31 g)	140	**50**	14
Honey	2 (28 g)	120	**40**	9
Hydrox Chocolate Sandwich				
Creme	3 (31 g)	150	**60**	18
Reduced-fat	3 (31 g)	130	**35**	9
Lemon Cooler	5 (30 g)	140	**50**	14
Oatmeal	3 (35 g)	170	**60**	14
Iced	2 (29 g)	130	**45**	27
Oh! Berry Strawberry Wafer	8 (28 g)	100	**0**	0
Peanut Butter Sugar Wafer	4 (32 g)	170	**80**	18
Sugar Wafer	3 (26 g)	130	**60**	14
Sunshine Classic				
Chocolate Chip	1 (19 g)	100	**50**	23
Chocolate Chip Shortbread	1 (19 g)	100	**60**	18
Chocolate Chip with Walnuts	1 (19 g)	100	**50**	23
Chocolate Chocolate Chip	1 (19 g)	90	**50**	18
Vanilla Wafer	7 (31 g)	150	**60**	14
Vienna Finger	2 (29 g)	140	**50**	14
Reduced-fat	2 (29 g)	130	**30**	5
Twix cookies				
Chocolate Caramel	1 (29 g)	140	**60**	23
Chocolate Peanut Butter	1 (25 g)	130	**70**	27
Weight Watchers Smart Snackers cookies				
Chocolate Chip	2 (30 g)	140	**45**	18
Chocolate Sandwich	3 (31 g)	140	**35**	9
Oatmeal Raisin	2 (30 g)	140	**15**	0
Vanilla Sandwich	3 (31 g)	120	**25**	9
Cookies and Bars, Mixes				
Apple Streusel (Pillsbury)	1 bar	150	**50**	14
Cheesecake Bar				
Lemon (Pillsbury)	1 bar	170	**90**	32
Strawberry Swirl (Betty Crocker)	1 bar	210	**110**	32
Oreo Bar (Pillsbury)	1 bar	150	**50**	14

SWEETS

| FOOD | AMOUNT | CALORIES | | |
		TOTAL	FAT	SAT-FAT
Cookies, Ready-to-Make				
Chocolate Chip (Pillsbury)	2	140	**60**	14
Sugar (Pillsbury)	2	130	**45**	14
Danish Pastry				
Almond or pecan	1 (55 g)	220	**100**	18
Blueberry	1 (55 g)	190	**80**	18
Cheese	1 (110 g)	380	**170**	45
Cherry Cheese	1 (100 g)	360	**140**	45
Coconut	1 (55 g)	210	**80**	27
Danish Ring				
Pecan	⅛ ring (57 g)	230	**100**	23
Walnut	⅛ ring (55 g)	240	**120**	23
Danish Twist (Entenmann's)				
Cinnamon	⅙ danish (61 g)	260	**130**	27
Raspberry	⅙ danish (53 g)	220	**100**	27
Lemon-filled	1 (100 g)	350	**140**	32
Orange Danish (Pillsbury, ready-to-make)	1 (41 g)	140	**50**	14
Donuts				
Bakery				
Apple raisin rosebud	1 (55 g)	220	**90**	23
Carrot cake	1 (80 g)	340	**160**	41
Chocolate-iced yellow cake	1 (55 g)	230	**90**	27
Cinnamon rosebud	1 (64 g)	260	**110**	36
Custard creme–filled	1 (65 g)	240	**130**	63
Glazed (Krispy Kreme)	1 (38 g)	180	**100**	27
Glazed yeast-raised	1 (55 g)	240	**130**	36
Honey wheat	1 (80 g)	340	**150**	36
Lemon custard–filled	1 (65 g)	190	**140**	36
Old-fashioned	1 (62 g)	270	**140**	36
Sour cream	1 (80 g)	340	**160**	36
Entenmann's				
Crumb-Topped donuts	1 (60 g)	260	**110**	27
Devil's Food Crumb	1 (60 g)	250	**110**	32
Rich Frosted	1 (57 g)	280	**170**	54
Hostess				
Cinnamon Donettes	4 (61 g)	240	**90**	36
Frosted	1 (40 g)	180	**100**	63
Powdered Donettes	4 (61 g)	250	**100**	36
Little Debbie				
Donut Sticks	1 stick (47 g)	210	**110**	27

SWEETS

FOOD	AMOUNT	CALORIES		
		TOTAL	FAT	SAT-FAT
Dumplings, Turnovers, and Strudel				
Apple Dumpling (Pepperidge Farm)	1 (85 g)	290	**99**	23
Apple-filled pastry	1 (64 g)	190	**45**	9
Apple fritter	1 (70 g)	300	**130**	32
Apple strudel	1 piece (64 g)	200	**90**	27
Apple turnover (Pepperidge Farm)	1 (89 g)	330	**130**	27
Apricot-filled pastry	1 roll (64 g)	200	**50**	9
Apricot strudel	1 piece (64 g)	220	**100**	27
Custard-filled pastry	1 (64 g)	190	**40**	9
Peach Dumpling (Pepperidge Farm)	1 (85 g)	320	**99**	23
Toaster Strudel Pillsbury (all flavors)	1 (54 g)	180	**60**	14
Frosting				
Betty Crocker				
Creamy Deluxe, Vanilla	2 tbsp	140	**45**	14
Frosting Partner				
Cream cheese frosting/ strawberry topping	2 tbsp	130	**35**	14
Dark chocolate frosting/ raspberry topping	2 tbsp	130	**45**	14
Milk chocolate frosting/ fudge topping	2 tbsp	140	**50**	23
Vanilla frosting/lemon topping	2 tbsp	130	**35**	14
Duncan Hines				
Caramel	2 tbsp	140	**50**	14
Vanilla, Raspberries, and Cream	2 tbsp	140	**50**	14
Pillsbury				
Chocolate Fudge	2 tbsp	140	**50**	14
Milk Chocolate	2 tbsp	140	**50**	14
Frozen Custard				
Kohr Brothers				
Light, Vanilla and Chocolate	4 fl oz	130	**50**	36
Frozen Yogurt, Grocery Store Freezer Compartment				
Ben and Jerry's				
Cherry Garcia	½ cup	170	**30**	18

SWEETS

FOOD	AMOUNT	CALORIES		
		TOTAL	FAT	SAT-FAT
Breyers				
Chocolate Chip Cookie Dough	½ cup	170	**45**	18
Colombo				
Shoppe Style				
Bavarian Chocolate Chunk	½ cup	170	**50**	27
Cappuccino Coffee Bean	½ cup	170	**40**	23
Caramel Pecan Chunk	½ cup	170	**40**	18
Chocolate Chip Cookie Dough	½ cup	170	**45**	27
Old World Chocolate	½ cup	120	**15**	9
Toffee Bar Crunch	½ cup	180	**60**	36
Vanilla Chocolate Twist	½ cup	120	**15**	9
White Chocolate Almond	½ cup	200	**70**	45
Slender Scoops, all flavors	½ cup	90–100	**0**	0
Dannon				
Light Nonfat, all flavors	½ cup	80–90	**0**	0
Pure Indulgence				
Crunchy Expresso	½ cup	160	**40**	27
Vanilla	½ cup	130	**20**	9
Elan Low-Fat				
Vanilla	½ cup	130	**25**	14
Häagen-Dazs				
Chocolate	½ cup	160	**25**	14
Coffee	½ cup	160	**25**	14
Strawberry Cheesecake Craze	½ cup	220	**70**	36
Vanilla	½ cup	160	**25**	14
Häagen-Dazs Bars				
Piña Colada	1 bar (70 g)	90	**10**	5
Raspberry and Vanilla	1 bar (71 g)	90	**10**	0
Kemp's				
Chocolate	½ cup	110	**25**	18
Fudge Marble	½ cup	110	**0**	0
Peach	½ cup	90	**0**	0
Pralines and Caramel	½ cup	150	**35**	18
Strawberry	½ cup	90	**0**	0
Vanilla	½ cup	120	**25**	18
Stonyfield Farm				
Chocolate Mint Chip	4 fl oz	140	**30**	27
Decaf French Roast	4 fl oz	100	**0**	0

SWEETS

FOOD	AMOUNT	CALORIES		
		TOTAL	FAT	SAT-FAT
Double Raspberry	4 fl oz	120	**0**	0
Mocha Almond Fudge	4 fl oz	150	**35**	0
Very Vanilla	4 fl oz	100	**0**	0
TCBY				
Honey Almond Vanilla	½ cup	150	**25**	14
Strawberry White Chocolate				
Almond Crunch	½ cup	130	**20**	14
Triple Chocolate Brownie	½ cup	150	**25**	14
TCBY Yog-A-Bar				
Vanilla	1 bar (63 g)	160	**80**	54
Vanilla Crunch	1 bar (67 g)	200	**110**	63
Vanilla with Heath Toffee	1 bar (67 g)	190	**100**	63

Frozen Yogurt, Yogurt or Ice Cream Shop

Colombo (These figures are for 1 fl oz. Ask the server for the number of ounces in your serving.)

FOOD	AMOUNT	TOTAL	FAT	SAT-FAT
Lite (nonfat)	1 fl oz	25	**0**	0
Low-fat	1 fl oz	28	**4**	2
Peanut butter low-fat	1 fl oz	30	**6**	1
ICBIY				
Nonfat	sm (6¾ fl oz)	135	**0**	0
	med (9⅓ fl oz)	187	**0**	0
	lg (12 fl oz)	240	**0**	0
Original	sm (6¾ fl oz)	182	**43**	NA
	med (9⅓ fl oz)	251	**59**	NA
	lg (12 fl oz)	324	**76**	NA
TCBY				
Nonfat	sm (5 fl oz)	138	**0**	0
	med (7 fl oz)	193	**0**	0
	lg (9 fl oz)	248	**0**	0
Original	sm (5 fl oz)	163	**38**	23
	med (7 fl oz)	228	**53**	32
	lg (9 fl oz)	293	**68**	41

Ice Cream
Ben & Jerry's

FOOD	AMOUNT	TOTAL	FAT	SAT-FAT
Ice Cream				
Aztec Harvests Coffee	½ cup	250	**130**	90
Deep Dark Chocolate	½ cup	250	**130**	81
Double Chocolate Fudge				
Swirl	½ cup	250	**140**	81
Mocha Fudge	½ cup	250	**150**	81
Vanilla	½ cup	230	**150**	90

SWEETS

FOOD	AMOUNT	CALORIES		
		TOTAL	FAT	SAT-FAT
Ben & Jerry's				
Ice Cream (*cont.*)				
Vanilla Bean	½ cup	230	**150**	90
White Russian	½ cup	240	**140**	90
Peace Pops				
Chocolate Chip Cookie				
Dough	1 (145 g)	510	**270**	117
English Toffee Crunch	1 (135 g)	420	**250**	162
Breyers				
Strawberry	½ cup	130	**60**	36
Viennetta				
Chocolate	1 slice	190	**100**	72
All other flavors	1 slice	190	**100**	63
Dove Bar				
Dark Chocolate Chocolate	1 (79 g)	270	**150**	99
Dark Chocolate Vanilla	1 (78 g)	260	**150**	99
French Vanilla Bite-Size	5 (103 g)	370	**210**	135
Milk Chocolate Vanilla	1 (77 g)	260	**150**	99
Vanilla	1 (98 g)	230	**200**	126
Edy's Grand				
Ice Cream				
Cherry Chocolate Chip	½ cup	150	**80**	45
Chocolate	½ cup	140	**80**	45
Chocolate Chip Cookie				
Dough	½ cup	170	**80**	45
Chocolate Fudge Sundae	½ cup	140	**70**	36
Cookies 'n Cream	½ cup	160	**80**	45
Crunchy Cone	½ cup	160	**80**	54
Ice Cream Sandwich	½ cup	150	**70**	45
Malt Ball 'n Fudge	½ cup	150	**70**	45
Strawberry	½ cup	120	**50**	36
Vanilla Bean	½ cup	150	**80**	54
Light Ice Cream				
Almond Praline	½ cup	110	**35**	18
Cheesecake Chunk	½ cup	120	**45**	27
Chocolate Chip Cookie				
Dough	½ cup	120	**40**	23
Chocolate Fudge Mousse	½ cup	110	**35**	23
Cookies 'n Cream	½ cup	110	**40**	23
French Silk	½ cup	120	**45**	27
Rocky Road	½ cup	120	**40**	23

SWEETS

FOOD	AMOUNT	CALORIES		
		TOTAL	FAT	SAT-FAT
Tangerine Dream	½ cup	100	35	18
Vanilla	½ cup	100	35	23
Eskimo Pie				
Chocolate-Coated Vanilla				
Bar	1 bar (75 ml)	150	90	54
Eskimo Pie	2½ fl oz (75 ml)	150	90	54
with Crisped Rice	1 bar (52 g)	160	100	54
Sandwich	1 (96 ml)	170	60	18
Good Humor				
Candy Center Crunch	1 bar (88.7 ml)	260	170	126
Chocolate Chip Cookie				
Sandwich	1 (118 ml)	300	120	72
Chocolate Eclair	1 bar (89 ml)	170	80	27
King Cone	1 cone (136 ml)	300	90	54
Original Ice Cream Bar	1 bar (89 ml)	190	90	72
Popsicle (Twister)	1 piece (52 ml)	45	0	0
Sidewalk Sundae	1 cone (118 ml)	280	140	90
Strawberry Shortcake	1 bar (89 ml)	160	80	36
Toasted Almond	1 bar (89 ml)	190	80	36
Häagen-Dazs				
Exträas				
Caramel Cone Explosion	1 bar (93 g)	350	210	126
Iced Cappuccino	1 bar (96 g)	330	220	126
Strawberry Cheesecake				
Craze	½ cup	290	160	90
Ice Cream				
Butter Pecan	½ cup	320	220	99
Chocolate	½ cup	270	160	99
Chocolate Chocolate Chip	½ cup	300	180	108
Coffee	½ cup	270	160	99
Cookies and Cream	½ cup	270	160	99
Macadamia Brittle	½ cup	300	180	99
Rum Raisin	½ cup	270	160	90
Strawberry	½ cup	250	150	90
Vanilla Fudge	½ cup	280	160	99
Vanilla Swiss Almond	½ cup	310	190	99
Ice Cream Bar				
Vanilla and Almonds	1 bar (106 g)	370	240	126
Vanilla and Dark				
Chocolate	1 bar (112 g)	390	240	162

SWEETS

FOOD	AMOUNT	CALORIES		
		TOTAL	FAT	SAT-FAT
Häagen-Dazs				
Ice Cream Bar (*cont.*)				
Vanilla and Milk				
Chocolate	1 bar (100 g)	330	**220**	126
Sherbet				
Raspberry Sorbet and				
Cream	½ cup	190	**80**	45
Heath				
Ice Cream Bar	1 bar (49 g)	160	**110**	72
Healthy Choice Low-Fat				
Ice Cream				
Cappuccino Chocolate				
Chunk	½ cup	120	**20**	9
Fudge Brownie	½ cup	120	**20**	9
Peanut Butter Cookie				
Dough 'n Fudge	½ cup	120	**20**	9
Praline and Caramel	½ cup	130	**20**	5
Rocky Road	½ cup	140	**20**	9
Vanilla	½ cup	100	**20**	14
Klondike				
Chocolate	1 piece (148 ml)	280	**180**	126
Gold	5 fl oz (148 ml)	390	**230**	135
Krispy	1 piece (148 ml)	300	**180**	117
Krunch	1 piece (89 ml)	200	**110**	72
Lite				
Original	1 piece (74 ml)	110	**50**	36
Sandwiches	1 piece (83 ml)	100	**20**	14
Vanilla (The Original)	1 piece (148 ml)	290	**180**	126
Vanilla Ice Cream Sandwich	1 piece (148 ml)	250	**80**	54
Lucerne				
Vanilla Ice Cream	½ cup	150	**70**	45
Mattus' Low-Fat Ice Cream				
Caramel Crunch	½ cup	190	**27**	9
Chocolate	½ cup	160	**27**	18
Chocolate Chocolate Cookie	½ cup	170	**27**	18
Coffee	½ cup	170	**27**	18
Cookies and Cream	½ cup	190	**27**	9
Honey Vanilla	½ cup	160	**27**	18
Len and Cherries	½ cup	170	**27**	9
Vanilla	½ cup	170	**27**	18

SWEETS

| FOOD | AMOUNT | CALORIES | | |
		TOTAL	FAT	SAT-FAT
Milky Way				
Ice Cream Bar, Dark	1 bar (51 g)	170	**80**	36
Low Fat Milk Shake	1 cup	220	**30**	18
Nestlé				
Bon Bon	9 pieces (103 g)	370	**230**	135
Cool Creation				
Ice Pop	1 pop (65 g)	50	**0**	0
Mickey Mouse Ice Cream				
Bar	1 bar (44 g)	110	**60**	27
Special Movie Edition Ice				
Cream Cone	1 cone (85 g)	280	**120**	81
Surprise Ice Pop	1 pop (64 g)	60	**0**	0
Crunch				
reduced-fat	1 bar (50 g)	130	**60**	45
Vanilla	1 bar (60 g)	200	**120**	81
Drumstick Sundae Cone				
Vanilla	1 cone (103 g)	350	**180**	99
Vanilla Caramel	1 cone (108 g)	360	**180**	108
Flintstones Push-Up				
Cool Cream Sherbet Treat	1 tube (60 g)	90	**20**	9
Original Sherbet Treat	1 tube (64 g)	100	**20**	9
Pebbles Ice Cream Treat	1 tube (50 g)	120	**60**	36
Snickers				
Ice Cream Bar	4 bars (108 g)	390	**220**	81
Trix				
Pops	1 bar (53 g)	40	**0**	0
Weight Watchers				
Chocolate Mousse	2 bars (82 g)	70	**10**	5
English Toffee Crunch Bar	1 bar (41 g)	120	**60**	32
Orange Vanilla Treat	2 bars (80 g)	70	**10**	5
Vanilla Sandwich Bar	1 bar (68 g)	160	**35**	18
Weight Watchers Sweet Celebrations				
Brownie à la Mode	1 dessert (91 g)	190	**40**	9
Chocolate Chip Cookie				
Dough Sundae	½ cup (77 g)	180	**35**	14
Double Fudge Brownie				
Parfait	1 parfait (109 g)	190	**25**	18
Praline Toffee Crunch Parfait	1 parfait (104 g)	190	**25**	18

SWEETS

FOOD	AMOUNT	CALORIES		
		TOTAL	FAT	SAT-FAT
Ice Cream Cones				
Cake	1 cone	16	9	<9
Sugar	1 cone	60	9	<9
Ice Cream Toppings				
Hershey's				
Candy Bar Sprinkles	2 tbsp	140	45	27
Chocolate Chips	1 oz	140	72	45
Coconut	2 tbsp	58	37	33
Reese's Sprinkles	2 tbsp	160	70	45
Juice Bars				
Fruit 'n Juice, all flavors				
(Dole)	1 bar	70	0	0
Fruit Juice Bar, all flavors				
(Dole)	1 bar	45	0	0
Pies (Bakery, Homemade, or Restaurant)				
Apple	⅙ pie (104 g)	280	120	36
Boston cream	1/12 pie	370	153	83
Cherry	⅙ pie (104 g)	310	120	32
Cherry Beehive (Entenmann's)	⅕ pie (130 g)	270	0	0
Coconut custard	¼ pie (139 g)	410	200	81
Dutch apple	⅙ pie (104 g)	290	110	27
Lemon meringue	⅙ pie (113 g)	290	120	36
Peach	⅙ pie (104 g)	300	100	23
Pecan	⅙ pie (113 g)	440	200	45
Sweet potato	⅙ pie (104 g)	270	80	23
Snack Pies				
Hostess				
Apple Fruit	1 pie (122 g)	410	170	81
Blueberry Fruit	1 pie (122 g)	400	150	72
Cherry Fruit	1 pie (122 g)	430	170	81
Tastykake				
Chocolate-Iced Tasty-Klair	1 pie (113 g)	410	180	45
French Apple	1 pie (120 g)	360	110	27
Pies, Frozen				
Mrs. Smith's				
Bake and Serve				
Apple	⅙ pie (123 g)	270	100	18
Apple Cranberry	⅙ pie (123 g)	280	100	18
Blackberry	⅙ pie (123 g)	280	100	18

SWEETS

FOOD	AMOUNT	CALORIES		
		TOTAL	FAT	SAT-FAT
Bake and Serve (*cont.*)				
Blueberry	⅙ pie (123 g)	260	**100**	18
Cherry	⅙ pie (123 g)	270	**100**	18
Coconut Custard	⅕ pie (142 g)	280	**110**	45
Dutch Apple Crumb	⅙ pie (123 g)	310	**110**	23
Mince	⅙ pie (123 g)	300	**100**	18
Pumpkin Custard	¹⁄₁₀ pie (130 g)	230	**60**	18
Handy-to-Serve				
Pecan	⅕ pie (136 g)	520	**210**	36
Old-Fashioned				
Apple	⅛ pie (131 g)	370	**160**	32
Cherry	⅛ pie (131 g)	320	**120**	23
Peach	⅛ pie (131 g)	310	**120**	23
Ready-to-Serve				
Apple	⅕ pie (69 g)	310	**120**	23
Boston Creme	⅛ pie (131 g)	170	**50**	14
French Silk Chocolate	⅕ pie (136 g)	410	**190**	54
Lemon Meringue	⅕ pie (136 g)	300	**70**	18
Pecan	⅕ pie (136 g)	520	**210**	36
Thaw and Serve				
Banana Cream	¼ pie (96 g)	250	**80**	23
Chocolate Cream	¼ pie (96 g)	290	**130**	36
Lemon Cream	¼ pie (96 g)	270	**120**	27
Thaw and Serve Smart-Style				
All fruit flavors	⅙ pie (95 g)	180	**25**	5
Blueberries and Cheese Yogurt	⅙ pie (80 g)	160	**45**	14
Peaches and Cheese Yogurt	⅙ pie (80 g)	170	**45**	14
Strawberries and Banana Yogurt	⅙ pie (80 g)	160	**27**	5
Sara Lee				
Chocolate Cream	⅕ pie (136 g)	500	**280**	144
Coconut Cream	⅕ pie (136 g)	480	**280**	126
Lemon Meringue	⅙ pie (142 g)	350	**100**	23
Pie, Mixes				
No Bake Chocolate Silk Pie (Jell-O)	⅙ pie (45 g)	310	**140**	54
Pie Crusts				
Graham Cracker (Keebler Ready)	⅛ 9″ crust	110	**45**	9

SWEETS

FOOD	AMOUNT	CALORIES		
		TOTAL	FAT	SAT-FAT
Hershey's Chocolate (Keebler Ready)	⅛ 9" crust	110	**45**	9
2 pie-crust shell				
Mrs. Smith's	⅛ 9" crust	80	**35**	9
Richford	⅛ 9" crust	80	**45**	18
2 pie-crust shell, deep-dish pie				
Mrs. Smith's	⅛ 9" crust	90	**50**	9
Puddings				
Chocolate				
Fat-free	4 oz	100	**0**	0
Hershey's Kisses	4 oz	180	**50**	14
Jell-O	4 oz	160	**45**	18
Snack Pack (Hunt's), all flavors	4 oz	150–160	**50**	14
Tapioca (Swiss Miss)	4 oz	140	**35**	9
Vanilla (Swiss Miss)	4 oz	160	**50**	14
Puddings, Restaurant				
Caramel bavarian cream	½ cup	246	**128**	73
Chocolate mousse	½ cup	324	**199**	115
Crème caramel	1 cup	303	**125**	27
Custard, baked	1 cup	305	**125**	61
Sugars, Syrups, etc.				
Honey	1 tbsp	65	**0**	0
Jams, Jellies, and Preserves	1 tbsp	55	**0**	0
Molasses	1 tbsp	43	**0**	0
Sugar				
Brown, firmly packed	1 tbsp	51	**0**	0
	½ cup	410	**0**	0
White				
Granulated	1 tsp	16	**0**	0
	½ cup	385	**0**	0
Powdered, sifted	1 cup	385	**0**	0
Syrups				
Chocolate (Hershey's)	2 tbsp	100	**9**	0
Corn	1 tbsp	61	**0**	0
Maple	1 tbsp	61	**0**	0

SWEETS

FOOD	AMOUNT	CALORIES TOTAL	FAT	SAT-FAT
Miscellaneous				
Baklava (Apollo)	4½ pieces (125 g)	540	**280**	45
Carob Chips	1 oz (2⅔ tbsp)	140	**63**	52
Chocolate				
baking, unsweetened	1 oz	145	**135**	81
chips	1 oz	140	**72**	45
semi-sweet	30 chips (15 g)	70	**35**	23
Chocolate Eclairs	1	239	**122**	40
Custard cream puffs	1	303	**163**	63
Escalloped Apples (Stouffer's)	⅔ cup	180	**25**	0
Gelatin dessert	½ cup	70	**0**	0
Puff Pastry, frozen (Pepperidge Farm)				
Sheets	⅙ sheet (41 g)	200	**100**	23
Shells	1 shell (47 g)	230	**130**	27

VEGETABLES AND VEGETABLE PRODUCTS

See also **FROZEN, MICROWAVE, AND REFRIGERATED FOODS.**

FOOD	AMOUNT	CALORIES TOTAL	FAT	SAT-FAT
Alfalfa seeds, sprouted, fresh	1 cup	10	**0**	0
Artichoke				
fresh	1 medium	65	**0**	0
	1 large	83	**0**	0
cooked	1 medium	53	**0**	0
hearts				
canned in water	½ cup	35	**0**	0
marinated, undrained	½ cup	190	**135**	18
Asparagus				
fresh	½ cup	15	**0**	0
	4 spears	13	**0**	0
cooked	½ cup	22	**0**	0
	4 spears	15	**0**	0
Baked beans, canned				
Brown Sugar and Bacon (Campbell's)	½ cup	170	**25**	9

VEGETABLES AND VEGETABLE PRODUCTS

		CALORIES		
FOOD	AMOUNT	TOTAL	FAT	SAT-FAT
Baked beans, canned (*cont.*)				
Plain or Vegetarian	½ cup	117	**5**	2
in Tomato Sauce				
(Campbell's)	½ cup	130	**20**	9
Pork 'n Beans (Hanover)	½ cup	120	**15**	5
with beef	½ cup	160	**42**	20
with franks	½ cup	184	**76**	27
with pork	½ cup	134	**18**	7
and sweet sauce	½ cup	141	**17**	7
and tomato sauce	½ cup	124	**12**	5
Bamboo shoots				
fresh	1 cup	41	**0**	0
cooked	1 cup	15	**0**	0
canned	1 cup	25	**0**	0
Beans				
Black				
dry	1 cup	661	**25**	6
boiled	1 cup	227	**8**	2
Great Northern				
dry	1 cup	621	**19**	6
boiled	1 cup	210	**7**	2
canned	1 cup	300	**9**	3
Kidney				
dry	1 cup	613	**14**	2
boiled	1 cup	225	**8**	1
canned	1 cup	208	**7**	1
Kidney, California red				
dry	1 cup	607	**0**	0
boiled	1 cup	219	**0**	0
Kidney, red				
dry	1 cup	619	**18**	3
boiled	1 cup	225	**8**	1
canned	1 cup	216	**8**	1
Kidney, royal red				
dry	1 cup	605	**7**	1
boiled	1 cup	218	**3**	0
Lima, baby				
fresh	1 cup	216	**6**	1
boiled	1 cup	188	**5**	1
Lima, large				
fresh	1 cup	176	**11**	3

VEGETABLES AND VEGETABLE PRODUCTS

FOOD	AMOUNT	CALORIES TOTAL	FAT	SAT-FAT
Beans				
Lima, large (*cont.*)				
boiled	1 cup	208	**6**	1
canned	1 cup	186	**4**	1
Navy				
dry	1 cup	697	**24**	6
boiled	1 cup	259	**9**	2
canned	1 cup	296	**10**	3
Pink				
dry	1 cup	721	**21**	6
boiled	1 cup	252	**7**	2
Pinto				
dry	1 cup	656	**20**	4
boiled	1 cup	235	**8**	2
canned	1 cup	186	**7**	1
Refried				
canned (Del Monte)	1 cup	260	**32**	10
Mexican restaurant	¾ cup	375	**146**	60
Snap				
fresh	1 cup	34	**0**	0
cooked	1 cup	44	**0**	0
canned	1 cup	36	**0**	0
Soy				
dry	1 cup	774	**334**	48
boiled	1 cup	298	**139**	20
Soy products				
miso	1 cup	565	**150**	22
tofu	1 piece (2½ × 2¾ × 1 in)	88	**50**	7
White, small				
dry	1 cup	723	**23**	4
boiled	1 cup	253	**10**	1
Yellow				
fresh	1 cup	676	**46**	12
boiled	1 cup	254	**17**	4
Beets				
fresh	1 cup slices	60	**0**	0
	2 beets	71	**0**	0
cooked	1 cup slices	52	**0**	0
	2 beets	31	**0**	0
canned, drained	1 cup	54	**0**	0

VEGETABLES AND VEGETABLE PRODUCTS

		CALORIES		
FOOD	AMOUNT	TOTAL	FAT	SAT-FAT
Black-eyed or cowpeas, cooked	1 cup	190	0	0
Broadbeans				
fresh	1 cup	511	21	3
boiled	1 cup	186	6	1
canned	1 cup	183	5	0
Broccoli				
fresh	1 cup chopped	24	0	0
	1 spear	42	0	0
cooked	1 cup chopped	46	0	0
	1 spear	53	0	0
Brussels sprouts, cooked	1 cup	60	0	0
	1 sprout	8	0	0
Cabbage				
fresh	1 cup shredded	16	0	0
	1 head	215	0	0
cooked	1 cup shredded	32	0	0
	1 head	270	0	0
Cabbage, Chinese				
fresh	1 cup shredded	9	0	0
cooked	1 cup shredded	20	0	0
Cabbage, red				
fresh	1 cup shredded	19	0	0
cooked	1 cup shredded	32	0	0
Cabbage, Savoy				
fresh	1 cup shredded	19	0	0
cooked	1 cup shredded	35	0	0
Carob flour	1 tbsp	14	0	0
Carrots				
fresh	1	31	0	0
	1 cup shredded	48	0	0
cooked	1 cup sliced	70	0	0
Carrot juice	1 cup	98	0	0
Cauliflower, fresh or cooked	3 flowerets	13	0	0
	1 cup pieces	24	0	0
Celery, fresh	1 stalk	6	0	0
	1 cup dices	18	0	0
Chard, Swiss				
fresh	1 cup chopped	6	0	0
	1 leaf	9	0	0
cooked	1 cup chopped	35	0	0

VEGETABLES AND VEGETABLE PRODUCTS

		CALORIES		
FOOD	**AMOUNT**	**TOTAL**	**FAT**	**SAT-FAT**
Chickpeas or garbanzos				
dry	1 cup	729	**109**	11
boiled	1 cup	269	**38**	4
canned	½ cup	110	**18**	3
Chili with beans, canned	1 cup	286	**126**	54
Coleslaw (*see also* **FAST FOODS**)				
made with mayonnaise	1 cup	171	**161**	34
Collard greens, cooked	1 cup chopped	27	**0**	0
Corn				
cooked	1 ear	85	**9**	1
	1 cup kernels	178	**15**	3
canned, cream style	1 cup	186	**10**	1
popped (*see* **SNACKS**)				
Cucumber, fresh	1 cucumber	39	**0**	0
	1 cup slices	14	**0**	0
Dandelion greens				
fresh	1 cup chopped	25	**0**	0
cooked	1 cup chopped	35	**0**	0
Eggplant				
fresh	1 eggplant	27	**0**	0
cooked	1 cup cubes	27	**0**	0
Endive, fresh	1 cup chopped	8	**0**	0
	1 head	86	**0**	0
Garlic, fresh	1 clove	4	**0**	0
Kale				
fresh	1 cup chopped	33	**0**	0
cooked	1 cup chopped	41	**0**	0
Leeks				
fresh	1	76	**0**	0
	¼ cup	16	**0**	0
cooked	1	38	**0**	0
	¼ cup	8	**0**	0
Lentils				
dry	1 cup	649	**17**	2
boiled	1 cup	231	**7**	1
Lettuce, fresh				
Boston butterhead	1 head (5-in)	21	**0**	0
crisphead, iceberg	1 head (6-in)	70	**0**	0
	1 wedge	20	**0**	0
	1 cup chopped	5	**0**	0

VEGETABLES AND VEGETABLE PRODUCTS

		CALORIES		
FOOD	AMOUNT	TOTAL	FAT	SAT-FAT
Lettuce, fresh (*cont.*)				
looseleaf, romaine	1 cup	10	0	0
Mushrooms				
fresh, sliced or chopped	1 cup	20	0	0
	1 lb	127	0	0
cooked	1 cup	42	0	0
canned	1 cup	38	0	0
Mushrooms, shiitake				
dried	4	44	0	0
cooked	4	44	0	
	1 cup	80	0	0
Okra				
fresh	8 pods	36	0	0
	1 cup	38	0	0
cooked	8 pods	27	0	0
	1 cup	50	0	0
Onions				
fresh	1 cup	54	0	0
cooked	1 cup	58	0	0
fried onion rings, frozen	7 rings	285	168	54
Onions, green, fresh	1 cup	26	0	0
Parsley, fresh	10 sprigs	3	0	0
Parsnips				
fresh	1 cup	100	0	0
cooked	1 cup	126	0	0
Peas, green				
fresh	1 cup	118	0	0
cooked	1 cup	134	0	0
Peas, split				
fresh	1 cup	671	21	0
boiled	1 cup	231	7	0
Peas and carrots, canned	1 cup	96	6	0
Peas and onions, canned	1 cup	122	8	0
Peppers				
hot chili, fresh	1	18	0	0
	½ cup	30	0	0
jalapeño	½ cup	17	0	0
sweet, fresh	1	18	0	0
	½ cup	12	0	0
sweet, cooked	1	13	0	0
	½ cup	12	0	0

VEGETABLES AND VEGETABLE PRODUCTS

		CALORIES		
FOOD	AMOUNT	TOTAL	FAT	SAT-FAT
Potatoes				
au gratin	1 cup	320	**167**	104
baked in skin	1 (2/lb)	145	**0**	0
	1 lb	325	**0**	0
boiled in skin	1	173	**0**	0
	1 (3/lb)	104	**0**	0
	1 cup	118	**0**	0
	1 lb	345	**0**	0
boiled, pared before cooking	1 (2/lb)	146	**0**	0
	1 (3/lb)	88	**0**	0
	1 cup	101	**0**	0
	1 lb	295	**0**	0
Fried, frozen				
French fries (*see also* **FAST FOODS**)				
Act II Microwave	1 box (88 g)	240	**110**	23
Ore Ida potatoes				
Crispers	17 (84 g)	220	**110**	18
Dinner Fries	8 (84 g)	110	**30**	9
Golden Crinkles	16 (84 g)	120	**35**	9
Tater Tots	9 (84 g)	160	**70**	14
Zesties	12 (84 g)	160	**80**	14
Potato puff	1	16	**7**	3
	½ cup	138	**60**	28
Frozen, other preparations				
hashed brown	½ cup ·	170	**81**	38
mashed				
with whole milk	½ cup	81	**6**	3
with whole milk and butter	½ cup	111	**40**	22
Ore Ida potatoes				
Mashed, butter flavor	½ cup	80	**20**	5
Onion Tater Tots	9 (84 g)	150	**60**	14
Potato Wedges with skins	9 (84 g)	110	**25**	9
Potatoes O'Brien	¾ cup	60	**0**	0
Twice-Baked				
Cheddar cheese	1 (140 g)	200	**80**	27
Sour Cream and Chives	1 (140 g)	180	**60**	36
Potato chips (*see* **SNACK FOODS**)				

VEGETABLES AND VEGETABLE PRODUCTS

		CALORIES		
FOOD	AMOUNT	TOTAL	FAT	SAT-FAT
Potatoes (*cont.*)				
Potato pancakes	1	495	**113**	31
Potato salad	½ cup	180	**92**	16
Potato sticks (*see* **SNACK FOODS**)				
Scalloped, from dry mix	1 cup	230	**99**	25
Pumpkin, cooked	1 cup	49	**0**	0
Radishes, fresh	10	7	**0**	0
	½ cup	10	**0**	0
Sauerkraut, canned	1 cup	44	**0**	0
Shallots, fresh	1 tbsp	7	**0**	0
Spinach				
fresh	1 cup	6	**0**	0
	10-oz pkg	46	**0**	0
cooked	1 cup	41	**0**	0
Spinach soufflé, made with whole milk, eggs, cheese, butter	1 cup	218	**165**	64
Squash				
summer (crookneck, zucchini)				
fresh	1 cup	26	**0**	0
cooked	1 cup	36	**0**	0
winter (acorn, butternut)				
fresh	1 squash	172	**0**	0
	1 cup	43	**0**	0
cooked	1 cup	79	**0**	0
Succotash, cooked	1 cup	222	**14**	1
Sweet potatoes				
baked in skin	1 (5 × 2″)	118	**0**	0
	½ cup mashed	103	**0**	0
boiled without skin	1 cup mashed	344	**0**	0
Tomatoes				
fresh	1	24	**0**	0
	1 cup	35	**0**	0
cooked	1 cup	60	**0**	0
canned in tomato juice	1 cup	67	**0**	0
Tomato juice, canned	1 cup	42	**0**	0
Tomato products, canned				
marinara sauce	1 cup	171	**75**	11
paste	1 tbsp	14	**0**	0
purée	1 cup	102	**0**	0

VEGETABLES AND VEGETABLE PRODUCTS

		CALORIES		
FOOD	AMOUNT	TOTAL	FAT	SAT-FAT
Tomato products, canned (*cont.*)				
sauce (*see also* **SAUCES, GRAVIES, AND DIPS**)	1 cup	74	**0**	0
spaghetti sauce (*see* **SAUCES, GRAVIES, AND DIPS**)				
Turnips, cooked	1 cup cubes	28	**0**	0
Vegetable juice cocktail, canned	1 cup	44	**0**	0
Water chestnuts, canned	1 cup	70	**0**	0
Yam, cooked	1 cup	158	**0**	0
Zucchini				
fresh	1 cup	26	**0**	0
cooked	1 cup	36	**0**	0

MISCELLANEOUS

		CALORIES		
FOOD	AMOUNT	TOTAL	FAT	SAT-FAT
Baking powder	1 tbsp	5	**0**	0
Carob flour	1 tsp	14	**0**	0
Cocoa powder	1 tsp	5	**0**	0
Cocoa powder	1 tbsp	14	**5**	0
Curry powder	1 tsp	5	**0**	0
Garlic powder	1 tsp	10	**0**	0
Gelatin, dry	1 envelope	25	**0**	0
Ketchup	1 tbsp	15	**0**	0
Mustard	1 tsp	5	**0**	0
Olives, green	4 medium	15	**15**	2
Olives, ripe	3 small or 2 large	15	**15**	3
Oregano	1 tsp	5	**0**	0
Paparika	1 tsp	5	**0**	0
Pickles				
dill	1 medium	5	**0**	0
gherkin	1	20	**0**	0
sweet	1	20	**0**	0
Vinegar	1 tbsp	0	**0**	0
Yeast, all types	1 tbsp	20	**0**	0

Food Tables Index

This index was designed to help you find some of the harder-to-locate foods in these tables as well as those foods that appear in several different categories.

GLOSSARY

APPENDIXES

REFERENCES

INDEX

TABLE OF
EQUIVALENT
MEASURES

Glossary

Adipose tissue. Tissue in which fat is stored.

Aerobic exercise. Steady, repetitive exercise that uses the large muscles and requires a steady supply of oxygen — in contrast to exercise that requires bursts of activity separated by periods of rest. Examples of aerobic exercises include walking, swimming, running, and biking. Aerobic exercise burns more fat than active sports, which burn more carbohydrate.

Basal metabolic rate (BMR). The rate at which energy is used when the body is completely at rest to maintain such vital functions as breathing, heartbeat, and digestion.

Burning or oxidation. The chemical process of combining substances (carbohydrates, fats, proteins in foods) with oxygen, resulting in the release of stored energy.

Calorie. A unit of heat or energy produced by burning (oxidizing) nutrients. Carbohydrates and proteins contain 4 calories per gram; fats, 9 calories per gram; and alcohol, 7 calories per gram.

Carbohydrate. One of the three major energy-containing nutrients in foods; the others are protein and fat. Carbohydrates are simple (sugars) or complex (starches); each type contains 4 calories per gram.

Cholesterol. A fatlike substance found in the cell membranes of all animals, including humans. Cholesterol is transported in the bloodstream. Some of it is manufactured by the body and some comes from the foods of animal origin that we eat. A healthy level of cholesterol for adults is below 200 mg/dL. A higher level is often associated with increased risk of heart disease.

Complex carbohydrate. One of the two major types of carbohydrates, which include starches. They are found in whole-grain and cereal products and vegetables. In their natural state complex carbohydrates are accompanied by dietary fiber.

Dietetic. A term used to describe a food that has been nutritionally altered in some way. "Dietetic" can mean less sodium, less fat, less sugar, or fewer calories. If a food is intended for weight loss, it must meet requirements for low-calorie or reduced-calorie claims. If not for weight loss, its label must state its special dietary purpose.

Energy. Power to do work. The energy in foods is measured in calories. A high-energy food is a high-calorie food. Energy expenditure, as in exercise, is quantified in terms of calories expended or burned.

Fat. One of the three major energy-containing nutrients in foods; the others are carbohydrates and proteins. Fat is an oily substance that is found in many foods, especially oils, dairy products, and meat products. Fat is the major form of storing energy in the body. Fat stores in the adipose tissue total 140,000 or more calories. Fat contains 9 calories per gram.

Fat Budget. The number of calories from ingested fat that are allowed per day to reach and maintain a person's desirable and healthy weight. Fat Budget is based on a percentage of minimum total calorie intake (BMR).

Fattening. A term commonly used to describe any substance that contributes to making a person fat. Many foods (often starchy ones) have been mislabeled "fattening." Truly, the most fattening substance is fat.

Fiber, dietary. A nondigestible substance found in plant products. It can be insoluble, like wheat fiber, or soluble, like oat bran, pectin (in fruits), and guar gum (in beans). Both types of fiber provide bulk and moderate the absorption of nutrients. Insoluble fibers help regularity, whereas soluble fibers reduce blood cholesterol.

Glucose. A simple carbohydrate or sugar found in foods and in the body; the preferred fuel for quick energy and the only fuel used by the brain.

Glycogen. The storage form of carbohydrate in the body; long chains of glucose linked end to end. Glycogen stores, which total about 800 calories, occur in liver, muscle, and other tissues.

Gram. A metric measure of weight. One ounce equals 28.35 grams. Nutrients are listed in grams on food labels: a gram of fat contains 9 calories; a gram of protein or carbohydrate contains 4 calories.

Hidden fat. Fat in foods that is not visible. Hidden fats include oils used in frying or baking and fat naturally present in foods, such as butterfat in cheese and whole milk, fat marbled throughout beef, or fat in the skin of poultry.

Ideal or desirable weight. Weight associated with general good health and lowest mortality rates.

Lean body mass. The metabolically active tissue in the body, primarily composed of muscle. The greater a person's lean body mass, the higher the metabolic rate and the greater protection against weight gain.

Lite or light. A product advertised as light must contain one-third fewer calories or half as much fat as the regular product. The nutrition information on the label should be used to determine how much fat the product contains and thus how it can be fit into your Fat Budget.

Low-fat. A term used to imply that a food is acceptable for a weight reduction diet. Foods labeled low-fat, such as 2% low-fat milk, may actually contain substantial amounts of fat. To be sure a product can fit in your Fat Budget, check the fat content on the food label.

Metabolism. The sum of the chemical changes that occur to substances in the body. Much of metabolism is the conversion of food into living tissue and energy.

Monounsaturated fat. One of the three types of fat commonly found in foods.

Monounsaturated fats help to reduce blood cholesterol levels. The richest source of monounsaturated fat is olive oil. Like all other fats, monounsaturated fat has 9 calories per gram.

Nitrites. Substances used to preserve, color, and flavor meat products. In the body, nitrites can be converted into nitrosamines, which have been shown to cause cancer.

Nondairy. A term commonly used for imitation dairy foods that contain no dairy products, such as imitation creamers, sour creams, and whipped toppings. While these products do not contain cholesterol, they do contain fat, often highly saturated fat like coconut oil. Check the nutrition information on labels to determine how much fat is present.

Nutrients. Substances in foods (carbohydrates, proteins, and fats) that contain energy and are building blocks for making living tissue. Also includes substances needed for normal bodily functioning, such as minerals and vitamins.

Obesity. Excess accumulation of body fat. Obese is defined as 20 percent to 40 percent over ideal weight, massively obese as greater than 40 percent over ideal weight.

Oxidation. See burning.

Polyunsaturated fat. One of the three types of fat commonly found in foods. Polyunsaturated fat helps to lower blood cholesterol, but in excess can lower the "good" cholesterol in the blood and has been associated with an increased risk of cancer. The most common sources of polyunsaturated fats are corn, sunflower, and safflower oils. Like all other fats, polyunsaturated fat has 9 calories per gram.

Protein. One of the nutrients in foods that provides energy and building blocks for making essential body constituents such as muscle, enzymes, and cell membranes.

Reduced-calorie. A term regulated by the Food and Drug Administration that means a product is at least one-quarter lower in calories than the food with which it is being compared. It does not necessarily mean that the product is low in fat. Consult the nutrition information on labels for fat content.

Saturated fat. One of the three types of fat commonly found in foods, saturated fat has a powerful effect on raising blood cholesterol levels. The most common sources of saturated fats are butterfat; beef, veal, lamb, and chicken fat; cocoa butter; hydrogenated vegetable oil; and the tropical oils (coconut, palm kernel, and palm). Like all other fats, saturated fat has 9 calories per gram.

Simple carbohydrate. One of the two major types of carbohydrate, also known as sugar. In contrast to complex carbohydrates, simple carbohydrates are not usually associated with any nutritionally beneficial substances and are often said to contain empty calories.

Sugar. Any carbohydrate with a sweet taste.

Thermogenesis or thermogenic effect of food. The process of producing heat. Carbohydrates in foods we eat increase the metabolic rate and produce a thermogenic effect.

Vegetable oil. The fat from plant products. Some vegetable oils are mostly unsaturated and are liquid at room temperature (olive, corn, sunflower) and some are mostly saturated and are solid at room temperature (coconut, palm kernel, palm). All vegetable oils are 100 percent fat and have 9 calories per gram.

Appendix A:
The Nitty-Gritty of How to Keep a Food Record

Now you are ready to get started on the road to leanness. Your first activity is to discover which foods have been making you fat. If you are like most people who want to lose weight, you know that you are eating some fattening foods. What you don't know is exactly how much fat is in the foods you eat or which foods are loaded with fat. That is why you are going to keep a food record — an activity you will find rewarding, insightful, and even a little bit fun.

These records are for YOU — not your spouse, your mother, your brother, your doctor, your dietitian — just for you, and they must be exact and accurate. They must reflect *exactly* what you eat, not what you think you *should* have eaten. Beautiful imaginary food records have no effect on weight loss. If you eat 3 chunky chocolate chip cookies, record 3 cookies, not 1 or 2. Okay. You regret your overindulgence. But being sorry won't put the cookies back in the package or take the fat out of your fat stores. If you don't record what you eat, you fool only yourself, not your body. Your body accurately and honestly records everything you put into it. On the other hand, if you write down the 120 fat calories you consumed, you can balance your fat intake for the rest of the day or the next by eating less fat.

Don't become frantic about your food diary. Your first records may reflect what got you into this mess in the first place. Don't feel guilty. Everyone used to wolf down hot dogs and french fries with no thought. We called whole milk a calcium-rich food and steak a high-protein food. Who knew?

More likely, cutting fat won't be a problem, but struggling to eat above your minimum total caloric intake may be. As the days and weeks progress and you ease into *Choose to Lose*, your records will reflect a diet lower in fat and higher in complex carbohydrates. But it

448

takes time. Don't expect to change your entire diet overnight. Experience shows that changes made more gradually are more apt to last.

> If you are interested in purchasing a Choose to Lose Passbook to keep track of your food intake, see the order form at the end of the book.

KEEPING GOOD RECORDS

Time

Record What You Eat When You Eat It. Write down what you eat when you eat it. Don't fill in your record at the end of the day. You're bound to forget what you don't want to remember. Recording the time helps you see patterns in your eating. The fact that you ate breakfast at 8 A.M. and then didn't eat again until 3 P.M. may give you a clue as to why you blew your Fat Budget on a late lunch of a double cheeseburger, milk shake, and fries.

Food and Amount

List All Foods Separately and List Amounts Accurately. Measure everything. Be accurate. Don't write down *just* "cream cheese." Write down the amount you ate — "cream cheese, 2 tablespoons." Don't write down *simply* "chicken breast." Write down "chicken breast with skin, batter-fried." Don't write down merely "roast beef sub." Ask the sandwich man how much roast beef and how much mayonnaise he gave you. (He'll know — his boss makes sure he gives everyone an exact amount.) Write down "6-inch sub roll, 4 ounces roast beef, 1 tablespoon mayonnaise." These details are important. If you eat out, ask the waiter what's in the cream sauce and how much butter is on the swordfish, the potato, vegetables, or toast.

For "Hints on Measuring and Recording What You Measured," see pages 453–56.

Total Calories

When people cut down on fat, they often cut down on total calories. This is unhealthy. When you reduce your fat intake, you must be sure to increase your intake of complex carbohydrates, fruit, and low- or

Sample Food Record

TIME	FOOD	AMOUNT	TOTAL CALORIES	TOTAL CAL SUBTOTAL	FAT CALORIES	FAT SUBTOTAL
9 A.M.	Cream cheese	2 tbsp				
1 P.M.	Chicken breast with skin, batter-fried	1 breast				
6 P.M.	Roast beef sub					
	roast beef	4 oz				
	6" sub roll	1				
	mayonnaise	1 tbsp				

nonfat dairy products. If you don't eat enough of these low-fat foods, you will miss the vitamins, minerals, and fiber they provide, your basal metabolic rate will slow down, and you will be hungry.

On the other hand, grossly eating over your minimum total caloric intake indicates that you are also probably eating over your Fat Budget.

You know if you are eating too many or too few total calories only if you keep track.

Your total caloric intake should be greater than the number you determined in Chapter 2. Remember: That number is a floor. It is the number of calories you need to sustain your body if you are completely at rest. Since you are active, you need more calories to fuel your activity. How much more depends on how much physical activity you do. For most people 400 to 600 total calories more than the minimum total caloric level will suffice. But don't worry. If you eat a few hundred more calories in addition as fiber-rich carbohydrates, they will be burned off. They will not be stored as fat. You need to eat to lose. Fat calories — not total calories — make you fat.

Use the Food Tables (look under the heading Total Calories) and labels on packages to determine the total calories of the foods you have eaten. Make sure that you adjust the total calories for the amount you eat relative to the serving size listed. For example, the portion size for Cheddar cheese is 1 ounce. The total calories for 1 ounce of Cheddar cheese are 114. If you eat 3 ounces of Cheddar cheese you record 3 × 114 = 342 total calories.

Fat Calories

Use the Food Tables (look under the heading Fat Calories) and labels on packages to determine the fat calories of the food you have eaten.

Make sure that you adjust the fat calories for the amount you eat relative to the serving size listed. For example, the portion size listed for chuck steak is 1 ounce. The fat calories for 1 ounce of chuck, lean and fat, are 78. No one eats 1 ounce of meat. If you ate 5 ounces of chuck, you would record 5 × 78 = 390 fat calories.

If you cannot find the exact food you have eaten in the Food Tables (first try using the Food Table Index, pages 438–41), find a similar food and record its fat calories. For example, if you ate veal parmigiana in a restaurant, you might check out the veal parmigiana entries (not low-fat) in the Frozen and Microwave Food section of the Food Tables.

If you have eaten a mixed dish such as chicken stir-fry, you should estimate the sum of the fat calories for the individual ingredients. For example, chicken stir-fry might contain one chicken breast without skin (13 fat calories), a tablespoon of corn oil (120 fat calories), green pepper, onion, and garlic (0 fat calories).

Or look in a cookbook (not low-fat) for the dish you ate and figure out the fat calories per serving (see page 139).

Food Labels. Read Chapter 8 on food labels. Take heed. Not only must you determine the calories of fat per serving from the nutrition label, you must adjust for the number of servings you eat. For example, according to the label, 1 ounce of light cream cheese contains 36 fat calories. If you eat 1 ounce, record 36 fat calories. If you eat 1½ ounces, record 54 (1.5 × 36 = 54).

Entering the Information. If you ate cereal with 2% milk for breakfast, start by entering the amount of cereal you ate. Read the nutrition label on the cereal box to determine the total calories and fat calories for that amount. Your first food entry would look like this.

TIME	FOOD	AMOUNT	TOTAL CALORIES	TOTAL CAL SUBTOTAL	FAT CALORIES	FAT SUBTOTAL
8 A.M.	Apple Cinnamon Cheerios	¾ cup	120		25	

Fat Subtotal. You should keep a running tally of your fat intake. This makes you aware of the amount of fat you have "spent" and the amount you have left in your Fat Budget. You can look at your fat subtotal and easily judge the fat impact of any food you are planning to eat.

For your first entry of the day, in the column labeled Fat Subtotal, repeat the number of fat calories you entered in the Fat Calories column.

TIME	FOOD	AMOUNT	TOTAL CALORIES	TOTAL CAL SUBTOTAL	FAT CALORIES	FAT SUBTOTAL
8 A.M.	Apple Cinnamon Cheerios	¾ cup	120		25	25

Total Calorie Subtotal

You will also want to keep a running tally of your total calories to make sure you are eating *enough* total calories.

For your first entry of the day, in the column labeled Total Cal Subtotal, repeat the number of total calories you entered in the Total Calories column.

TIME	FOOD	AMOUNT	TOTAL CALORIES	TOTAL CAL SUBTOTAL	FAT CALORIES	FAT SUBTOTAL
8 A.M.	Apple Cinnamon Cheerios	¾ cup	120	120	25	25

For your second entry, record food as 2% milk, amount as 1 cup, total calories as 121, and fat calories as 42. Add the fat calories for your second entry to the previous Fat Subtotal to calculate the new Fat Subtotal (42 + 25 = 67) and add its total calories to the previous total calorie subtotal to calculate the new total calorie subtotal (121 + 120 = 241).

TIME	FOOD	AMOUNT	TOTAL CALORIES	TOTAL CAL SUBTOTAL	FAT CALORIES	FAT SUBTOTAL
8 A.M.	Apple Cinnamon Cheerios	¾ cup	120	120	25	25
	2% milk	1 cup	121	241	42	67

Final Subtotals

At the end of the day compare your fat intake (last entry of your Fat Subtotal) for the day with your Fat Budget. Is your fat consumption way over budget? But is it closer to budget than yesterday? What foods contributed the most fat to the day's intake? Can you eat these in smaller amounts, less often, not at all, or make low-fat substitutions? Look at your total caloric intake for the day (last entry of your Total Cal Subtotal). Have you been eating enough total calories? Are you at least 400 total calories over your minimum total caloric intake?

Minimum Basic Nutritional Requirements

You want to be sure that you are not only reducing fat and eating enough total calories, but that you are eating a balanced diet (see Chapter 12, page 169). To ensure that you are satisfying the minimum basic nutritional requirements, copy these recommended number of servings for each food category at the bottom of your food record each day. (They are printed in the Choose to Lose Passbook.)

Fruits (2–4):_____   **Vegetables (3–5):**_____   **Grains (6–11):**_____   **Dairy (2–3):**_____

You will find definitions for these servings on page 175. Check over your food record and record your intake in the space provided. If you are not meeting your minimal basic nutritional requirements, make an effort to add the necessary foods to your diet. This is supremely important. **Not only do these foods supply the vitamins, minerals, and fiber you need, they make you feel full and thus less likely to binge on high-fat or empty-calorie foods.**

HINTS ON MEASURING AND RECORDING WHAT YOU MEASURED

Liquids

Most Liquids. Use measuring cups and spoons to measure the amount of a liquid you use.

This table of equivalent measures should help you record liquids:*

```
1 cup = 8 fluid ounces
½ cup = 4 fluid ounces
¼ cup = 2 fluid ounces
2 tablespoons = 1 fluid ounce
```

Solid Food

Meat. Read the meat package label or use a kitchen scale to measure the weight (in ounces) of *beef, lamb, pork, veal, poultry,* and *fish.* Record the weight of meat in ounces. Indicate if the meat was raw or cooked when it was weighed and if the fat is included or has been trimmed. If necessary, use the following estimates:

```
¼ cup meat = 1 ounce meat
Chicken breast half = 3 ounces
4 ounces raw meat without bone = 3 ounces cooked
6 ounces raw meat with bone = 3 ounces cooked
```

Bread should be recorded by slice.

Crackers and cookies should be recorded by unit (i.e., 5 crackers).

Cereals**, cottage cheese***, creams, fats, frozen desserts, canned fish, sliced fruit, grains, milks, nuts†, pasta, puddings (not canned), rice, salad dressings, sauces and gravies, snacks, soups, vegetables. Use measuring cups and spoons to measure and record these foods.

Candy, cheese, cold cuts, nuts, yogurt, frozen yogurt. Read the label on the package or use a scale to measure the weight (in ounces). Save packages with nutrition labeling for use later. Record weight of food in ounces.

Cakes and pies should be recorded by fraction of whole dessert (i.e., ¹⁄₁₀ cake).

---

*See page 473 for a more complete table of equivalent measures.
**If you have a scale, you may also weigh and record cereal in ounces.
***Cottage cheese and ricotta should be measured by measuring cup rather than weighed.
†You may also weigh and record nuts in ounces or count and record the number of nuts you eat.

Frozen food should be recorded by package or the fraction of the package you eat. If possible, save packages with labels for future reference.

Fast food should be recorded by unit, piece, serving, order, or slice, except for shakes, which are measured in fluid ounces.

Here's a summary chart that lists foods and the unit used to measure them.

Summary Chart

FOOD/BEVERAGE	UNIT	EXAMPLES
Dairy/Eggs		
Butter	pat, teaspoon, tablespoon	
Cheese, hard, soft	ounce	2 oz Cheddar
Cheese, curd type	cup	½ c ricotta
Cream	tablespoon	1 tbsp table cream
Milk	cup	1 c skim milk
Yogurt	fluid ounce	8 fl oz nonfat vanilla yogurt
	cup	1 c nonfat plain yogurt
Egg	1 egg	
	1 egg white	
	1 egg yolk	
Fast Foods	number	1 cheeseburger
	order	1 order fried shrimp
	ounce	12 oz shake
	piece	1 chicken breast
	serving	1 serving coleslaw
	slice or fraction of whole*	3 slices, 12-inch pepperoni pizza
Fats and Oils		
Margarine	teaspoon, tablespoon	2 tsp Promise
Oils	teaspoon, tablespoon	1 tbsp olive
Salad dressings	teaspoon, tablespoon	1 tbsp Russian
Fish and Shellfish	ounce	4 oz orange roughy

*Specify diameter of whole (i.e., pizza, 14-inch diameter).

FOOD/BEVERAGE	UNIT	EXAMPLES
Frozen and Microwave	Depends on product	Use information on food labels
Fruits and Fruit Juices	piece cup	1 apple ½ c applesauce
Grain Products Bagel Bread Cereal Cracker Pasta/rice Popcorn Roll	 number slice cup ounce number cup cup number	 1 bagel 2 slices rye ⅔ cup Wheatena 1 oz Cheerios 1 Wheat Thin ¾ c macaroni, cooked 5½ cups air-popped 1 poppy seed
Meats	ounce	5 oz round steak, with fat
Nuts and Seeds	ounce tablespoon number of kernels cup	1 oz pecans 2 tbsp peanut butter 12 cashews ½ c sunflower seeds
Poultry	piece ounce	½ chicken breast 3 ounces white meat turkey
Sauces, Gravies, and Dips	tablespoon cup	3 tbsp mushroom gravy ½ c cream sauce
Sausages and Cold Cuts	ounce slice link	4 oz turkey bologna 3 slices salami 1 link smoked sausage
Soups	cup	1½ c tomato soup
Sweets Cakes Cookies, bars Pie Sugar, jelly	 fraction of whole number fraction of whole teaspoon, tablespoon	 1/12 chocolate cake 1 sugar cookie ⅙ pumpkin pie 1 tsp grape jam
Vegetables	cup number	½ c spinach 1 carrot

Appendix B:
Recalculating Fat Calories of Recipes

RECALCULATING FAT CALORIES

If you wish to reduce further the fat content of *Choose to Lose* recipes, the following directions will help you determine the new lower number of fat calories.

1. Figure out how many fat calories you are eliminating from the recipe.

---

1 tablespoon of olive oil contains 119 calories;
1 tablespoon of margarine contains 90 fat calories*.

For example, a recipe for Curried Turkey calls for 3 tablespoons of olive oil. You decide to use only 2 tablespoons instead. You are eliminating 1 tablespoon of olive oil (119 fat calories).

2. Look at the fat calories per serving for the recipe. In this example, Curried Turkey contains 60 fat calories per serving. To figure out the fat calories for the entire recipe, multiply the number of servings (6) by the number of fat calories in each serving (60).

$$6 \times 60 = 360 \text{ fat calories}$$

---

*The margarine used in *Choose to Lose* recipes is Promise, which contains 90 fat calories per tablespoon.

3. Subtract the fat calories you eliminated (119) from the total fat calories of the recipe (360).

$$360 - 119 = 241$$

4. The fat calories for the entire Curried Turkey recipe with the olive oil eliminated are 241. To get the new fat calories per serving, divide 241 by the number of servings (6).

$$241 \div 6 = 40$$

The Curried Turkey with reduced fat contains about 40 fat calories per serving.

References

Chapter 1

Acheson, K. J., Y. Schutz, T. Bessard, K. Anantharaman, J. P. Flatt, and E. Jéquier. "Glycogen Storage Capacity and de Novo Lipogenesis During Massive Carbohydrate Overfeeding in Man." *American Journal of Clinical Nutrition* 48 (1988):240–247.

Barrows, K., and J. T. Snook. "Effect of a High-Protein, Very-Low-Calorie Diet on Resting Metabolism, Thyroid Hormones, and Energy Expenditure in Obese Middle-Aged Women." *American Journal of Clinical Nutrition* 45 (1987):391–398.

Bray, G. A. "Obesity — A Disease of Nutrient or Energy Balance?" *Nutrition Reviews* 45 (1987):33–43.

"Can Eating the 'Right' Food Cut Your Risk of Cancer?" *Tufts University Diet and Nutrition Letter* 6 (1988):2–6.

Donato, K., and D. M. Hegsted. "Efficiency of Utilization of Various Sources of Energy for Growth." *Proceedings of the National Academy of Sciences* 82 (1985):4866–4870.

Dougherty, R. M., A. K. H. Fong, and J. M. Iacono. "Nutrient Content of the Diet When the Fat Is Reduced." *American Journal of Clinical Nutrition* 48 (1988):970–979.

Dreon, D. M., B. Frey-Hewitt, N. Ellsworth, et al. "Dietary Fat: Carbohydrate Ratio and Obesity in Middle-Aged Men." *American Journal of Clinical Nutrition* 47 (1988):995–1000.

Elliot, D. L., L. Goldberg, K. S. Kuehl, and W. M. Bennett. "Sustained Depressions of the Resting Metabolic Rate after Massive Weight Loss." *American Journal of Clinical Nutrition* 49 (1989):93–96.

Flatt, J. P. "Dietary Fat, Carbohydrate Balance, and Weight Maintenance: Effects of Exercise." *American Journal of Clinical Nutrition* 45 (1987):296–306.

———. "Differences in the Regulation of Carbohydrate and Fat Metabolism and Their Implications for Body Weight Maintenance." *Hormones, Thermogenesis, and Obesity.* Edited by Henry Lardy and Frederick Stratman. New York: Elsevier Science Publishing, 1989.

————. "Effect of Carbohydrate and Fat Intake on Postprandial Substrate Oxidation and Storage." *Topics in Clinical Nutrition* 2(2) (1987):15–27.

————. "Importance of Nutrient Balance in Body Weight Regulation." *Diabetes/ Metabolism Reviews* 4(6) (1988):571–581.

————. "Metabolic Feedback on Food Intake Among ad Libitum Fed Mice." *International Journal of Obesity* 9 (1985):A33.

Flatt, J. P., E. Ravussin, K. J. Acheson, and E. Jéquier. "Effects of Dietary Fat on Postprandial Substrate Oxidation and on Carbohydrate and Fat Balances." *Journal of Clinical Investigation* 76 (1985):1019–1024.

Gray, D. S., J. S. Fisler, and G. A. Bray. "Effects of Repeated Weight Loss and Regain on Body Composition in Obese Rats." *American Journal of Clinical Nutrition* 47 (1988):393–399.

Hammer, R. L., C. A. Barrier, E. S. Roundy, J. M. Bradford, and A. G. Fisher. "Calorie Restricted Low-Fat Diet and Exercise in Obese Women." *American Journal of Clinical Nutrition* 49 (1989):77–85.

Hultman, E., and L. H. Nilsson. "Factors Influencing Carbohydrate Metabolism in Man." *Nutrition Metabolism* 18 (Suppl. 1) (1975):45–64.

Katch, F., and W. D. McArdle. *Nutrition, Weight Control, and Exercise.* Philadelphia: Lea & Febiger, 1988.

Lissner, L., D. A. Levitsky, B. J. Strupp, et al. "Dietary Fat and the Regulation of Energy Intake in Human Subjects." *American Journal of Clinical Nutrition* 46 (1987):886–892.

Manson, J. E., M. J. Stampfer, C. H. Hennekens, and W. C. Willett. "Body Weight and Longevity." *Journal of the American Medical Association* 257 (1987):353–358.

Mattes, R. D. "Fat Preference and Adherence to a Reduced-Fat Diet." *American Journal of Clinical Nutrition* 57 (1993):373–381.

Mattes, R. D., C. B. Pierce, and M. I. Friedman. "Daily Caloric Intake of Normal-Weight Adults: Response to Changes in Dietary Energy Density of a Luncheon Meal." *American Journal of Clinical Nutrition* 48 (1988):214–219.

Romieu, I., W. C. Willett, M. J. Stampfer, G. A. Colditz, et al. "Energy Intake and Other Determinants of Relative Weight." *American Journal of Clinical Nutrition* 47 (1988):406–412.

Schutz, Y., J. P. Flatt, and Eric Jéquier. "Failure of Dietary Fat Intake to Promote Fat Oxidation: A Factor Favoring the Development of Obesity." *American Journal of Clinical Nutrition* 50 (1989):307–14.

Steen, S. N., R. A. Oppliger, and K. D. Brownell. "Metabolic Effects of Repeated Weight Loss and Regain in Adolescent Wrestlers." *Journal of the American Medical Association* 260 (1988):47–50.

Chapter 2

Dennison, D. *The DINE System: The Nutritional Plan for Better Health.* St. Louis: C. V. Mosby, 1982.

Chapter 4

National Center for Health Statistics. *Anthropometric Reference Data and Prevalence of Overweight, United States 1976–1980*. DHHS Publication no. 87-1688. Washington, D.C.: Government Printing Office, 1987.

U.S. Department of Health and Human Services. "Health Implications of Obesity." *National Institutes of Health Consensus Development Conference Statement*. Vol. 5, no. 9, 1985. National Institutes of Health, Office of Medical Applications of Research, Building 1, Room 216, Bethesda, MD 20205.

U.S. Department of Health and Human Services. *The Surgeon General's Report on Nutrition and Health*. DHHS (PHS) Publication No. 88-50210. Washington, D.C.: Government Printing Office, 1988.

The fat tables are based on data from the following sources:

U.S. Department of Agriculture. *Composition of Foods*. Agriculture Handbook No. 8. Washington, D.C.: Government Printing Office, sec. 1–16, rev. 1976–1989.

U.S. Department of Agriculture. *Nutritive Value of American Foods in Common Units*. Agriculture Handbook No. 456. Washington, D.C.: Government Printing Office, November 1975.

Chapter 10

Stunkard, A. J., and H. C. Berthold. "What Is Behavior Therapy? A Very Short Description of Behavioral Weight Control." *American Journal of Clinical Nutrition* 41 (1985):821–823.

Stunkard, A. J., T. T. Foch, and Z. Hrubec. "A Twin Study of Human Obesity." *Journal of the American Medical Association* 256 (1986):51–54.

Stunkard, A. J., T. I. A. Sorenson, C. Hanis, et al. "An Adoption Study of Human Obesity." *New England Journal of Medicine* 314 (1986):193–198.

Chapter 11

Ballor, D. L., V. L. Katch, M. D. Becque, and C. R. Marks. "Resistance Weight Training during Caloric Restriction Enhances Lean Body Weight Maintenance." *American Journal of Clinical Nutrition* 47 (1988):19–25.

Cooper, Kenneth. *The New Aerobics*. New York: Bantam Books, 1983.

Cooper, Kenneth, and Mildred Cooper. *The New Aerobics for Women*. New York: Bantam Books, 1988.

Hammer, R. L., and C. A. Barrier, E. S. Roundy, J. M. Bradford, and A. G. Fisher. "Calorie Restricted Low-Fat ⌐ ⌐ Exercise in Obese Women." *American Journal of Clinical Nutrition* 49 (19. ,.77–85.

Hill, J. O., P. B. Sparling, T. W. Shields, and P. A. Heller. "Effects of Exercise and Food Restriction on Body Composition and Metabolic Rate in Obese Women." *American Journal of Clinical Nutrition* 46 (1987):622–630.

Katch, F., and W. D. McArdle. *Nutrition, Weight Control, and Exercise*. Philadelphia: Lea & Febiger, 1988.

Rippe, J. M., A. Ward, J. P. Porcari, and P. S. Freedson. "Walking for Health and Fitness." *Journal of the American Medical Association* 259 (1988):2720–2724.

U.S. Department of Health and Human Services, Public Health Service. *Exercise and Your Heart.* National Institutes of Health Publication No. 18-1677, 1981.

Chapter 12

Dougherty, R. M., A. K. H. Fong, and J. M. Iacono. "Nutrient Content of the Diet When the Fat Is Reduced." *American Journal of Clinical Nutrition* 48 (1988): 970–979.

Goor, R., and N. Goor. *Eater's Choice: A Food Lover's Guide to Lower Cholesterol,* rev. ed. Boston: Houghton Mifflin, 1995.

James, W. P. T., M. E. J. Lean, and G. McNeill. "Dietary Recommendations after Weight Loss: How to Avoid Relapse of Obesity." *American Journal of Clinical Nutrition* 45 (1987):1135–1141.

Index

Table of Equivalent Measures

Volume Measures

1 gallon	4 quarts
1 quart	4 cups 2 pints
1 pint	2 cups
1 cup	8 fluid ounces 16 tablespoons
½ cup	4 fluid ounces 8 tablespoons
⅓ cup	5 tablespoons + 1 teaspoon
¼ cup	2 fluid ounces 4 tablespoons
2 tablespoons	1 fluid ounce
1 tablespoon	3 teaspoons ½ fluid ounce

Weight Measures

1 pound	16 ounces 454 grams
3.5 ounces	100 grams
1 ounce	28.35 grams

EATER'S CHOICE®
A Food Lover's Guide to Lower Cholesterol
by DR. RON GOOR and NANCY GOOR
Houghton Mifflin Company, 1987, 1989, 1992, 1995

FOURTH EDITION!!

Now that you are following Choose to Lose, you know that it is important to EAT lots of DELICIOUS, LOW-FAT FOOD to LOSE WEIGHT and MAINTAIN your weight loss. This is where *EATER'S CHOICE* comes in. YOU NEED LOTS OF WONDERFUL RECIPES — SCRUMPTIOUS, EASY-TO-MAKE, LOW-FAT RECIPES to keep you full and satisfied.

NATIONAL BESTSELLER
FOURTH EDITION, COMPLETELY REVISED
EATER'S CHOICE
A FOOD LOVER'S GUIDE TO LOWER CHOLESTEROL
• A simple method to reduce your risk of heart disease by up to 60 percent
• 290 delicious recipes low in fat
• New food labels demystified
Dr. Ron Goor & Nancy Goor

TRY THESE FOR STARTERS:

- Cauliflower Soup, Tortilla Soup, Sour Cherry Soup, Vegetable Soup Provençal, Apple-Squash Soup, and more . . .
- Cajun Chicken, Apricot Chicken Divine, Turkey with Capers, Turkey Mexique, Oriental Fish Kebabs, Broiled Ginger Fish, Shrimp Curry, and more . . .
- Chili Non Carne, Focaccia, Asparagus Pasta, Calzone, Potato Skins, Indian Rice, Onion Flat Bread, Key Lime Pie, and much more!

HOT OFF THE PRESS — The Fourth Edition has:

- 290 delicious low-sat-fat recipes!
- Fat calories for Eater's Choice recipes
- Chapter on children and cholesterol
- Everything you ever wanted to know about diet, cholesterol, and heart disease, including updated information on trans fats, reversal of coronary heart disease, cholesterol-lowering drugs, etc.

EATER'S CHOICE is available at local bookstores, or use the order form below

----

SHIP TO: **ORDER FORM**

Print clearly or type

Name _____

Address _____

City _____ State _____ Zip _____

CHOOSE TO LOSE COMPANIONS	QUANTITY	PRICE EACH	TOTAL PRICE
Passbook		$4.50	
Balance Book Refills		.75	
Choose to Lose SKILL-BUILDER*		9.00	
Choose to Lose book (Revised Edition)		13.95	
Eater's Choice book (4th edition)		15.95	

Send check or money order to:
Choose to Lose
P.O. Box 2053
Rockville, MD 20847-2053

5% tax (MD residents)
Postage and handling ... 2 00
TOTAL ORDER ... $

I would like book(s) dedicated to:
* Requires Passbook. At least 2 Refills are useful.

CHOOSE TO LOSE
COMPANIONS
Put Choose to Lose to work for you!

PASSBOOK

The key to losing weight is to stay within your Fat Budget. This convenient pocket-size passbook (like a checkbook) with a handsome vinyl cover contains everything you need to keep track of your fat intake:

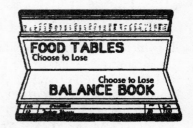

- Abbreviated **FOOD TABLES** listing total and fat calories for hundreds of foods
- **BALANCE BOOK** for keeping a two-week record of fat calories and total calories of the foods you eat, the time you spend exercising, and how you are meeting your basic nutritional requirements.

SKILL-BUILDER

The next-best thing to taking the Choose to Lose Weight Loss Program* is the Choose to Lose Skill-Builder workbook. Based on the success of thousands of people who have taken the Choose to Lose Weight Loss Program throughout the country, Dr. Ron Goor and Nancy Goor have developed a Skill-Builder workbook to help you master the skills you learned in the *Choose to Lose* book. This fun, interactive workbook helps you take control of your diet and your life.

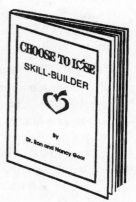

THE CHOOSE TO LOSE SKILL-BUILDER will help you master these skills:

- Keeping a food record so you know *exactly* how much fat you are eating, so you can find the biggest offenders in your diet and make better choices, so you can fit in your high-fat favorites and save for splurges;
- Deciphering food labels so you can cut through the hype, be savvy about serving sizes, and make choices that will fit comfortably into your Fat Budget;
- Ordering low-fat items from restaurant menus;
- Ensuring that you eat a healthful, balanced diet;
- Modifying recipes to make them low in fat.

* *Call 301-897-9360 to learn if the Choose to Lose Program is offered in your community.*